VICTORIAN SOCIAL MEDICINE

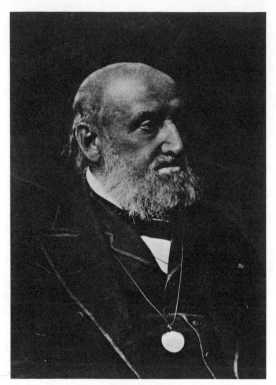

William Farr

JOHN M. EYLER

VICTORIAN
SOCIAL MEDICINE

THE IDEAS AND METHODS
OF WILLIAM FARR

The Johns Hopkins University Press
Baltimore and London

This book has been brought to publication with the generous assistance of the Andrew W. Mellon Foundation.

The Johns Hopkins University Press, Baltimore, Maryland 21218
The Johns Hopkins Press Ltd., London

Library of Congress Catalog Number 79-7560
ISBN 0-8018-2246-7
Library of Congress Cataloging in Publication data will be found on the last printed page of this book.

Frontispiece: William Farr (From a negative by Lombardi, Pall Mall)

For my parents,
Marvin and Catherine Eyler

CONTENTS

PREFACE

Historical interest in William Farr is of two kinds. Farr's work not only played an important part in the development of Victorian state medicine but also helped establish a basic methodology for such modern technical fields as epidemiology, vital statistics, and demography. Seen in this light, Farr's career belongs to the history of science and medicine as usually conceived. We are concerned in part to analyze the evolution of Farr's statistical methods and their application in the study of medical and economic problems.

On the other hand, Farr has broader historical interest. Because of the circumstances in which he worked and his qualities as an author, Farr's writings offer an excellent chance to study the character and interplay of a number of Victorian attitudes about health and their relationship to human welfare and social change. Farr was keenly interested in the sciences, especially in those sciences that dealt with aggregates. He was convinced that quantitative approaches would both advance medicine and assist the process of social reform. He was one of an important group of Victorian social activists who believed that the reform of society might be made scientific. Statistics would become the positive science of the state. Through the quantitative analysis of current circumstances and problems the means of effecting progressive, orderly social change could be found.

Within this program questions of health and disease had unusual importance. According to men of Farr's opinion, health was not only a state of physical well-being but also a reflection of the broader social and political circumstances in which men lived. Its inverses, disease and death, were therefore indices of an underlying social pathology whose quantitative measures, morbidity and mortality, were of political as well as medical interest. In Farr's writings we can explore the relation of Victorian ideas about the causes of disease and human misery to assumptions about economic and political processes and realities. In Farr's wide-ranging pronouncements on the Poor Law, on eugenics, on the Malthusian debate, on insurance, on human capital, we have a rare opportunity to examine the medical face of Victorian liberalism.

A study of Farr complements those of Edwin Chadwick, John Simon, and Florence Nightingale. Farr shared many of the same interests of his three contemporaries, but his perspective was novel. He was both more critical and technically more precise than Chadwick or Nightingale. Simultaneously his writings exhibit both a greater breadth of interest and a sensibility more finely tuned by human sympathy and social ideology than are to be found in John Simon's publications. Farr's secure civil service position granted him a period of tenure and an opportunity for candor rare among medical men in public service. For these reasons he is a unique spokesman of Victorian ideals in social medicine.

This book is not a personal biography. In several sections, especially in Chapter One, I have merely summarized the major events of Farr's career and commented on what new material has come to light since the standard biographical sketches were written. My purpose is to analyze Farr's ideas and methods in order to illuminate aspects of Victorian medicine, social science, and social thought. My purpose is both to interpret Farr's work as a product of historical forces—scientific, medical, and social—and to suggest how his writings illustrate the Victorian mind at work on difficult problems of human welfare.

In preparing this work I have received the help and support of many individuals and institutions, especially the following: I must thank Victor Hilts for first encouraging me to study Farr. Financial support came from the Josiah Macy, Jr., Foundation and from the National Institutes of Health. With the help of their fellowships I was able to continue my research and to broaden my acquaintance with the history of medicine. I am indebted to Barbara Rosenkrantz, James Cassedy, Saul Benison, William Coleman, and the late George Rosen for the interest they have shown in my work. I have also been fortunate in having a pleasant and stimulating academic environment at the University of Minnesota. Leonard G. Wilson and other members and friends of the History of Medicine Department, the staff of the Biomedical Library, and in particular, Judith Overmier and Cheryl Owens of the Owen H. Wangensteen Historical Library of Biology and Medicine have been helpful in many ways. Lora Beth Norton and Helen Mammen typed the manuscript. James Cassedy read it and offered important suggestions.

Final thanks are for Audrey, my wife, for patience and moral support, for essential help on style and organization, and for her sense of humor. She needed the latter. I needed all of the above.

VICTORIAN SOCIAL MEDICINE

ONE

WILLIAM FARR
DURING THE 1830s

THE REFORM CAUSE IN MEDICINE

Of the events in William Farr's early life and training we have only the barest outline.[1] He was born November 30, 1807, in Shropshire. First child of a farm laborer, he was, because of the family's extreme poverty, apprenticed at age eight to Joseph Pryce of Dorrington, near Shrewsbury, indentured to learn the "art and mystery of husbandry."[2] Pryce, however, recognized the boy's unusual curiosity and ability and provided him with some education. After some attendance at local day schools, supplemented by tutoring from a Dissenting minister, Farr began to teach himself and by the age of sixteen he had gained reasonable competence in Latin, French, and Italian and had begun to study Hebrew. The elderly Pryce encouraged him, remained his patron, and thus helped him leave the working class—the only member of his family to do so—to enter a profession.

Farr's medical education began in May 1826, when he was nineteen years old. He associated himself with the staff of the Salop Infirmary in Shrewsbury and for two years commuted six days a week from Dorrington, a distance of about seven miles each way. He studied medicine with a physician, served as a dresser to a surgeon, and was "nominally apprenticed" to an apothecary. This was good basic medical training for a provincial student of the 1820s, and it might have been followed by further training in the hospitals of London or by attendance at a Scottish university[3] had Farr not followed a more unusual course for an English student by taking further training in Paris. A legacy of £500, inherited on Pryce's death in November 1828, made his Parisian study possible. This was the first of two bequests for that amount received by Farr. The second came from his physician-preceptor, Dr. Webster, in 1837, along with the physician's library. In April 1829 he set out for the French capital.

In Paris Farr came in contact with some of the leading clinical teachers of his day. He was clearly impressed with what he found there. Years later, references to his experiences in the Parisian clinics appear in his writings. In the 1860s, for example, he recalled attending the lectures of Guillaume Dupuytren, head surgeon at the Hôtel Dieu, and observing

1

the treatment of the wounded from the Revolution of 1830 at that famous hospital;[4] he also recalled being among a group of English and American students to study typhoid fever under Pierre Louis at La Pitié.[5] In the next decade he commented that when he had been a student, Magendie pointed out to him how the cause of death of old patients at the Saltpetri-ère was often due to pneumonia, which could only be detected by percussion on the chest.[6]

Farr may have benefited enormously from his study in Paris. The Paris school was at the time the leader in clinical medicine, but in addition it pioneered in the teaching of subjects that Farr later made his special province: hygiene and medical statistics.[7] Both Farr's contemporaries and more recent commentators have suggested that he became interested in these subjects while at Paris.[8]

The Revolution of 1830 brought Farr's days in Paris to an end. After a brief tour in Switzerland he returned to England. For the next two years he attended medical lectures at University College, London, and returned to Shrewsbury for six months to replace the House Surgeon who had taken leave of absence to seek further qualifications.[9] In March 1832 he passed the examination of the Society of Apothecaries, and early the next year married and tried to establish a practice on Fitzroy Square, London.[10]

Times were difficult for Farr. He had acquired a good education, but he had neither the prestigious credentials, the connections, nor the social graces to attract patients. As a young apothecary, he stood at the bottom of a highly stratified and very competitive profession.[11] He apparently found general practice unrewarding, and for intellectual satisfaction, as well as supplementary income, he turned to medical journalism. Several of his articles appeared in the *Lancet* in the 1830s. Beginning in 1835 he served as a medical editor. He helped edit the *British Medical Almanack*, an annual review of the medical profession, and prepared for these volumes an original series of articles on vital statistics and on the history of the medical profession.[12] He also began the more ambitious scheme of editing his own journal, *British Annals of Medicine, Pharmacy, Vital Statistics, and General Science.*[13] This weekly journal continued for only nine months, January to August 1837. It published articles on a wide range of subjects, especially clinical and pathological reports, reprinted portions of continental works, and carried book reviews, notices of meetings, and editorials on the state of the profession and of medical science. Farr wrote six major articles for his journal as well: two on medical reform[14] and four on vital statistics.[15]

These comparatively rare journals provide our earliest evidence of Farr's intellectual life. What they reveal is a mind keenly aware of political and social phenomena, a preoccupation which at this time was directed to medical affairs. Even the *British Medical Almanack,* ostensibly an annual digest of mere facts, exhibits these concerns. Farr was interested in how power and wealth were distributed in the medical profession. In this almanac he collected information on the structure and regulation of the profession: on the requirements of medical licensing bodies; on medical schools' curricula, requirements, and fees; on the facilities, medical and surgical staffs and patient populations of British hospitals; and on the activities of medical societies.

He had already decided that medicine had two aspects. It was both a body of knowledge—a science—and a social institution. It is significant that in the medical history he wrote in 1839 he chose to emphasize the latter. He carefully labeled it a history of the medical profession.

The History of Medicine is strictly the history of the facts and principles which have been successively discovered in that science; the History of the English Medical Profession is here understood to imply the history of a social institution, established to preserve the health and to alleviate the physical sufferings of the nation. The state of Medical Science is only one of the elements of the inquiry; for the problem is—given a certain quantity of science, how has that science been brought into contact with the people, by what class of persons, by what institutions, and with what effect. . . .[16]

In the middle thirties Farr believed his profession stood at the threshold of a new era. "There is, in short, a general *movement* in the profession. Medical men live less for themselves, and more for mankind."[17] He spoke of an intellectual awakening and a quickening of social conscience to be found especially among the ordinary practitioners whose forum was the newly established Provincial Medical and Surgical Association, the antecedent of the British Medical Association.[18] Medicine, he believed, would soon be reformed from within and was about to play a role in the reformation of industrial society. His writings in this decade are preoccupied with both the restructuring of the medical profession and with medicine's potential value to society, especially in matters of hygiene and prevention. We shall consider Farr's comments on both issues in turn, because they offer our surest indication of the origin and interplay of some of his basic ideas.

Editorial after editorial in the *British Annals of Medicine* is devoted to the need for changes in the regulation of the medical profession. At issue was the long-standing and growing dissatisfaction of ordinary British practitioners with the traditional hierarchical structure of their profession and its governance by the London elite through the three ancient medical corporations: the Royal College of Physicians, the Royal College of Surgeons, and the Worshipful Society of Apothecaries.[19] Within the chorus of complaints Farr's voice was particularly strident. During these years, in fact, he kept company with the extreme group of metropolitan medical reformers, including the radical Thomas Wakley, who formed the first British Medical Association.[20] These medical men called for sweeping changes in the profession, changes that would unify the various ranks of medical men into one profession and divest the elite of their corporate privileges. Farr apparently hoped to make his journal a rallying point for medical reform and to establish a readership among the disgruntled and professionally frustrated general practitioners. It is no coincidence that his indictment of the medical establishment is reminiscent of that by his more prominent colleague, Thomas Wakley.

Perhaps the most significant feature of these editorials in the *British Annals of Medicine* is their use of the logic and rhetoric of political reform.[21] At an early age Farr had imbibed the precepts of political liberalism, and he used them to analyze his own profession. He portrayed the reform of medicine as the counterpart of the reform of government and institutions just under way in Britain. It was comparatively easy to portray the medical corporations as unreformed pockets of privilege, mindless traditionalism and autocratic goverance, "floating down from antiquity like icebergs, freezing and darkly frowning on the life and freedom of these sunnier times."[22]

Like the unreformed municipal corporations the medical corporations governed autocratically and irresponsibly. "Some hundred physicians, 21 London surgeons, and a trading band of Apothecaries, set at defiance and rule in unrestrained license over all the physicians, surgeons, and general practitioners of the empire. . . ."[23] In so doing they denied the principle of self government recently affirmed in the Great Reform Bill and in the Municipal Corporations Act and were consequently out of harmony with the aspirations of the age.

The principle of self-government is so well understood in this country that it needs no illustration. If it were necessary to show that their own interests may be more safely intrusted to a body of men themselves than to other individuals, we should refer to the present corporations. The Council of the College of Surgeons has never lost sight for a moment of its own interests, or of the interests of the entire profession, so far as they were involved in its own; but whenever the interests of the 8000 have been in any way opposed to the interests of the 21, those of the latter have invariably been consulted. This is no accident; it is no crime peculiar to the men who have sat on the Council; it is a law of human nature capable of calculation and prediction. Large bodies of men, like masses of matter, always obey the same laws. If the Council of 21 in Lincoln's-inn-fields had this alternative submitted to their decision:—"Shall the Council or the 8000 members of the College be thrown into the Thames?" the reply may be predicted; nor would the reply be different if the question were submitted to any other 21 men, indiscriminately taken, who happened to be equally bad swimmers.[24]

Farr called on his readers to send letters and petitions to Parliament. The cause was no mere struggle for recognition and influence. It was part of a greater fight for freedom and justice. Mean objectives or small motives were to be brushed aside before the tide of liberal reform.

When men demand the repeal of moral grievances, nothing is more common than for their adversaries, if closely pressed, to address themselves to the lowest feelings of our nature. A slave or an Irishman demands emancipation; he is immediately asked whether emancipation will give him a wife or a potato more than he possesses? A German desires to express his opinions through a free press; Metternich tells him to mind his business, a free press is neither meat nor drink. Medical men complain that they are shut out in England from all privileges of self-government, and all the honours of office; the monopolists ask them whether these vain things are fees.[25]

It was matters of education, certification, and recognition that attracted Farr's special attention in these editorials on the profession. He attributed to the Council of the Royal College of Physicians the lowest and most selfish motives for changing the requirements for its license and demanding retroactively a longer period of study than any Scottish university required for its M.D.[26] The licensing examination of Apothecaries Hall, the broad portal to general practice, came in for sharpest criticism. His demands here were radical. He suggested that Parliament abolish the Society of Apothecaries and establish in its place a Hall of Pharmacy whose main responsibility would be to regulate the drug trade, not to control general practice.[27] He was, in fact, suspicious of any regulation by boards: "Better far would it be for the medical profession and the public, that people should be left, as in the legal profession, to find out talent themselves, than remain at the mercy of meddling Boards, which, like paternal governments, are always tyrannical, and more pernicious than anarchy."[28]

Under the existing professional arrangements, rewards and recognition were dispensed according to privilege, social background, and general education, not according to technical qualifications. The fact that graduates of Oxford and Cambridge obtained professional places as a matter of course, although they might have had very deficient medical training, was a very sore point among dissatisfied, ordinary practitioners such as Farr. "It is evident that even now little more is indispensable in the English M.D., than a smattering of Greek, Latin, Heathen Mythology, and Christianity."[29] In their education in modern subjects, particularly in the sciences, the academically trained ordinary practitioners could claim superiority over their professional betters. The reformers recognized this fact and often included the demand for greater recognition of the sciences in their reform package.

Like Charles Babbage before him, Farr warned of the decline of English science. "The endowments and fellowships of Oxford and Cambridge are the prey of rich, indolent men; and he [the British scientist] is driven by necessity, as Liebig remarked, to serve Mammon. If a physician, he publishes a book upon new medicines, a treatise upon nervous affections, a book upon the diseases of females, or some other fortune-fraught theme, and is thus seduced, by corrupt institutions, from the path his genius might have illustrated under happier influences."[30]

Medical knowledge, Farr claimed, was rooted in the sciences. Medical education must acknowledge this fact. In commenting upon contemporary discussion of the medical curriculum at London University, Farr outlined briefly Auguste Comte's classification of the sciences, and he argued that study of mathematics, astronomy, physics, chemistry, physiology, and social physics should precede medical studies.[31] Medical students must be taught both the value of minute observation and how to undertake it. Farr believed that the establishment of the Clinical Report Society at Guy's Hospital was a valuable improvement in English medical education.[32] This society, like its French predecessor, La Société Médicale d'Observation, was a student society in which members presented clinical reports for criticism. Farr hoped to see similar groups established at other English hospital schools. Practitioners should be encouraged to continue studying science. His *British Medical Almanack* offered short practical summaries of recent discoveries. The *British Annals of Medicine* presented more complete reports on recent scientific work, most significantly a serialized publication begun in May 1837 of the first part of the Baly translation of Johannes Mueller's *Handbuch der Physiologie*. Farr recommended that his readers study Mueller's physiology, forming clubs if necessary in order to purchase a good microscope.[33]

Empirical investigation was the only way, Farr believed, that medical knowledge would be advanced. The enemy of medical progress was the hypothetical or speculative reasoning of physicians. "It is time to tell such persons that these vague speculations, opinions, assertions, are worth nothing, and that they can only advance science by registering facts, employing the microscope, by chemical analysis, weighing, measuring phenomena, determining their relations, and by applying that mighty instrument of natural science—arithmetic, mathematics."[34]

Besides the reform of the training and governing of medical men, these early works of Farr exhibit a deep interest in hygiene. His concern with hygiene was fundamental, and seems to have sprung from both his vision of science, a vision which included the notion that the systematic application of the tools of science would be a vehicle for social reform, and from his drive to find means whereby medicine could participate in social amelioration. His earliest publications, two of a series of lectures he gave in his home and which later appeared in the *Lancet*,[35] are devoted to hygiene. Neither is highly original. Both use ancient history for illustrative purposes. The first relies on the hygienic codes of the ancient Hebrews and Spartans; the second uses the Hippocratic treatises. He portrayed Moses as a pioneer hygienist who turned a people debased and degenerated by slavery into a triumphant race. The harsh Spartan law, he explained, also served a hygienic end. Farr clearly believed that mankind had the means of controlling his future well-being. Hygiene was the science which would make this goal possible. It was the way not only of preserving individual health and prolonging individual life, but, more importantly, of increasing the health and vigor of whole nations and "developing the human faculties, and raising them to their greatest possible degree of organic perfection."[36] His parting shot to those in his profession who might fear that the advance of public hygiene would mean diminished practice reiterated his insistence on medicine's public responsibility.

Gentlemen, I know that you—I know that our generous profession—will not, for a moment, harbour sentiments base. We exist, as a body, to promote the public health, and if the persistence of our craft is at variance with the public good, in the name of God let it be abolished,—let us betake ourselves to something else. Happily our interests are the interests of the community: in proportion to the health and strength and knowledge of England, it has flourished, and will flourish, and in its prosperity or reverses we shall participate.[37]

These two lectures also are suggestive of the origin of Farr's ideas. They offer on the one hand some evidence of the influence of Farr's Paris study. In later life he recalled that the Paris medical school pioneered the teaching of hygiene. He contrasted the situation in Paris of the thirties, where Andral's lectures regularly attracted nearly a thousand voluntary students, with the state of affairs during his student days in England, where hygiene formed no part of a medical education nor of the knowledge required of military medical officers.[38] These lectures reveal a skepticism about therapeutics common among certain members of the Paris school. Farr cited an authority, Hennen, who claimed that deaths among the Russian, French, and English troops in the Ionian islands were nearly equal, in spite of the substantial differences in the therapeutics the English and French physicians there employed.[39] While therapeutics seemed to make little difference in the health of armies, differences in hygiene were enormously important. A wise commander, Farr pointed out, could keep his troops in health by judicious choice of camp sites and regulations. Failure in this line, however, brought poor health in spite of abundant supplies of drugs.

An environmental perspective strongly reminiscent of Hippocrates replaced to some extent the emphasis on therapeutics. Like certain members of the Paris school, Farr expressed admiration for Hippocrates, emphasizing in particular the seasonal and geographic influences on health and the regularity of disease processes described in the Hippocratic treatises: *Airs, Waters, and Places* and *Epidemics I and III*. But Farr went further and tried to use Hippocrates to defend other trends in Parisian medicine. Engaging in a bit of historical pipe-dreaming, he claimed that if the father of Western medicine were alive in 1835, he would appreciate the true significance of the discoveries of the Parisian pathological anatomists and their British counterparts: Laennec, Louis, Carswell, and Baillie.[40]

Farr's first two publications also show that by 1835 he had begun to study vital statistics.[41] In the first lecture he used estimates of death rates by the Cambridge-trained actuary, Thomas Rowe Edmonds, and by Sir Francis D'Ivernois and the official vital statistics of Sweden. In the second he made use of mortality figures for the British army in the Mediterranean. The second lecture is especially interesting because it contains a numerical effort to demonstrate the regularity of disease phenomena. In attempting to answer modern critics of the Hippocratic doctrines of critical days and crises, Farr showed that the crises in acute diseases occurred in a regular pattern. This regularity was not apparent when one considered the number of crises that occurred on successive days of the disease, but a regular rise and fall of crises was obvious when the case histories were arranged into weekly periods. For this demonstration Farr used the 41 cases in *Epidemics I* and *III* and 296 cases of fever reported by Dr. Latham.[42] It is clear, however, that his statistical study was just beginning. His methods were rudimentary, and he lacked the command of the sources that typifies his works of only a few years later.

Over the next two or three years Farr's knowledge of vital statistics grew quickly, and he began to publish articles on statistical subjects in both journals he edited.[43] He had come to realize that vital statistics was a most powerful ally of hygiene. He made his *British Annals of Medicine* one of the first British medical periodicals to devote particular attention to statistics. In the first volume he explained that the journal's purpose would be like that of the *Annales d'hygiène publiques et de médecine légale* but even broader. It would extend to "all the laws of vitality capable of being observed in masses of men, expressible in numbers," and he mentioned as particular subjects of attention state medicine, public health, the census and vital registration, and insurance and benefit societies.[44]

Farr emerged as an accomplished statistician in 1837 with the publication of his section on vital statistics for McCulloch's statistical digest of the British Empire.[45] A classic summary of the state of English knowledge of vital statistics in the middle 1830s, it established Farr as a statistical authority. Nearly fifty years later Noel Humphreys still recommended it to students.[46] In preparing this chapter Farr did a remarkable job of synthesizing material from widely diverse sources. He relied on British and foreign medical journals. Of particular importance to this and to most of his other major studies was a series of articles by Edmonds in the *Lancet* in 1835 and 1836.[47] He also used work stimulated by the needs of the insurance business: the evidence collected on the experience of the Friendly Societies by both the Highland Society and by the Select Committee on Friendly Societies of 1825, Joshua Milne's *Treatise on Annuities*, and the records of the Equitable Society on the causes of death among its policy holders. For his section on sickness, Farr relied on records for select groups of men: the military, members of the Friendly Societies, and employees of the East India Company, as well as on the testimony submitted to the Factory Commission. His information in this instance was current and put to imaginative use. In his final section on the causes of death at various ages, he was on much less reliable factual ground, and he had to use the notoriously inaccurate London Bills of Mortality and the death records Dr. John Heysham collected for Carlisle, 1779–1787.

All told, this article suggests that Farr was well-versed in the available data and methods of vital statistics by 1837. His use of this material was creative but tempered by some recognition of the limitations of the figures he possessed. Despite these merits, however, Farr's chapter in McCulloch's volume displays the glaring deficiencies of the vital statistics in the period before national registration of births, deaths, and marriages. He had information for special groups of people, crude local life tables, records and studies of the experience of insurance companies and benefit societies, testimony before governmental investigatory bodies, and a few good local surveys. What was missing was direct information on the sicknesses and deaths of the mass of the English population. When such mortality data became available, it served as the basis of most of his professional activities. It was, in fact, while Farr was composing this article that the Registration Act of 1836 was passed. In two footnotes he remarked on its importance for the future of vital statistics, especially on the value of the provision for recording the cause of death.[48] It seems entirely plausible that he already had his eye on a position in the newly established General Register Office where he could professionally cultivate his unusual combination of interests.

Farr joined the staff of the General Register Office in 1839.[49] He made a career of the appointment, serving forty years under two registrars general, first as compiler of abstracts and then as superintendent of the Statistical Department. The appointment marked a major change in his activity. He abandoned practice altogether and became a less frequent contributor to medical journals. But his major ideas remained unchanged, merely evolving and finding new outlets. He remained deeply committed to the cause of reform. Most important in the context of this chapter is the fact that Farr retained his affiliation and sympathy with the medical profession. He had, consequently, a perspective at times rather different from that of many lay sanitarians and social reformers with whom he collaborated.

His faith in the sciences never wavered. While he undertook neither experimental nor clinical research himself, he remained well-read in the medical sciences throughout his career. His major works demonstrate a surprising command of contemporary scientific and medical literature, especially of etiological research and disease theory. Examples are plentiful. He noticed Jacob Henle's theory of contagion the same year Henle's work appeared.[50] In discussing mortality in childbirth, he mentioned Oliver Wendell Holmes's "The Contagiousness of Puerperal Fever" the same year this famous address was printed.[51] In his monograph on the 1866 cholera epidemic he included a discussion of contemporary research by pathologists, chemists, and microscopists, mentioning in particular the work of John Burdon-Sanderson, Louis Pasteur, Lionel S. Beale, Filippo Pacini, J. B. A. Dumas, Rudolf Virchow, and Robert Angus Smith.[52] Although he undoubtedly depended upon reviews and later upon the annual reports of the Medical Officer of the Privy Council to keep up-to-date, the fact remains that he had a keen scientific curiosity and eclectic mental habits.

It is abundantly clear as well that Farr considered his own statistical work part of the British empirical medical tradition, a tradition represented by Thomas Sydenham and by the latter's eighteenth century descendants: John Heysham, William Herberden, Thomas Short, John Haygarth, and John Pringle.[53] In the works of these British doctors Farr found a recognition of the value of hygiene, an environmental theory of disease compatible with his own, and a rudimentary use of medical statistics. The accuracy of Farr's historical judgment is not at issue here. It is significant, however, that he was familiar with the work of his British predecessors and felt indebted to them. This fact alone should make us cautious of attributing too much importance to the French influence. In his official reports he frequently began a section with a historical introduction.[54] These sketches demonstrate wide reading and an intimate familiarity with the medical tradition of his country. As an example, consider his second statistical nosology. In presenting this official classification of diseases Farr cited some 115 medical authorities.[55] The vast majority of these were British. What today would be considered minor British figures are listed along with the more famous French physicians, Laennec, Andral, Louis, and Villermé.

While the focus of Farr's reform interest shifted to social problems—public health in particular—as he joined the civil service, he did not forget the interests of rank-in-file practitioners. He repeatedly showed concern for the public recognition of medical expertise and service. While still a journalist he joined the clamor in the medical profession against the niggardly way the Poor Law authorities rewarded their medical officers, and demanded that such medical men in public service be paid on a scale commensurate with what they might earn by attending artisans in private practice.[56] As Farr became a government expert on medical statistics he began to use the prestige of his office to encourage the election of medical men as coroners and the appointment of properly qualified medical officers of health.[57] He argued, as Thomas Wakley had a decade earlier, that the ignorance of coroners often made their inquests shams and left crime undetected.[58] But Farr added to that argument the need of medical opinion in assuring that mortality statistics were accurately collected locally.

As his reputation grew, William Farr participated in the medical world at higher institutional levels. He became a recognized authority on public health, as well as on vital statistics. His expertise was acknowledged by the British Medical Association. Farr was made president of the Section of State Medicine in 1869, succeeding John Simon and Henry Wyldbore Rumsey.[59] He also was a member of the important Joint Committee on State Medicine of the British Medical Association and the Social Science Association of 1868 that was instrumental in getting the Royal Sanitary Commission appointed. The recommendations of that commission led to valuable health legislation in the last three decades of the nineteenth century.[60]

Farr also served on various medical committees and boards in his later career. He was, for example, a member of the Scientific Committee appointed by the General Board of Health to investigate the cholera epidemic of 1853-1854.[61] He served on this committee with such prominent medical men as John Simon and Neil Arnott. He also served as an examiner for the diplomas in sanitary science or public health and hygiene that were established in the universities and recognized by the General Medical Council in the 1870s. Among his papers are schedules for examinations he took part in at London University in 1875 and at Oxford in 1877.[62] His questions for the former examination have been preserved and offer valuable insight into the state of knowledge of statistics expected among medical officers of health.

Throughout his career in the civil service the medical profession claimed him as its own. Among the numerous honors and symbols of recognition he received during his lifetime a number came from medical societies and faculties. He was awarded honorary M.D. degrees by New York University in 1847 and by Trinity College, Dublin, a decade later. Also in 1857 he was elected Honorary Fellow of the Royal Medical and Chirurgical Society. He became an Honorary Fellow of King and Queen's College of Physicians, Dublin, in 1867. In 1880 he received the Gold Medal of the British Medical Association. But Farr's later work, work on which this recognition was based, was built on a conceptual framework constructed in the 1830s, an intellectual structure medical in nature and infused with liberal reform ideas. This basis gave Farr's endeavors much of their characteristic stamp. In considering Farr's statistical career then we must bear in mind his medical training and his peculiar position in the medical profession. He achieved a reputation and an influence quite incommensurate with his professional credentials. He became a government expert on matters of public health, yet he remained independent of the central health authority. When he began to consider social problems in the late thirties, his medical perspective remained and tempered both his reform ideas and his statistical approach.

TWO

STATISTICS

A SCIENCE OF SOCIAL REFORM

The Statistical Movement of the Thirties:
Numbers to Serve Reformers

British interest in statistics was at an all time high when William Farr began to study the science in his Grafton Street house. This is not to say the subject was new in England. There had been important isolated studies in the eighteenth and early nineteenth centuries. Mid-seventeenth-century London had also witnessed a flash of enthusiasm for vital statistics and political arithmetic. But in the 1830s the interest took on new proportions. As G. M. Young has explained: "It was the business of the thirties to transfer the treatment of affairs from a polemical to a statistical basis, from Humbug to Humdrum. In 1830 there were hardly any figures to work on. Even the census was far from perfect. . . . But statistical inquiry, fostered very largely by the development of the Insurance business, was a passion of the times."[1] Other historians have called the 1830s and 1840s an era of enthusiasm for statistics and have described the evolution of a statistical movement in Britain that culminated in the birth of government statistical offices and in the founding of private statistical societies.[2]

Although the ground was prepared before his arrival, the English visit of the Belgian astronomer and statistician Adolphe Quetelet served as a catalyst for this movement. Quetelet attended the third meeting of the British Association for the Advancement of Science in 1833, and his presence encouraged a group of interested men to press for the creation of a statistical section, Section F. The next year the Statistical Society of London was founded by the same group. Although the London society was eventually to dominate the field, it was neither the first nor initially the most productive. Honors on both counts go to the Manchester Statistical Society, established in 1833.[3] In the 1830s statistical societies also existed briefly in such cities as Bristol, Liverpool, Birmingham, Newcastle, Leeds, Glasgow, and Dublin.

In spite of some obvious differences between the London and the provincial bodies, there was remarkable similarity in their membership and activities. The founders were prominent men of affairs. In Manchester, for example, the influential banker Benjamin Heywood was "the

13

archetype of the Society's early membership: a liberal Whig, Unitarian, reform-minded, devoted to the cause of national education, and active in many charitable organizations."[4] Heywood's colleagues in the early society were business or professional men: textile manufacturers, bankers, physicians, mutually acquainted and already active in such local organizations as the Manchester Literary and Philosophical Society.

The Statistical Society of London was founded by London Whigs, many of whom had well-developed interests in political economy. Besides Charles Babbage, who at the time was involved in Whig politics, there were Richard Jones, professor of political economy at King's College, London; John Elliot Drinkwater, a rising young lawyer in liberal Whig circles; Colonel William Henry Sykes, former statistical reporter to the government in Bombay; Henry Hallam, Whig historian; Nassau Senior, political economist at the Poor Law Commission; and, something of an exception in this company, Thomas Malthus, who died soon after the founding. As M. J. Cullen has well illustrated, the founders were not rebels but were members of the reforming establishment.[5] They succeeded in launching a prestigious organization but, as events were to prove, they had neither the time nor the experience to make the society thrive intellectually. In the early years attendance at meetings dwindled, and it proved difficult to find contributors. This was at a time when the Manchester Society was most active. By the early 1840s, at a time when the Manchester Society had begun to decline and the other provincial societies had vanished, the Statistical Society of London was revived. Younger men whose careers in the civil service or in the insurance business involved the handling of quantitative data joined the society in larger numbers. A small group of these professional statisticians, actuaries, and administrators proved to be the core of the society in the middle decades of the nineteenth century.[6] William Farr was one of these. He joined the society in 1839 and remained an active member for the rest of his life, sitting on the council for over forty years and serving at various times as treasurer, vice-president, and president.[7] It was to this body, one of his principal forums, that he read his papers on economic subjects as well as summary papers on vital statistics.

The London society and Section F were professional homes for Farr and for the other members of the first generation of British career statisticians. Statistics had, of course, at the time no place in the universities.[8] The statistical societies, especially the London society, provided what support there was for this new science outside government. They provided a place for the exchange of ideas, a publication outlet, and at first some financial support for research. They helped advance the cause of statistics in other ways as well. Of particular interest to us here are the programmatic statements the London society issued. These helped to define statistics for contemporaries, and for us they are useful ways of discovering what Victorians expected of this subject.

The founders of the Statistical Society of London issued three major explanations of the society's purpose and of the nature of the subject it would cultivate. These were: the *Prospectus* of the society, issued under the auspices of the British Association in 1833; the "Introduction" to the first volume of the Statistical Society's journal that appeared in 1838; and the sixth report of the council, which was published in 1840.[9] These documents insisted that statistics was not merely a method but a separate science. "It was not to perfect the mere art of 'tabulating,' that it [the Statistical Society] was embodied;—it was not to make us hewers and drawers to those engaged on any edifice of physical science;—but it was that we should ourselves be the architects of a science or sciences. . ."[10] The founders of the statistical movement believed that the essence of science was empirical investigation. The pursuit of statistics was in their view entirely a matter of the accumulation and arrangement of facts. "Like other sciences, that of Statistics seeks to deduce from well-established facts certain general principles which interest and affect mankind; it uses the same instruments of comparison, calculation, and deduction: but its peculiarity is that it proceeds wholly by the accumulation and comparison of facts, and does not admit of any kind of speculation; it aims, like other sciences, at truth, and advances, *pari passu*, with its development."[11] The pursuit of facts would banish speculation, opinion, and even theory. As the *Prospectus* put it, "The Statistical Society will consider it to be the first and most essential rule of its conduct to exclude carefully all *opinions* from its transactions and publications—to confine its attention rigorously to facts,—and, as far as it may be found possible, to facts which can be stated numerically and arranged in tables."[12]

This stubborn insistence on an exclusively empirical approach led the framers of the journal "Introduction" to exclude even the consideration of cause and effect. "The Science of Statistics differs from Political Economy, because, although it has the same end in view, it does not discuss causes, nor reason upon probable effects; it seeks only to collect, arrange, and compare, that class of facts which alone can form the basis of correct conclusions with respect to social and political government."[13]

By the time the Council wrote its sixth report two years later some suspicion had arisen that the case had been overstated. While it still gave pre-eminence to observation, the council now acknowledged that hypothesis and conjecture had a place in the science of statistics, if only in guiding the individual researcher in the direction that would prove most useful. In any event, however, a scientific society had no business deciding on the truth of a theory. "They [scientific societies] do not vote upon systems, and decide the truth by majorities, but simply open the way for its demonstration by facts."[14]

On the face of it the founders seemed to have chosen an entirely inappropriate methodology for the subject they elected to pursue. Statistics, its British practitioners of the 1830s believed, was to be the most thoroughly applied and socially relevant of the sciences. It was to serve as a link between the other sciences and practical affairs.[15] In other words it had as its province an area in which opinion, theory, and speculation had full sway. What the founders seemed to have had in mind was the creation of a science of government, the principles of which would be discovered outside the realm of partisan dissention and arise from the accumulation of simple, irrefutable social facts. The statistician, or "statist," as he was called, was to be the scientific expert in matters of policy, the one who spoke from a knowledge of facts, not from mere conviction. Statistics so understood was a master science encompassing the results of other sciences and directing them to human need.

Statistics, by their very name, are defined to be the observations necessary to the social or moral sciences, to the sciences of the *statist*, to whom the statesman and the legislator must resort for the principles on which to legislate and govern. These sciences are equally distinct from the purely physical, the purely mathematical, and the purely metaphysical, though the mathematical must lend aid to their pursuit. . . . The Statist does not undertake to pursue geology, or meteorology, or geography, or botany, or zoology, as separate and complete sciences; but selects from the facts which these elucidate, such as may bear on the welfare of the human race in our present state of knowledge; in fine, he contemplates only those facts known to science which are also cognizable by art. For his is the science of the arts of civil life. . . .[16]

The founders' classification of the components of their subject reveals this bias toward the study of the "arts of civil life." The *Prospectus* listed four major divisions in statistics: economic, political, medical, and moral and intellectual. The sixth report of the council offered a slightly different classification: physical geography and appropriation, production, instruction, protection, consumption and enjoyment (including health).

It is hardly surprising then that the early statistical societies devoted much of their attention to determining the state of English society. Studies of the living conditions of the urban poor were especially common. In 1833 employed agents of the Manchester Statistical Society began a series of investigations. Over the following three years they surveyed education, housing, and other features of working class life. The London society and some of the provincial societies sponsored similar investigations in the 1830s.[17] Although these social surveys proved too expensive to sustain, interest in the early societies continued to focus on questions of social welfare. The official history of the London society states that the "condition of England question," that is the social and moral condition of the wage-earning population, dominated the organization's attention in the first decade of its existence, and that three-fifths of the papers presented in those ten years were in one way or another related to this issue.[18] T. S. Ashton in his centenary history of the Manchester Statistical Society makes a similar point. In Manchester even in the later years, 1853–1875, roughly a third of the papers read to the society dealt with sanitary or Poor Law subjects.[19]

It was primarily this interest in the state of the poor that seems to have united the members of the statistical societies and to explain the rapid spread of the statistical movement in the 1830s.[20] There is a link between the advent of the movement and the later developments of social policy in Britain.

. . . the stench of urban poverty drove thoughtful, vigorous, unsentimental middle-class people—doctors, bankers, those experienced in insurance, and the like—to the study of social pathology. These successors to the early political arithmeticians and to the later, isolated labours of Davies, Eden and Colquhoun organized themselves up and down the country in statistical and philosophical societies for the investigation of the accumulating consequences of urban and technological growth. Their local investigations into the educational, physical and criminal conditions of town populations served as pilot surveys for the great national inquiries of the forties. Their membership provided the nucleus of later royal commissioners and inspectorial public servants. During the thirties new intellectual and professional attitudes were established and they derived from medicine rather than from religion. . . . And alongside the vast and growing apparatus of sentimental charity through which the upper classes discharged warm advice and cold comforts at the poor, there developed central and local agencies equipped to make realistic assessments of the social costs of urban industrialism.[21]

But despite its influence on subsequent events, the complex of ideas underlying the statistical movement seems to the late twentieth-century observer a most curious mixture of incompatible elements. It was a program dedicated to finding solutions to urgent social problems but one which abjured opinion and politics. It was a separate science, a social science, which rejected both theory and discussion of cause and effect. Finally it was a science of individual facts and observation which showed remarkable indifference to mathematics.

The loud claims of objectivity seem to have been seized as an answer to a fundamental problem: How might the statistical societies harness social and political concerns without at the same time appearing to be merely political organizations and without abandoning their claims as scientific societies?[22] In this circumstance one might expect to find mathematical methods emphasized in the statistical program of the thirties. But such was not the case. We have already seen the council state that statistics is distinct from mathematical science, although it might use the tools of mathematics. Among the members of the statistical societies we look in vain for anyone with more than modest mathematical ability. Charles Babbage would have been something of an exception, but rather early he ceased to be active in the movement. Prior to Francis Galton there was probably no one in the Statistical Society of London who understood the mathematical significance of Quetelet's demonstration of the law of error. No one, of course, rivaled the sophistication of Laplace. The statistician of the early nineteenth century was not expected to be highly trained in mathematics. His function was to collect and arrange useful data. The abstract mathematical side of statistics received almost no attention in early Victorian Britain.

To understand this attitude toward and the interest in statistics by public-minded men, men educated in the classics or medicine or experienced in commerce or manufacturing, one must consider the immediate past of statistics, especially on the continent.[23] The Victorian statisticians were familiar with that tradition, as the definition and derivation of the term "statistics" offered in the introduction to volume one of the London society's journal indicates.[24] The introduction explains that the word "statistics" was derived from the German word *"Staat,"* and that the purpose of statistics was to bring together facts which would "illustrate the condition and prospects of society." This was the purpose of statistics as taught in the German universities of the eighteenth century, and it was best represented in the work of Gottfried Achenwall, Göttingen professor of law and politics. Statistics as taught in the German universities was the comparative description of states and countries, which might take as its purview a wide range of facts concerning population, geography, climate, natural resources, trade, manufacturing, military strength, education, religious observance, and constitutional provisions. The subject was regarded as a useful tool for governing and was frequently taught in conjunction with law. Most of the students intended to become civil servants. The first known course of lectures in statistics was offered at the University of Brunswick in 1660. By the middle of the eighteenth century statistics of this sort was being taught in several German universities.

The subject as understood in Germany was not essentially mathematical. Numerical or tabular data might be employed, but facts might also be recorded, using descriptive language. There was little or no mathematical manipulation of data. So far removed was German academic statistics from computation and numerical reasoning, that historians have detected a conflict in late eighteenth-century Germany between two rival schools: statistics in the Achenwallian tradition and political arithmetic, which was inspired by the work of the seventeenth-century English writers, John Graunt and William Petty.[25] The major point of difference between the two schools was the more rigid insistence by the political arithmeticians on the use of numbers. These proponents of the numerical method gradually won the day, but the academic tradition continued to be influential. Perhaps because of that tradition, statistics in the early nineteenth century was more commonly defined by subject matter than by method. The statistician or statist was, according to that tradition, one interested in the objective study of the problems of the state. He might be expected to use numbers because they facilitated measurement and comparison, but he was not expected to possess a high level of mathematical skill.

Tradition, then, helped to sanction the way early Victorians defined statistics and to explain why men of little mathematical ability did not shy away. In other ways as well, the climate of opinion in early Victorian England encouraged men of liberal education and public interest to study statistics. Two intellectual traditions seem especially relevant. Although neither can be held responsible for the statistical movement, each in its own way probably helped to determine the character of the movement. The first of these is the concurrent revival of interest in the works of Francis Bacon.[26] A complete edition of the works of Bacon with a new biography appeared during the years 1825–1834, and another edition came out between 1857 and 1859. Macaulay's essay on Bacon in the *Edinburgh Review* of July 1837[27] stimulated wide interest and gave Bacon's philosophy a Whiggish interpretation. A more critical defense that was also influential was John Herschel's *Discourse on the Study of Natural Philosophy* of 1831. Bacon, of course, had seriously underestimated the value of mathematics, and he had advocated neither statistics nor political arithmetic; nevertheless, his writings appealed to the men who founded the statistical societies. They seem to have valued Bacon's defense of modernity, his "rationalistic vision of the orderly and progressive reconstruction of society on a scientific basis through discovery of the operation of social laws," his faith in material progress and his assumption that this progress would be accompanied by moral and intellectual improvement, and his emphasis on inductive reasoning.[28] Especially as interpreted by Macaulay, Bacon's philosophy was congenial to Whig sensibilities, particularly to the individuals who joined the statistical societies. Here was a proper English authority who appeared to defend these cherished beliefs.

The first generation of British statisticians was undoubtedly acquainted with at least the Whig interpretation of Bacon. References to the father of the inductive method occur in various places in the early papers of the London Statistical Society. An unusually explicit attempt to link statistics to Bacon was made by a leading member of the Society, William A. Guy, professor of forensic medicine at King's College, London. The assertion was made in 1865, at a time when the society was to some extent reevaluating its understanding of statistics. Guy defended the early Victorian understanding of statistics, although in a slightly more sophisticated manner than would have been necessary in the thirties. Then regarding statistical technique he wrote: "We largely use the true Baconian method of induction, and Lord Bacon's own favorite instrument the *Tabula inveniendi*."[29] While it is probably true that Bacon was more frequently cited than read, his authority certainly helped bolster the early vision of statists with its emphasis on simple empiricism and its concern with social and material progress.

Although Whig interpreters of Bacon like Macaulay might criticize such Utilitarians as Jeremy Bentham or James Mill for deriving the principles of human nature and government from reflection, not observation, and for constructing a "frivolous" and "useless" philosophy,[30] there were elements in the Utilitarian tradition that were congenial to the statistical movement. A recent historian has shown that as Bentham grew older, he turned more and more from the general principles of the philosophes toward the collection and publication of social and political intelligence.[31] He envisioned statistics as a tool for reform and as a "newly cultivated branch of *Geography*, having for its subject the quantities and qualities of the matter of *population. . . wealth. . .* and *political strength*."[32] Ackenwall would have had no reason to disagree with this definition. Bentham also hoped to turn this knowledge to useful ends by establishing a science, ultimately a numerical science of legislation, a science less akin to the physical sciences than to the applied sciences, an "art-and-science," like medicine. He believed statistics was to the moral sciences what experiment was to the physical sciences. Statistics would eventually enable a legislator to calculate the social consequences of proposed legislation by using a social calculus, yet to be developed from the principles of human nature and accurate knowledge of social realities.[33] Ignorant political tampering by uninformed legislators was to be avoided at all costs. Legislative and judicial reform, Bentham held, must be directed by accurate knowledge.

Neither the goal nor the medical analogy was highly original. The founders of the Statistical Society of London agreed and chose a similar mode of expression.

By this cultivation [of statistics of all sorts] only can we arrive at a knowledge of the physiology of societies, and comprehend the paroxysms of disease which they sometimes exhibit in a state of violence, or the exhilaration of health, which displays itself in a state of peace. Empirical treatment of symptoms, without this knowledge, must be as vain in its effects upon the body politic as upon the human frame; for it has no guide but "opinions," under which name may be couched the wildest or the most rational notions, the truth or fallacy of which is as yet equally unsusceptible of proof from scientific data.[34]

Scattered references in the early numbers of the *Journal of the Statistical Society of London* suggest that members were acquainted with at least the outlines of Bentham's ideas and found mottoes or slogans in his writings, just as in Bacon's. One example will suffice. The author, W. R. Deverell, in introducing his paper has claimed that vital statistics is the primary subject of statistical science. He continues: "facts are statistical only inasmuch as they can be shewn to have a direct relation to the ostensible end for which social union is established—the greatest happiness of the greatest number; and that, all national and even local legislation can be just and equitable only as it proceeds upon the general average principles obtained from statistical documents."[35]

Bentham himself had tried to encourage the collection of statistics. He suggested the creation of a population register in 1782, and in the following decades tried rather unsuccessfully to collect data by circulating questionnaires. As early as 1801 he had begun work on a new vocabulary for statistics which he hoped would put it on a scientific footing, and in 1832, the year of his death, he endorsed preliminary plans for a statistical society for London.[36]

In the early nineteenth century there were good reasons for the insistence that the legislator and civil servant be better informed. The state of official ignorance was enormous and shocked middle class professional and commercial men no less than it shocked Bentham. The Napoleonic Wars had helped demonstrate the government's failure to mind its own business. In the war years Bentham discovered both that the government did not know the number of paupers receiving relief, and that it could not even account for the amount of money in circulation.[37] Matters had improved somewhat by the fourth decade of the nineteenth century. There was a national census, and several government offices were beginning to collect statistics. However, even the 1831 census revealed the kind of errors that dissolved confidence in official statistics. That census gave the acreage of England twice, with the disagreement between the two figures as large as the area of Berkshire. At the same time imports continued to be evaluated according to official values which were based upon the prices of 1690.[38]

It is no wonder then that rationalistic, reform-minded men might insist that the collection of accurate social data precede reform and might greet with enthusiasm any program which promised to build a useful science of social facts. Following the Reform Bill of 1832, the political climate was conducive to both the enactment of a certain range of social reforms and the collection of an unprecedented amount of official information. The parliamentary commission may be taken as a symbol of the age in this respect.[39] These investigations increased in number after

the Reform Bill and came in the normal course of events to precede major legislation. Many of them collected statistical information and several employed statistical society members as investigators. It seems that both the commissions and the collection of statistics were seized upon as tools by those members of the newly reconstituted political establishment interested in reform.

Thus we come to another peculiar aspect of the statistical movement, the one that M. J. Cullen and Philip Abrams have featured in their recent interpretations: the way the statistical program filled the political and ideological needs of its founders. Cullen and Abrams have demonstrated very well that many of the early statistical studies were anything but objective and that the statistical reports were sometimes no more than propaganda disguised as fact.[40] The prohibition of theory and opinion, trumpeted so loudly in the public statements issued by the societies, was ignored from the very beginning. It was impossible to separate fact from theory. The claims of objectivity seem to have been rather a way of disarming political opponents, of capturing attention, and of bringing the reform message before influential classes. Cullen has offered a useful analysis of the early statisticians' ideals.[41] Especially in the provinces, the leading members were concerned with justifying the factory system against its critics. The first study the Manchester Statistical Society undertook was a refutation of the findings of Michael Sadler's Factory Commission. The industrialist statisticians quite naturally opposed factory legislation. They blamed urbanization, not industrialism, for the misery of the industrial towns. Their solution to the condition-of-England question was "the creation of a virtuous and quiescent working class. Humanitariansism, class interest, and statistics made a powerful reforming brew."[42] Education and moral reform were among the chosen instruments for obtaining this end. The moralistic explanation of the causes of poverty and human misery these men offered argued against state intervention. But as Cullen illustrates, there was a fundamental tension in the position taken by the statisticians. They also believed that the urban environment was to blame for the plight of the working class. Most believed that in matters of education and sanitation effective public action was necessary before a decent, moral society could be created. It was in these two areas, where their own position favored environmentalist explanations of present conditions and interventionist solutions, that the statisticians concentrated their early efforts. Especially in the provincial cities, statistics was accepted as a tool for this limited vision of social reform. Although valuable information on social life was obtained, the studies were rigged, perhaps often unconsciously, to serve these ends.

Abrams has stressed the relation of statistics to political economy.[43] Political economy postulates, Abrams suggests, the essential unity of in-

terests and blames misinformation and hasty generalization for conflicts. Yet in the thirties the problem of maintaining a consensus and defending the fundamentals of the creed was acute. "The problem was to keep political economy practical without plunging into self-destructive scrutiny of its own fundamental positions."[44] Thus statistical inquiry not only provided factual weapons for political battles, it also served to postpone any thoroughgoing assessment of ideology. Looking forward to the last two decades of the century, Abrams finds that statisticians clung most doggedly to political economy, while others, interested in the problems of society, abandoned such doctrines.[45]

He also finds in the provinces that additional motivation came from the fear of working class revolt and the need to redefine the proper roles of charity and, more generally, of the provincial elite in the new industrial society. One might claim that the statistical societies existed in part to serve the same purposes of amelioration as the Social Science Association of the 1860s and 1870s. What McGregor has said of that national body applies to some extent to the statistical societies as well. They "existed to save society from the twin perils of aristocratic government and the doctrines propagated by Owen and St. Simon. From the thirties onwards middle-class people were continuously digging channels by which working class demands could be drained away from the foundations of property."[46]

Farr's Political Liberalism

In many important ways William Farr was a characteristic member of the statistical movement, especially of the London group. He was a professional man of liberal reform sympathies with civil service connections. He shared most of the social and political biases that typified that group and defended the ideals and institutions associated with high Victorian liberalism: free trade, private property, representative government, self-help, respectability, and family life. While he occasionally adopted a highly moralistic tone which tended to blur the distinction between the physical or physiological and the moral or conventional, he usually sought physical or environmental causes and remedies for social problems. It was a principal axiom of his social and medical investigations that the misery of the urban poor was due to remediable physical defects in the environment of modern cities. The results of such defects appeared both in ill health or premature death and in human behavior. As we shall see, his disease theory was capable of explaining many of the physiological consequences. The moral consequences he discussed much less frequently, insisting when he did that their miserable circumstances had a brutalizing effect on the poor, sharpening competitive instincts and passions and encouraging vice.[47]

Cullen was quite correct to observe that Farr was one of the "best Victorian rationalist reforming minds" and "one of the clearest exponents of a considered environmentalist theory."[48] But the tension Cullen observed in the statistical movement at large—that between a moralistic explanation of human suffering with a concomitant demand for minimum state interference and an environmentalist explanation of other social problems with a demand for public action—is to be found in Farr's writings as well. We see this ambivalence in his attitudes toward pauperism, a particularly thorny problem for Victorian liberals. Farr's views on this subject reflect his attitudes toward social reform.

Like many public-minded, middle class men, Farr was worried about the existence of a pauper class. On a medical level alone it was a threat to society. He once blamed Irish immigrants for introducing and maintaining fevers in English cities.[49] The condition of the London underworld appalled him both professionally and morally. The metropolis, he wrote, "requires no harbours for criminals; no rookeries for the wilfully idle, drunken, and degraded. It does not want them; they infest its pure population with vermin, and zymotic diseases; it only accepts as fellow citizens the men who consent to abide by its hygienic laws."[50] But it was the sturdy beggar, the individual who was capable of working but who chose not to do so, that Victorians viewed with the greatest apprehension. Paupers of this sort were both a threat to social order and a continual reminder of a moral blight. Farr had no sympathy with such people, and supported a stern poor law policy against them.

. . . if the poor laws in this country existed to no greater an extent than in Scotland, the labouring population would not live a whit the worse; on the contrary, the rates—expended indiscriminately on the idle, reckless, vicious, as well as the good, but unfortunate—would be paid in wages to the industrious labourer, and saved by the prudent: while the worthless hereditary vagabond would eat the fruit of his evil ways in a precarious existence, and the bitterness of undeserved poverty—of helpless destitution—would be mitigated by the charity never inactive in the human heart.[51]

The Poor Law policy was a genuine dilemma. How could undeserved human suffering whose existence was unquestionable be relieved without at the same time creating a permanent dependent class and assuming the paternalism of an unreformed aristocratic government? Farr never found a solution, although he was sure he knew the goal. The Poor Law, he explained, should exist only temporarily. It was fit only for an intermediary state of civilization, between the time when men were slaves and were cared for like domestic animals, and the future when liberal government would have performed its duty "to call forth their [the poor's] energies, teach them to provide for their own wants, and to take care of themselves."[52] Although he had reservations, especially in the 1830s, about the administration of the new Poor Law, he could defend the law throughout his life. "Without abuse," he observed in the 1870s, the Poor Law "is an insurance of life against death by starvation, and of property against communistic agitations."[53]

But Farr did not believe the Poor Law should be a means of punishment. The poor had both rights and a special claim on society. As he expressed it in an 1837 editorial: "We believe it now to be a prevalent opinion, among the majority of reflecting men, that the grand object of every good government should be to protect the weak from the tyranny or oppression of the more powerful. . . . Even under our reform government, we blush to say that the poor—the weak—who are always least able to defend themselves, have been, in the case of the new Poor-law, very harshly dealt with."[54] He went on to contrast Parliament's refusal to investigate the claims for each pension the government granted, with its swift passage of an act to deprive the poor of their "small pensions" unless they entered a work house.

Farr's writings give evidence of a genuine empathy with the misery of the deserving poor. This is most evident in his early career, in the 1830s and 1840s. But it shows up in later writings as well. Both Cullen and Greenwood have commented on it.[55] Even after making allowances for the sentimentality of his prose style and the occasional evidence of a morbid fascination with death, Farr's writings reveal a genuine sympathy for human suffering, absent in Edwin Chadwick and more professionally obscured in John Simon. Greenwood suggested this fellow feeling was bred in Farr's own difficulties in his childhood and his early career. Like numerous other Victorian general practitioners, Farr also gained an intimate familiarity with human misery in his practice among the poor.

Medical practitioners meet with many distressing cases of starvation in this metropolis. I will mention one. In the winter of 1838 I was requested in the middle of the night, to see a woman, who, it was said, was dying for want of help. I followed the messenger through a labyrinth of narrow passages, near Fitzroy market, and found in the corner of an attic a young woman, thinly clad, lying on a straw bed spread upon the floor. She had given birth to a child, then at her feet. Three children lay on the same bed, under a single rug. It was intensely cold. She had no fire, no candle, no food, and, if I recollect right, had not more than three halfpence in money to meet the exigencies of child-birth. The lodgers in the room below had been aroused by her groans.[56]

One further example will help illustrate his attitude toward the poor. It also shows his fundamental optimism about human nature and the possibility of genuine social improvement. He described a walking tour he took with the local registrar in a particularly miserable part of London's East End. He was shocked at the condition of the inhabitants:

"women, half naked, look drunk, and herd with the men; the children dirty, wasted, or ricketty—mischievous or wicked; the men swearers, liars, or thieves." He was tempted to despair of any chance of raising moral habits or improving the physical condition of such a population. But then a man went by with a collection box, and these same people gave freely, so that, as his guide told him, their sick and afflicted fellows could avoid the work house. Farr was touched. The incident confirmed his deepest hopes.

It was a ray of light in the darkest place. Here were the people who, to a superficial observation, appeared to have lost the vestiges of humanity, not only with self-dependence, but social affection and charity in their hearts—ready to divide their few pence with the sick and afflicted—with those a little more miserable than themselves—as freely as if they were fathers, sisters, brothers. God had left them charity; and if circumstances had obscured, they had neither paralyzed the intellect nor the heart. Who will venture then to despair—to pronounce these most miserable men inaccessible to the influence of enlightenment and humanity? If you talk to them of their interests, they can understand you; if you approach them to save their families from sickness and death, with a kind and generous liberality, bringing into their wretched courts and habitations what they may not now purchase—the necessaries and blessings of health—they can be grateful, for they also have succoured their fellows.[57]

That optimism was basic to Farr's position. Reform was possible, and it was possible without drastically altering traditional institutions or existing property relationships. While he could denounce the abuses of government or administration and condemn the lethargy of local authorities, he offered no radical explanations or solutions for the problems of his society. He realized privation might play a part in raising the death rates. In fact he clashed with the Poor Law commissioners and Chadwick over just this point. In his first letter to the registrar general, Farr had attributed sixty-three deaths in the metropolis over six months to starvation. While the subsequent correspondence shows he had been incautious with his details, he was undoubtedly right in substance in attributing some direct and more indirect importance to economic hardship.[58] However, the primary tendency of his observations in the first letter and more generally in his other writings, even during the economically hard late 1830s and 1840s, was to blame other factors, especially population density, the conditions of employment, and the impurity of the atmosphere for the high death rates of cities.[59]

Although he favored public intervention in many instances, he also believed in self-help, even in matters of public health. Intervention was needed to insure access to the minimum requirements of a decent life. But after that had been done, the cooperation of the poor was essential, and much could be done by their own efforts—encouraged by the examples of temperance and hygiene which the middle class could provide in lectures, health tracts, and medical advice in the popular press.[60] He hoped ultimately to make the poor independent of state assistance in medical affairs no less than in financial matters.

In spite of the fact that he expressed the ideal of self-help, the result of his investigations was usually the advocacy of an enlarged role for the state. This was due in part to his experience with the statistical evidence and to his frustration with the tardiness of improvement. It also grew out of his sympathy with needless suffering and his conviction that deaths caused by human neglect or ignorance demanded enlightened public action. In the midst of the 1841 smallpox epidemic and about the same time that he argued that public health reform involved minimum public action followed by self-help, he expressed the case for intervention this way:

Is not a case for public interference, then, clearly made out? Should not an energetic effort be made to save these lives, amounting to *several thousands*, from small-pox? They are helpless children, the great majority of them have not numbered fifteen years; but that can be no reason for abandoning them to their fate,— to the hot fever, the blistering pains, the defacing hands of this sad malady. They are, in many instances, the neglected offspring of the poor,—which again only gives them a stronger claim on the humanity, justice, and protection of society.[61]

Despite his ideal of the relations between the individual and the state, he was driven by both his facts and his heart into the role of advocate for positive state action. The use he made of his statistics in that advocacy is subject for later comment.

Farr's attitudes were certainly not unique. He falls within the broad spectrum of Victorian liberal opinion. He found like-minded men in the early statistical society. He also found them a bit later in the Social Science Association. This fashionable body existed from 1857 to 1886, and served as a national forum for a wide range of reform platforms.[62] It popularized these reform demands among the governing classes and brought pressure on Parliament. For a while it was quite successful. Farr was a founding member of the association and he was on its council and executive committee for many years. The health section claimed most of the attention he gave this society. He once presided over this section, and it was here that he read some of his most popular versions of his findings. He was one of many who belonged to both the Social Science Association and the Statistical Society of London. In many ways these societies may be regarded as two embodiments of the same impulses. But it might be more correct to say that the Social Science Association adopted the most popular and practical of reform concerns, when the Statistical Society of London began to devote more of its attention to technical problems and to economic questions.

Farr on the Nature of Statistics

Farr was in agreement with the founders of the statistical societies on the nature of statistics no less than on social goals. In fact he was a rather late defender of the early Victorian idea of statistics. The opening of his presidential address to the Statistical Society of London in 1872 might have been written thirty-five years earlier.

Statistics—that is the science of States—the science of men living in political communities, was never in such demand as it is in the present day; and the supply promises to be equal to the demand. Politics is no longer the art of Letting things alone, nor the game of audacious Revolution for the sake of change; so politics, like war, has to submit to the spirit of the age, and to call in the aid of science: for the art of government can only be practised with success when it is grounded on a knowledge of the people governed, derived from exact observation.[63]

Elsewhere he defined statistics as the bookkeeping or accounting of the state and its subject as comprised of two great divisions: population and property.[64]

More revealing still is his 1877 defense of the British Association's Section F against the attacks of Francis Galton.[65] Galton criticized the statistical section for its lack of rigor and for its disinterest in the mathematical basis of statistics and showed little sympathy with the general reform orientation of its leading members. Farr and older statistical enthusiasts like Chadwick defended Section F and the original view of statistics in terms of its social utility and past association with prominent men.[66] Nothing better illustrates the differences between the older and the younger generations of statisticians than the differences between Farr and Galton. Farr had little interest in mathematical theory. Mathematics for him was a tool, and the primary value of statistics was its application. Galton, of course, thought otherwise. The difference in interests between the two can be seen very clearly in the change that occurred in the reports of the British Association's Anthropometric Committee when its chairmanship changed from Farr to Galton in 1880. For five years under Farr's direction the committee had collected and printed its physical measurements for various occupational and social groups and noted simple relationships such as the comparison of mean values.[67] However, in the first report issued under his chairmanship, Galton published a theoretical discussion of probable error and introduced the concepts of mean, quartile, and decile as applied to a normal curve.[68] The work of the committee took on a mathematically more sophisticated tenor typical of the new generation of statistics.

But although he lacked Galton's mathematical interests and skill, Farr was never guilty of the excesses to be found in the formal pronouncements of the early Statistical Society of London. He rejected the mindless garnering of numbers and had nothing but scorn for the "empiric who throws heaps of tables in our faces, and asserts that he can prove anything by figures."[69] Although he had the utmost faith in the power of empirical investigation, he never assumed that the facts observation produced constituted the essence of science. In a medical editorial of 1837 he wrote: "facts, however numerous, do not constitute a science. Like innumerable grains of sand on the sea shore, single facts appear isolated, useless, shapeless; it is only when compared, when arranged in their natural relations, when crystallised by the intellect, that they constitute the eternal truths of science."[70] He insisted that the statistician adopt a critical approach, investigating the accuracy of his data, questioning the appropriateness of the units used, and attempting with the help of ratios, logarithms, and the calculus of probabilities to discover relationships and regularity in order to make predictions.[71] He also was never found advocating unattainable indifference to theory or to the political implications of the results of statistical investigation. Farr was always dedicated to making the results of statistical inquiries practical. In his later years, as president of the Statistical Society of London, he suggested that the time had come for the society to reconsider its determination to stand aside from partisan discussions, and he recommended that it take a more direct part in policy discussions.[72]

Part of the reason for Farr's more sophisticated understanding of statistics and his greater willingness to discuss the practical implications of statistics is to be found in his medical bias. As a professional group, medical men, especially physicians, showed an unusual interest in the early statistical societies. James Phillips Kay is only the most famous. Kay had first helped to found the Manchester Statistical Society. When he moved to London upon becoming assistant Poor Law commissioner, he joined the statistical society there. In London, of course, he had the company of other medical statisticians: William Guy, F. Bisset Hawkins, and William Farr being the most prominent among them. Not only were members of the medical profession attracted to the statistical societies, but, also health and medical problems played a very large role in the early deliberations of these societies.[73]

There were some very good reasons for the presence of the medical men and the discussion of health problems in the statistical societies. Public health was, of course, recognized as a fundamental component of the well-being of the working classes. It was also a subject that was comparatively easy to enumerate. Such was not the case with the study of the moral qualities, although some of the studies sponsored by the societies used such things as the cultivating of flowers, the number of prints on the wall, or the ability to sing a cheerful song as indices of respectability and morality.[74] Deaths, cases of sickness, or the amount spent on medical relief presented themselves more readily as useful indices.

There was also in the British medical profession a tradition of local investigation, connected with efforts to improve the condition of the poor. Physicians, especially those affiliated with dispensaries, were frequently the first professional people to gain extensive and direct experience with the lives of the poorest classes of cities.[75] Since the late eighteenth century the incidence of fever in the poorest parts of industrial cities had from time to time encouraged local investigations and some efforts at control by individual physicians or by voluntary boards of health. The profession was learning a principle it would make great use of for the future: there is a relation between the conditions of life and the incidence of endemic and epidemic diseases; fever was considered the paradigm disease. Some physicians had come to recognize that severe hardship and ill-health went hand-in-hand, and a few were learning that it was possible to prevent disease by the isolation of cases and by hygiene and sanitation.

Those trained in Edinburgh in the early nineteenth century like James Phillips Kay and Thomas Southwood Smith found some members of the medical faculty convinced that the high incidence of fever in cities was the result of poverty, and even found some who believed in the continental doctrine of medical police with its emphasis on state action to protect the public health.[76] Although English students seldom adopted the economic interpretation of disease or advocated the paternalism of medical police, several of these students became prominent in the public health movement in England, and were important advocates of environmentalist explanations of ill health and debility.

Physicians then who had absorbed the lessons of the past half century about the prevalence and prevention of fever had special reasons for joining the statistical societies. For them professional attitudes reinforced political and social ideology. James Phillips Kay, who had served in the Anscoats and Ardwick Dispensary in Manchester before becoming active in poor law administration and educational reform, accepted this social and environmental explanation of disease, and also shared the alarm of other statistical society members about the political consequences of the condition of the poor. Later he recalled that by the 1830s he became convinced that "the condition of the great mass of the people was one of the surest tests of the wisdom and efficiency of government, and the indispensable basis of the stability of institutions. . . . I not only became convinced of the necessity of a great reform which should bring into the front rank of topics for public discussion every question affecting the well-being of the manual labour class, but I entered eagerly into these discussions."[77]

But there was more to the doctors' interest in statistics. Statistics was seen by a number of medical men as a means of improving medical *reception in US?*

knowledge and practice. As early as 1829, in what is probably the first English textbook on vital statistics, F. Bisset Hawkins predicted that the application of statistics to medicine would provide a means of evaluating the effectiveness of various modes of treatment, of compiling accurate histories of disease, of establishing the effect of the conditions of life or labor on health, and of providing a basis for reliable prognosis.[78]

Doctors were more aware than their lay counterparts of the example of the physical sciences and of how poorly the medicine of their day compared in the precision of its methods and the accuracy of its predictions with those of the sciences. Two works published by medical men about 1840 recommended numerical or statistical methods to physicians on the analogy of the successful application of these methods in the sciences. One was William Guy's article in the *Journal of the Statistical Society of London* in 1839; the other was *Observations on the Application of Mathematics to the Science of Medicine* by Daniel and William Griffin.[79] These authors contrasted the casual methods used in medicine and the disagreements among physicians on fundamental questions with the methodological rigor and the extent of theoretical agreement in astronomy. The Griffins asked their readers to imagine an astronomer using words like "very frequent" or "sometimes," to imagine him dispensing with his tables to rely on memory for his information. The very idea was ludicrous. Both they and Guy suggested that the successful use of mathematics made astronomy an advanced science. They had no doubt that numerical methods could be successfully used in medicine, and as benefits of that application, they listed results like those Hawkins suggested a decade earlier.

Guy and the Griffins obviously were interested in more than finding practical benefits. Guy in fact blamed the excessively practical bent of most physicians and their preoccupation with individual cases for the backward state of medical knowledge. The only way to achieve greater certainty was to obtain knowledge of entire groups and of the probability of events. He suggested that even the essence of the art of medicine, the judgment of an experienced physician, was really the result of a rough calculation of chances, the type of calculation the numerical method would formalize and make more available to inexperienced practitioners. These authors did not accept the argument that the phenomena of life were too complex to be studied numerically. The Griffins offered the examples of Laplace and Roemer to illustrate that very complex astronomical problems could only be handled mathematically. They also referred to Pierre Louis's studies of the effects of bloodletting, although they did so with some apologies for the apparently "absurd conclusion" he reached by studying too few patients and by relying on the duration of cases as a measure of the value of treatment.[80] Both the Griffins and Guy also used the success of life insurance to illustrate that seemingly unpredictable events, like the duration of a human life, could be accurately forecast in the aggregate. Finally, in what seems to have been a comparatively rare use among the members of the Statistical Society of London of the example of Quetelet's best statistical work, Guy pointed to the constancy of certain social phenomena, such as the number of crimes committed annually or the percentage of accused criminals found guilty, to illustrate that even complex events that involve the human will become nearly as regular and predictable as physical phenomena when considered in large numbers.[81]

It was this realization, that statistics could discover order and regularity in complex events, that attracted the interest of certain medical men. Although Guy's mathematical vision was extremely short (he equated the numerical method with the "method of averages"), he recognized Quetelet's contribution in demonstrating the possibility of discovering such fundamental regularity. The discovery of such "laws" Guy took as the highest aim of statistics. Here again he used Quetelet as an example. The Belgian astronomer and statistician, Guy pointed out, had discovered that the "curve of viability," that is the regular change in the probability of living at different ages, resembled the way other things, such as the tendency to crime, changes with human age. As another example Guy cited the recent discovery of a statistical regularity in the case fatality for smallpox.[82] Guy did not name the author of that study, but a number of his listeners at the statistical society would have known that it was William Farr.[83]

Farr agreed wholeheartedly that the phenomena of life and death were law-abiding, and he believe rational medicine possible only when such vital laws were assumed.[84] The lawful nature of vital phenomena was a fundamental precept for him. Evidence came from a variety of sources. The most important was drawn from the insurance business. A life table illustrated that generations of men do, in fact, succeed each other in a regular way. He once described these changes as the march of a generation through life.[85] A certain number dies each year, and the number of either sex who will still be alive at some future age can be accurately predicted. The analogy of the life table is one he commonly employed. Early in his career Farr explained, "observation proves that generations succeed each other, develope their energies, are afflicted with sickness, and waste in the procession of their life, according to fixed laws; that the mortality and sickness of a people are constant in the same circumstances, or only revolve through a prescribed cycle, varying as the causes favourable or unfavourable to health preponderate."[86] This was a conviction he retained throughout his career, for it was essential to his entire program. Thirty-five years later he praised Halley for showing that "generations of men, like the heavenly bodies, have prescribed orbits, which analysis can trace."[87] To a challenge put forward in the French Academy of Medicine, that mathematical calculation and probability were not applicable to medicine, Farr responded: "If the Academy had sent M. Double and his metaphysical friends to the *Bourse*, or to the annuity and insurance offices of this country, he would have learned that the relations of vital phenomena *are* determined by the doctrine of probabilities; and that, so far from being the dream of theorists, the monied people of England have invested many millions of money, valued and exchanged on the principle that the duration of vital phenomena admits of calculation."[88]

This regularity and order in human life and behavior is what gave statistics its potential value as a tool for the study of man. The ability of statistics to discover laws in massed data in turn served to guarantee statistics the status of a science. Like other medical men in the statistical societies Farr looked to the sciences for example and justification. He reminded critics who pointed to the crudity of statistical calculation of the poor agreement between calculated atomic weights and careful chemical experiment.[89] Statistics was certainly no less a science than natural history or taxonomy, which used similar methods of observation and classification, but whose subject matter was inherently less interesting than the "laws of Human Life, and Mortality."[90] These laws of life touched human experience more directly than those of any other science and were of great interest "even if the knowledge of those laws gave men no more power over the course of human existence than the meteorologist wields over the storms of the atmosphere, or the astronomer over the revolutions of the heavens."[91]

The essential point, of course, for Farr was that the laws of life which statistics could discover did admit of very important applications: in medicine, in social amelioration, in commercial insurance. Medicine and public health were the first area of his statistical interest. In 1837 he employed a clever, if questionable, analogy to illustrate the value of numerical analysis. He contrasted the physiologist who studies the human body in its elementary units to the statistician who deals with groups of men. He suggested that although both studied the same laws and did complementary research, the immediate future lay with the statistician. Just as men had first discovered the laws of inert matter for gross bodies, not for particles, they would probably first discover the laws of life by studying nations, not individuals.[92] Even in 1870 when his interests had broadened enormously and his ideas evolved in several important ways, his faith on this point remained firm.

It is the duty of physicians, in recording facts respecting disease and death, to employ the same care as astronomers and meteorologists bestow on the observation of physical phenomena, and if that is done the observations will admit of the same kind of generalizations. And it must be evident, that as far as progress is concerned, these direct observations on the death, and life, and reproduction of the human race are of fundamental importance. The processes are complicated; life is enshrouded by an almost divine mystery; death is a kind of darkness; but it is a darkness which science can illumine.[93]

It is clear, then, why Farr was preoccupied with the discovery of statistical laws. Their discovery both guaranteed the scientific credibility of his endeavors and offered the hope of progress. Despite the importance of statisical laws, Farr used the term law fairly loosely. In investigating the possible relationship between food prices and mortality he described a "law regulating scarcities in England." In this case the law was a simple average, the discovery that between 1201 and 1600 there were seven famines and ten years of famine each century.[94] But in most instances the law was a mathematical expression which described how one set of values changed with time or circumstance. The density law he announced in 1878 may serve as an example.[95] In this case the law described how life expectancy in districts varied with the mean proximity between residents. Laws implied the power of prediction. But Farr was careful to warn his readers that statistical laws were somewhat different from physical laws. Statistical laws provided certainty only for large numbers. For any individual the probability of events was all that could be expected.[96]

Although Farr's most basic ideas about statistics remained unchanged throughout his long career, the focus of his interest enlarged as the statistical enterprise developed. As the popular interest in statistics waned in the socially less turbulent 1850s, economic subjects became more important.[97] With the formation of the International Statistical Congress in 1853 more regular channels for international statistical cooperation were created. Although he never abandoned his concern with the use of vital statistics for the improvement of public health, Farr was led by an early interest in life insurance to consider a number of economic problems, including civil service retirement schemes, taxation, and international coinage. He also became an advocate of international statistical cooperation: he corresponded with prominent foreign and colonial statisticians,[98] and played an active role in the International Statistical Congress.

The International Statistical Congress held nine sessions in various European capitals between 1853 and 1876; Farr was usually chosen a British delegate. He summarized the progress of official statistics in England for those meetings and reported to the registrar general on the congress's deliberations.[99] He was especially active at the 1860 meeting held in London. It was he who delivered the official invitation to hold the congress in the English capital.[100] As one of the secretaries, Farr helped plan the program, and he played a part in inviting leading figures such as the Prince Consort and Lord Brougham to assume honorary responsibilities in the congress.[101]

As Farr explained, the meetings of the congress gave evidence of the twin influences of Quetelet's social physics, and of the practical advances of British statistical administration.[102] Leaders of the congress like Farr regarded the organization as a means of facilitating the study of states by helping to bring together information about the economy, natural resources, population, and administration of European states in a form that allowed easy and strict comparison.[103] Farr's special areas of concern and activity in the congress were the creation of a uniform system of vital statistics to facilitate the international study of disease, and the establishment of a uniform decimal system of currency for statistical purposes. He designed a classification of diseases for international use based upon the nosology he had helped establish in Britain.[104] He also formulated a decimal currency system based on the British gold sovereign or a 25-franc piece.[105] In order to exploit the emerging mountain of statistics from the British Empire, Farr supported one further recommendation of the International Congress, the establishment in each country of a central board to coordinate all statistics taken in that country.[106] He believed this board should be a high-level policy-making organ, chaired by the Prime Minister, assisted by a prominent statist, and joined by M.P.s and colonial representatives. Its purpose would presumably be administration by statistical expertise.

He believed statistics would be of great value in policy-making at the highest level. He foresaw a place for statistics, not only in the domestic policy-making of his own country, but also in its political and military relations with the rest of the world. In a tone reminiscent of the Achenwall tradition of statistics, but with an analogy drawn from physics, Farr spoke of the statistician or statist helping the statesman tackle the unsolved problem of the balance of power. He saw the problem in these terms: "How are political powers to be measured, and how is the statesman to construct his parallelogram of forces? In past times France, the Emperor, and England were the principal powers; and the problem had then the complications of the three bodies in mechanics. . . . "[107] The solution, as might be expected, was the collection of crucial state information. In order to determine the European political equilibrium, national leaders needed to know: population, wealth, credit, size of military force, and the more complex elements in the war-making machine, like efficiency of administration and level of military genius. Farr attempted this unlikely program once during the Crimean War.[108] In that study he gave the population of the seven great powers, compared Britain and Russia in terms of the number of men of military age and the sizes of their armies and navies, and computed the sizes of the allied military forces and that of the Russian army. He chided Russia for having to learn from the armies of England and France in 1855 what she refused to learn in 1853 by failing to send delegates to the first statistical congress.[109]

Towards the end of his life Farr could muse on the progress of statistics in Europe—Russia had just announced her intention to begin a census, leaving the Turkish Empire as the last hold-out against progress, the last " 'unstatistical state' in Europe."[110] Elsewhere in the world the progress of science and enlightenment had been slower, but statistics and science would follow the colonial flags. Asia would be conquered for science from the north by Russia and from the south by England. Above all it lay with Britain to help remove the "Egyptian darkness" from Asia and Africa: "The English occupy, fortunately for science, a large portion of the finest parts of the world; and up to a certain point, as we know, they are, like every governing race, statistical. All the colonies have their own census; and some of them are prosecuting inquiries which have not yet been undertaken in England."[111] The arrangement may be new but the tune is very familiar. His science, as well as his religion and law, was to follow the European all over the globe. It was almost inevitable that those who believed in statistics as the science of states would add this discipline to the already ponderous weight of the white man's burden. The native was to be taught not only to vote, pray, and wear clothes, but to compute averages. What more telling evidence is needed that for men like Farr statistics had become an essential part of western culture?

THREE

THE GENERAL REGISTER OFFICE AND ENGLAND'S MORTALITY STATISTICS

Vital Data Before Civil Registration

The forces that had created the statistical societies were also bringing changes in the civil service.[1] In the 1830s statistical bureaus were established: the Statistical Department of the Board of Trade and the General Register Office (G.R.O.). Official statistics were also collected by other agencies, the Poor Law commissioners, the Army, and the census all playing a part. Therefore, the Registration Act of 1836 was only one of several reforms that brought statistical expertise to the civil service, but it is historically significant for several other reasons besides the creating of one of several new governmental statistical offices. From the viewpoint of administration it was an important link in the chain of social legislation that followed the 1832 Reform Bill, a complement to the new Poor Law and the Factory Act. From the perspective of the technical expert—physician, actuary, lawyer—the Registration Act marked the end of the first major campaign to remedy the long-acknowledged deficiencies of existing English vital statistics. Politically the act was a triumph for religious dissenters who chafed under the discrimination they suffered in the old system of keeping vital records.

The most important feature of that old system was its ecclesiastical character.[2] Ever since 1538, when the parish churches of England were required to keep records of baptisms, marriages, and burials, with the exception of two brief periods (1653–1660 and 1694–1704), the parish registers were records of ceremonies of the Church of England. As a source of vital statistics for the nation they suffered from several inherent deficiencies. They recorded baptisms, not births, and burials rather than deaths. In most instances dissenters were excluded, as were the religiously indifferent. Even poor Anglicans may not always have been included. Custom required a celebration at baptisms, and the registration of a baptism called for payment of a fee. Both expenses may have discouraged some churchmen from entering all their children in the baptism registers. As if these deficiencies were not enough, there was still another failing: the lack of supervision. In spite of Lord Burghley's recommendation of 1590 that the parish records be centralized in a single office and Anglican Church orders of 1597 and 1603 requiring that transcripts of the local records be sent annually to the bishops' offices, parish records for the entire nation were never effectively centralized and correlated. Parish registration remained a purely local affair, dependent on the diligence of minor church officials.

The inherent weaknesses of the system were magnified with the passage of time. Increasing "abuses" in the church such as pluralism and nonresidentism meant that local supervision of registration may have deteriorated, and the growth of dissent and the increasing inadequacy of church facilities, due in part to population growth and internal migration, meant that an ever larger segment of the population was excluded from the registers. .The parish register system "virtually collapsed" in the years 1790–1820.[3]

In spite of the casual way in which the parish registers were kept, they were regarded as important, especially to property-holding families. The records provided a means of proving personal relationships or tracing ancestry, and therefore were valuable in assuring inheritance and in gaining preferments for children in the professions or the trades. For these reasons during the eighteenth century dissenters, other than Baptists, were often baptized in the Anglican Church in order to have their names enrolled in the register. They would have preferred, of course, legal recognition of their own church records; they even lobbied for an extension of the stamp duty on the Anglican registers, a tax in effect from 1783 to 1794, in the hope that legal recognition would follow. They got the tax, but not the legal recognition.[4] Their discontent smoldered, only to resurface politically in the 1820s, when they helped pass the Registration Act of the next decade.

The other major source of vital statistics before the nineteenth century was the bills of mortality for several English cities. These bills were published by local companies; in London, by the Company of Parish Clerks. In London weekly bills for plague deaths appeared in 1592, and an Elizabethan order followed two years later that set up the machinery for their collection.[5] Following a brief lapse they were begun again when plague threatened in 1603. Thereafter they were published regularly. Like the parish registers the bills of mortality were based upon the experience of the parish churches, but unlike the parish records, the bills were published at the time of recording. The bills also differed in containing an entry for the cause of death. This information was supplied by local informers, usually untrained women, who would ascertain the cause of death and report to the clerk of the parish for a fee. Needless to say, little certainty can be placed in the precision of their identification or in the consistency of their nomenclature.

By the eighteenth century the inadequacies of the bills were recognized.[6] William Maitland, the topographer, called attention to the bills' imperfections and attempted to estimate the number of deaths omitted in 1729. Physicians were especially conscious of the defects in registering the cause of death. Thomas Short, John Fothergill, Thomas Percival, John Haygarth, and William Heberden (both father and son), all complained about the state of affairs and urged reform. In 1781 the physician William Black proposed the creation of a public office staffed by medically trained men to collect London's vital statistics. The Company of Parish Clerks also realized the need for change. On three occasions it tried to persuade Parliament to authorize such reforms as registering births and deaths, rather than baptisms and burials, and making notification compulsory. Nothing was done, and the existing system was allowed to continue in force.

Before the nineteenth century another major defect in British vital statistics was the absence of a census. There had, of course, been population estimates. These were made indirectly, usually from tax or military records. There had also been a few local enumerations, such as the ones of Carlisle which John Heysham undertook in 1780 and 1788. But although some smaller nations such as Iceland, Sweden, Norway, and Denmark had taken censuses earlier in the eighteenth century, England and other large continental powers like France refused to follow suit. In England, bills providing for the taking of a census at regular intervals were introduced in the House of Commons in 1753 and 1758, but defenders of traditional English liberties opposed them. William Thornton, a leading opponent, threatened to have his servants give any persistent census taker who appeared at his home the "discipline of the horse pond."[7] Both bills died in Parliament. Another reason for the reluctance to take or especially to publish a census was the feeling, born no doubt of mercantilist theory, that population figures were crucial state secrets. William Wales, for instance, feared that if a census showed the population of England to be smaller than was commonly thought, her enemies would be encouraged.[8] It was merely symptomatic of learned ignorance that the population debate of the later eighteenth century centered around this very basic question: whether the number of Englishmen had increased or decreased since the Glorious Revolution.[9]

That basic question, made more complicated by Malthus's doctrines, was in part responsible for the founding of the British census. More immediate reasons lay in the financial and manpower concerns of the government during the Napoleonic Wars and more immediately in the fears raised by the poor harvest of 1800.[10] The Population Act of 1800 established the machinery for the first four censuses, and vested authority for their supervision in John Rickman, clerk of the House of Commons, who had suggested as early as 1796 the political and economic advantages to be gained from an enumeration.[11] The censuses that Rickman supervised gathered information from two sources: direct enumerations conducted locally by overseers of the poor, and abstracts from the parish registers compiled by the clergy. For the 1801 census the overseers of the poor reported the number of houses in each parish, the number of these uninhabited, and the families living in each house. They also returned the size of the population, exclusive of soldiers and sailors, distinguishing males from females. Finally, the occupation of each person was required in one of three categories: agriculture, trade or manufacture, or neither of these. The other part of the census inquiry was designed to exploit the parish records to answer questions about population growth. The clergy in 1801 were required to return the number of males and females baptized and buried for every tenth year, 1700–1780, and for every year, 1781–1800. They also had to report the number of marriages registered each year, 1754–1800. Some changes were introduced in the next three censuses. Ages of the living were reported in only one of the first four censuses, the one for 1821, and that voluntarily. Better definitions of occupations were devised, although the returns were made for families, not for individuals, in 1811. In the census of 1831 the ages of the dead were compiled from the parish registers for the years 1813–1830. In all of these early enumerations, the returns were really local statistical summaries, in that information was not returned for named individuals.[12]

Statisticians became dissatisfied with several features of these early censuses. To be sure, some problems were unavoidable. Besides being tried on unproven principles, the census of 1801 was a rushed job. It was taken just ten weeks after the Population Bill received royal assent. This census and the other three Rickman supervised also suffered by inheriting all the imperfections of the parish records. He also realized that his local enumerators, although sincere, were often not intellectually equal to their task.[13] Rickman might have made better use of the means at his disposal had he been technically capable or more receptive to criticism. Although an able administrator, he was not a good statistician or demographer.[14] He was frequently inconsistent in technical matters, and although he had tried, he never really mastered such basic tools as the theory of probability or the principles of a life table. By the time preparations were being made for the 1831 census, he was coming in for some rather stiff criticism. The most outspoken came from John Ramsay McCulloch in the *Edinburgh Review* of 1829.[15] McCulloch criticized the supervision of the local enumerators, the classification Rickman used for occupations, and, for good measure, the preparation of London Bills of Mortality over which Rickman had no control. Rickman would not bend. In May of 1830, before a Parliamentary committee, he argued down Joshua Milne's suggestion for an improved census of ages, and he worked hard "to keep their [political economists'] nonsense out of the act."[16] It was 1841 before the census was substantially modified. By the time of that enumeration Rickman was dead, and the supervision of the census had also passed on to the General Register Office.

The 1841 census was the first modern British census.[17] For the first time, information for individuals was taken on printed household schedules that were completed by families all over England on a single night. This was also the first census supervised by a statistical bureau. The schedules were better planned and sought additional information for individuals. The office also tried to include people missed by previous censuses.

Farr spent much of his professional energy on the census. Beginning in 1841 he was on the committee of the Statistical Society of London that offered advice on taking the census.[18] He played a major role in the censuses of 1851, 1861, and 1871, when he was either an assistant commissioner of commissioner and one of the joint authors of the general reports.[19] Knowledgeable contemporaries claimed Farr exercised a decisive influence on these censuses and wrote a large part of the final reports.[20] One mark of his influence was the increased medical value of the census. The census of 1851, the first over which he exercised much influence, was also the first to include questions on physical disabilities, especially on the deaf, dumb, blind, and insane. These questions were repeated in 1861 and 1871 under Farr and under his successors until 1911.[21] From the household questionnaires Farr obtained information on the number of handicapped persons, their ages, their geographical distribution, their present or previous occupations, whether their conditions were congenital, and information about special institutions to serve their needs.[22]

Another census innovation which Farr put to greater immediate use was an improved return for occupations. Past returns had been of little statistical value because occupations were reported in very broad categories. For the 1851 census Farr introduced a new temporary classification of occupations.[23] The next two enumerations used an entirely new classification which Farr hoped would overcome some of the old ambiguities and provide an adequate basis for the scientific study of occupational disease.[24] He identified 431 occupations that he regarded as basic, and he reported the age of each person in five year groups under one of these 431 groups. To bring some order to the returns, the occupations were arranged in classes and orders. There were five classes: professional, domestic, commercial, agricultural, and industrial, to which he assigned Greek names, and a final class, indefinite or nonproductive. The classes were subdivided into eighteen orders. The six orders under the industrial class were differentiated primarily on the nature of the material used in manufacture, while the three orders of the unproductive class were designed to distinguish the independently wealthy from those with a useless skill or those on relief. Farr placed himself in class I, order I: government civil servants. Although subject to some criticism in the Statistical Society of London,[25] the scheme pleased Farr enough to encourage him to press its use on the International Statistical Congress.[26] It also provided basic facts for his major studies of occupational mortality for the decades of the 1850s and 1860s.[27]

Establishment of Civil Registration

By the early thirties critics of existing vital data had become more vocal, especially in their dissatisfaction with parochial registration. The most articulate were professional men who testified before the Select Committee on Parochial Registration which the Reformed Parliament established in 1833.[28] John Finlaison, the actuary of the National Debt Office, maintained that the defects of parochial registration made it impossible to determine the correct actuarial basis for government annuity schemes or for the operation of friendly societies. Antiquarians like Sir Thomas Phillipps testified to the poor care many registers had received, the difficulty in searching the registers, and the deliberate falsification some had suffered. Barristers and solicitors showed the legal importance of the registers and urged the creation of an improved system. The medical benefits of national civil registration were lauded by the editor of the *Medical Repository*, George Mann Burrows, who was led to testify to the political and moral advantages as well. Both he and the star witness, Adolphe Quetelet, told the Committee that England lagged far behind continental countries in its vital statistics.

In spite of the fact that such witnesses may have provided the expert testimony, the political force that brought the issue before Parliament was the grievances of dissenters.[29] Their complaints were of two sorts: first, their church records did not have legal status, and second, the terms of Hardwicke's Marriage Act of 1754 had brought the legal status of many dissenters' marriages into question. By the 1830s dissenters were prepared to take political action. It was John Wilks, leader of dissent in the House of Commons, who called for the Select Committee. He did so by stressing both the dissenters' claims to justice and the national need. Wilks chaired the committee and carefully guided its deliberations.[30] The conclusion reached was a predictable one: parochial registration ought to be superseded by a national system of civil registration.

Support came from other quarters: from the *London Medical Gazette*, from the Provincial Medical and Surgical Association, from the

British Association for the Advancement of Science, and from the legal profession.[31] After a series of parliamentary maneuvers, legislation of 1836 brought civil registration to England and Wales.[32] Although the staunchest proponents wanted a system for the compulsory registration of births, deaths, and marriages for all of Great Britain, in the face of Anglican opposition somewhat weaker measures were passed.[33] Two acts established the basic registration procedure: An Act for Marriages in England and An Act for Registering Births, Deaths, and Marriages in England.[34] The G.R.O., which these acts created, also interpreted the law and set up detailed procedures in a pamphlet it issued to its superintendent registrars.[35] The registration system was based upon the administration divisions recently established for the new Poor Law. By the first of March 1837 the guardians in all existing Poor Law unions were to have divided their districts into registration subdistricts, each under an appointed registrar of births and deaths. Those parts of England and Wales in which the new Poor Law was not yet in effect were to be divided into temporary registration districts and subdistricts. A total of 626 districts was formed in England and Wales.[36] Most districts consisted of a single union. The Act did not extend to Scotland and Ireland. Scotland got its own civil registration system in 1854, as did Ireland nine years later.[37]

The two thousand local registrars recorded the births and deaths that occurred in their subdistricts. Under the procedure that was developed, no fee was charged for registering a death or for registering a birth within six weeks. Between six weeks and six months a birth could be registered upon payment of 7s 6d. After six months a birth could no longer be registered unless it had occurred at sea. The registrars prepared each quarter a copy of the entries for births and deaths and presented their books and copies for certification to the superintendent registrar of their district. The registrars of births and deaths were paid according to their entries, 2s 6d for the first twenty and 1s for each additional birth or death registered. The superintendent registrars forwarded the certified copies to the General Registrar Office and received 2d for each entry made in their districts.

The superintendent registrar had a fairly desirable post. The Act provided that if qualified, the clerk of the Board of Guardians would become superintendent registrar also. This provision later proved a disappointment to the lower ranks of the medical profession. The position of superintendent registrar was considered a responsible one, and the incumbent was asked to deposit £100 with the registrar general as security. Besides appointing and supervising the registrars of births and deaths and forwarding the quarterly certified copies to the G.R.O., the superintendent registrar was responsible for indexing the registers of his union so that they might be consulted by the public. He also was the central official in the registration of marriages. It was he who issued notices of the intention to marry and marriage licenses and received the caveats of parties objecting to a forthcoming marriage. He also certified places of worship in his union where marriages might take place. In addition, he was authorized to have marriages performed in his presence, and he sent quarterly records of these marriages to the G.R.O. He derived additional income from fees for these services.

The birth register included entries for the date of birth, the child's names, the names of both parents, and the rank or profession of the father. Before 1927 only the registration of live births was required.[38] Originally parents suffered no penalty for failure to register a birth. In the marriage register the following information was required: date of marriage, the names of both parties, their ages (whether a minor or of age), marital status, their condition or profession, their residences at the time of marriage, and their fathers' names and professions. The registration procedure for marriages was quite elaborate and apt to be more expensive than for births and deaths. It was apparently regarded as a service to individuals, and no penalty was provided for failure to register.

It was the registration of deaths that received the greatest attention, legal, statistical, and demographic. The reason may be found in part in the medical and actuarial interest in the laws of mortality and morbidity. Public health questions also served to direct attention to the death registers. Although there seems to be no direct evidence for it, there may be something to the unusual suggestion of Arthur Newsholme that a major factor in marshaling support for civil registration was the mortality caused by the first visitation of Asiatic cholera, 1831–1832.[39] The death registers were certainly watched anxiously in subsequent epidemics both by public authorities and by the medical profession.

Attempts were made from the very beginning of civil registration to see that the death returns were complete.[40] It was only here that a penalty was imposed on private individuals for noncompliance. According to the original regulations, each death in England and Wales was to be registered with the local registrar within five days. Responsibility for the reporting lay with the family or persons in attendance of the dead person during the final illness or with anyone present at the time of death. In practice, the responsibility for registration lay with the person who would have to bury the deceased, since the registrar's certificate was authority for burial. Although a burial might legally take place without that certificate, the person officiating at the burial was subject to a £10 fine if he did not report the burial to the registrar within seven days. If a coroner's inquest was not involved, the informant supplied the required information about the deceased, identified himself, and signed or made his mark in the register. The required information concerning the deceased was date of death, name, age, sex, rank or profession, and cause of death.

Medically the entry for the cause of death was a most important feature of the Act. Doctors who had urged the creation of a national system of civil registration or had criticized the London bills of mortality emphasized the importance of providing accurate records of the cause of death. The British Medical Association (B.M.A.) consistently supported efforts to improve these records. At its first annual meeting, the Provincial Medical and Surgical Association, as the B.M.A. was then called, sent a memorial to the Select Committee on Parochial Registration urging measures to insure accurate records of the causes of death.[41] But in spite of such professional interest, the cause of death was not mentioned in the original bill. It seems to have been at Edwin Chadwick's urging that Lord Ellenborough made this addition. In his account of how the Registration Act was passed, Cullen tries to establish the origin of Chadwick's interest in the matter and finds it in Chadwick's hope to use the registration system as a means of placating the medical profession, with whom he was at loggerheads over the Poor Law medical services.[42] If the registration of the causes of death were required, a strong argument could be made, Chadwick realized, for appointing medical men to the places created by the act as registrars of births and deaths. This, he hoped, would weaken the medical opposition by providing additional income for Poor Law medical officers. The case is quite plausible and gains strength in the fact that many of these local positions were originally filled by medical men.[43] Other evidence, however, suggests that the profession was not so easily bought off. Besides sensing a cheap device to quell opposition, authors of medical editorials suggested it was beneath the dignity of a member of the profession to serve below a clerk of the guardians, and they claimed that medical men ought to fill the superior positions as superintendent registrars.[44] It is also important to remember that Chadwick's interest in the registration of death and its causes quickly outran these small political ends, as he realized the potential value such information might have for poor law administration and especially for sanitary reform.[45]

In spite of this interest in the cause of death, the provisions of the act for obtaining the information were quite lax. The informant could either report the cause of death as it had been related to him verbally by a physician, or he could simply give his own opinion on the matter. If a coroner's inquest were involved, the registrar entered the judgment of the jury on the cause of death. But the information received from coroners was often no more precise than that returned by laymen. In the early years of registration, coroners frequently listed as causes of death such phrases as "natural causes" or "visitation of God."[46]

At the center of the registration system was the G.R.O. in London.

The Registration Act gave the G.R.O. supervision of registration and required it to prepare a yearly abstract for Parliament and to issue copies of vital records. The office assumed other responsibilities and grew in size accordingly. It began issuing weekly reports for the metropolis in 1840. Quarterly reports for the nation began to appear in 1842. The G.R.O. from time to time also prepared special reports. Farr's reports on the cholera epidemics of 1848–1849 and 1866 and his third life table are early examples. Finally, beginning with the 1841 enumeration the G.R.O. had responsibility for the census of England and Wales. From a staff of five permanent members it grew to over eighty permanent and temporary employees in the first decade.[47] By that time Farr's department employed, besides Farr, three senior clerks, ten junior clerks, and ten temporary clerks who were working on the 1841 census. When Farr retired, the G.R.O. was employing a hundred permanent clerks.[48] By the time the first appointments to the office were being made. Chadwick had become keenly interested in the registration system. He had already issued instructions to the Poor Law guardians and had tried to establish a mechanism for studying epidemic disease and pauper sickness in the unions.[49] He took an interest in the staffing of the new office as well. He recommended Charles Babbage for the position of registrar general. The post, however, was filled according to the dictates of Whig patronage and went to the brother-in-law of Lord Clarendon and Lord John Russell, Thomas Lister, "a flatulent young novelist" and the "decorative headpiece" of the office.[50] Babbage, it seems, realized this would be the fate of the appointment and decided not to apply for it.[51] Chadwick remained interested in the G.R.O. In fact, when Lister died in 1842 Nassau Senior recommended that Chadwick become the second registrar general.[52]

Lister's replacement was also chosen by the dictates of patronage, but in this case the choice was a fortunate one. Major George Graham, brother-in-law of the home secretary, Sir James Graham, took office in 1842 and made a career of the post, serving until 1879. Graham had considerable administrative skill. Looking back from 1890, a most knowledgeable contemporary, Sir John Simon, had nothing but respect for Graham's organization, discipline, and pride of public service.[53] On taking office Graham trimmed the staff and ended the Whig placemanship his predecessor had practiced.[54] Thereafter he seems to have retained a firm grip on administrative affairs, and he saw to the routine work of the office. He left statistical matters to the statistical department, especially to its head, William Farr. Graham and Farr seem to have established a fruitful working relationship. This partnership led Major Greenwood to comment that although Babbage was a better mathematician than Graham, it was well that Graham became Registrar General since he saw that the office was well run and left the statistics and their interpretation to Farr.[55]

Farr's Role in the General Register Office

Farr had watched from outside while the Registration Act was being implemented, and although he welcomed national and civil registration, he was not entirely happy with the way things were going.[56] He did not like certain provisions of the act, particularly the connections it established between registration and the Poor Law administration. He was also critical of the facts that the registration of stillborn infants was not required and that no provision was made for having medical men certify the cause of death. The medical profession was expected to cooperate voluntarily, but it was promised little in return—not even a guarantee that the results of registration would be available for medical purposes. Farr was especially troubled by the first appointments to the G.R.O. His editorial of February 10, 1837, is devoted to this subject. Incompetent men were being appointed, he claimed, and the beginning of registration unnecessarily delayed. Registration was in fact postponed from the beginning of March to July of 1837.

The neophytes of the Registration-office demand through Lord John Russell four months longer to familiarize themselves with their duties: from all we have learnt, four years, as hinted in the House of Commons, would not suffice. Statistics require for their successful cultivation a particular turn of mind, a long preliminary education, and extensive practice; and is it not a fact, that Lord John Russell's brother-in-law, the Registrar-General, never produced any statistical paper, and, at the time he received the appointment, knew very little of statistical registration? Did not he propose to employ an able deputy, and was not a young gentleman thrust into this place from another quarter, who knew less of statistics than himself? . . . It is perhaps to be regretted that sinecures have been abolished. If they still existed, Ministers could give their relatives and followers salaries without obstructing the progress of science. . . .[57]

We do not know whether Farr regretted having written this editorial when he was asked to join those statistical neophytes. The chances are that he did not. He was never known for tact or understatement, and he may have thought he had given Lister his due by acknowledging the registrar general's talents as an author and by saying he would welcome Lister's appointment to a more appropriate post like Poet Laureate or *Romancier General*. Farr first joined the G.R.O. unofficially to head the statistical department, and his appointment to the permanent establishment came in July of 1839.[58] We do not know how he was chosen. Evidence suggests that several men recommended him who were familiar with his articles in medical journals and his chapter on vital statistics in McCulloch's volume. Dr. Neil Arnott apparently recommended Farr to Chadwick, who in turn brought him to the attention of Lister.[59] Sir James Clark may also have recommended him.[60]

Farr was at first a rather minor official, "to be seen and not heard," as Greenwood put it.[61] He had the comparatively modest first clerk's salary of £350, while his superior earned £1,000 annually.[62] But the value of Farr's technical knowledge was quite early recognized. He was the only one of the heads of the four divisions to have a special title "Compiler of Abstracts," and by 1846 his income had been raised to £505, making him the third highest paid member in the office.[63] Two of the other division heads then earned £390 and the third only £340. Under George Graham, Farr received quite exceptional treatment. He was given the title "Statistical Superintendent." His salary was gradually increased, so that it reached the statutory limit for his position: £600. Thereafter, at Graham's prompting it was raised above the current ceiling by a special Treasury grant. In 1855, when these grants began, his special allotment was £200, bringing his annual income to £800. By 1874 he was earning £800, plus a £300 Treasury grant, plus a £30 grant from London University.[64] That was a very generous civil service salary. The registrar general's salary was then only £1200. It cannot be fairly claimed, as the medical profession later tried to do, that the government had not recognized Farr's extraordinary importance to the office.

We can learn something of that importance in a memorandum that outlined the duties of the statistical superintendent.[65] Although the document is in a formal scribal hand very different from Farr's scrawl, internal evidence indicates that Farr composed the summary and did so around 1872. The duties listed were numerous and varied, and they included planning and supervising the office's abstracts and assisting in the preparation of the annual, quarterly, and weekly reports. The undertaking of special projects, such as the reports on the cholera or the English life tables, was also mentioned. The statistical superintendent was also to keep himself informed of foreign statistics and to be prepared to give evidence and testimony to Parliamentary committees. Farr pointed out that his responsibilities called for a knowledge of medicine and related sciences, practical mathematical ability, and knowledge of foreign languages, at least French, Italian, and German.

The document presents in fact a fair picture of Farr's official activities. Not surprisingly, in view of the fact that it may have been composed to support the request for a larger treasury grant, the memorandum portrays the statistical superintendent as a very responsible scientific figure. Farr suggested that any future occupant would need even better medical and scientific qualifications than he possessed. He also urged the creation of a "distinct title" for the office as a reward and reminded the government that in the future the statistical superintendent would probably be drawn from the class of "successful and eminent medical men" who earn £2,000 to £10,000 a year. Farr's professional expectations had certainly swollen since he entered the civil service. By the time he composed this document his professional reputation did in fact make him the peer of the famous and fashionable practitioners and of the politically influential physicians of his day.

Farr came to so dominate the workings of the G.R.O. and especially its publications that he was considered by some contemporaries to be the real registrar general.[66] There was certainly reason for this opinion. It was Farr who appeared before parliamentary committees. It was he and not George Graham who defended the registration of births and the census procedure from the criticism of William Lucas Sargant in the Statistical Society of London.[67] The impression has been furthered by twentieth-century historians. Under Lister, Finer claimed, "all the work of the Registry was done by William Farr."[68] While Farr was certainly responsible for the scientific content of the office's reports and was perhaps the most outspoken interpreter of the official mortality statistics, he was, of course, highly dependent on the efforts of a large staff of assistants and especially on George Graham's administrative abilities. Graham may have contributed to his comparative neglect by historians. In his last report he paid a gracious tribute to Farr. "To his scientific researches and reports," wrote Graham, "I attribute any reputation that may have accrued to the General Register Office of England and Wales from the time he accepted office in this Department."[69]

Yet the running of the G.R.O. had become a partnership. While they certainly had their differences, Graham and Farr complemented each other's abilities and interests. Farr was less cautious and more impatient for change. He must have badgered Graham on countless occasions about changes in procedure and various reforms he thought necessary. Although there seems little hope of establishing the nature of their working relationship in any detail, since many of the G.R.O. records have been destroyed,[70] two helpful letters of Graham to Farr survive. Both seem to have been written in response to Farr's proposals. Both show Graham slow to make changes, reluctant to put pressure on the government, and interested in guaranteeing the accomplishment of routine tasks. The first, dated June 6, 1866, deals with department affairs and ends rather gloomily. "Her Majesty's Government have frequently shown that they consider my opinion as to registration of Vaccination cases of no value whatsoever. They would probably entertain the same (probably just) opinion of my advice as to Registration of Deaths."[71] The second, of October 31, 1874, was written after Farr had made suggestions for changes in the registration and census schedules in order to make the procedures of England and Wales, Scotland, and Ireland compatible. While acknowledging the value of the idea, Graham replied such changes could only be tried after a great deal of discussion which could not then be undertaken, and he reminded his colleague that among other things the office was about to move into new quarters and also was about to implement the reforms authorized by the Registration Act of 1874. Furthermore, the work of the office was badly behind schedule. The annual abstract for 1872 would not appear before 1875, the *Supplement to the Thirty-fifth Annual Report* was far from complete, and the *Thirty-sixth Annual Report,* which should have been published March 31, 1875, was still unfinished.[72] We can imagine this scene repeated on other occasions.

Farr's eagerness for improvement, both scientific and social, made him one of the leading advocates of medical and public health reform in the civil service. He had a singular combination of abilities and interests for that role. At some distance of time John Simon drew a very sympathetic and objective picture of the qualities of the statistician with whom he had collaborated and occasionally disagreed. Mr. Farr, he wrote,

had a happy combination of qualities for the position to which he was named. Of liveliest intelligence, and with a mind which revelled in generalisation, well-instructed in theoretical medicine according to the earlier lights of the present century, and a master of the methods by which arithmetic is made argumentative, he had also considerable literary resources and powers; was a wide reader, for use and pleasure, in the books of many languages; was a practised writer, having for several years been active in journalistic and other authorship; and wrote with admirable directness and simplicity. Eminently he was the man to bring into statistical relief, and to make intelligible and instructive to the common mind, whatever broad lessons were latent in the life-and-death ledgers of that great counting-house: eminently, too, not a man to forget the practical human interest of such mathematics.[73]

Unlike Chadwick and Simon, who might influence events through administrative and legal means, Farr could exert influence only indirectly. The G.R.O. had no authority to undertake field investigations, or to offer advice, or to advocate specific reforms. The Victorian understanding of the duties of the office was stated very concisely in a report of a Treasury Committee of 1855: "The primary object of the Department is to record all the Births, Deaths, and Marriages in England and Wales, without distinction of class or religious persuasion, in order to furnish the means of tracing the descent of property, of calculating the expectation of life and the laws of mortality, and of ascertaining the state of disease and the operation of moral and physical causes on the health of the people and the progress of population."[74]

That Farr was able to make the office something more than a storehouse of vital information was due both to his own abilities and to the peculiar circumstances in which he was placed. His isolation from the wellsprings of political and administrative power also protected him from criticism and political reprisals. He was able to overcome some of the limitations of his position and of the Registration Act by exploiting his annual letter to the registrar general. These letters appeared in almost all of the forty-one *Annual Reports of the Registrar General* on which he worked, and they are among his most important writings. Ostensibly their purpose was to allow comment on the statistical and medical significance of the abstracts of the deaths and causes of death for the year. They really offered him a virtually free forum for discussion of sanitary reform, preventive medicine, and other topics. The special studies Farr supervised, such as his cholera reports, offered him even greater freedom.

Farr also had the advantages of having joined the civil service at a time when the structure and internal discipline of departments was comparatively loose. This permitted individual civil servants considerable freedom of expression. In the Whig ministry of 1830–1841 there were numerous examples of officials personally advocating political or administrative change and of even doing so by appealing over their superiors' heads directly to the public.[75] This freedom was curtailed by mid-century,[76] but because of his personal repute, and his position—principally the fact that he had the support of his chief—Farr continued to enjoy comparative independence. Medical men in the civil service were especially likely to express independent opinions. John Simon is the most famous example. Besides building up his medical enterprise in the Privy Council to unprecedented proportions by a unique combination of personal charm and masterful diplomacy, Simon actively participated in the sanitary agitation outside government. Royston Lambert, who has narrated Simon's administrative accomplishments, acknowledges that Farr was even more independent in not only taking part in the sanitary agitation but openly advocating reforms in his own department that his chief opposed.[77]

Farr had adopted this stance from the beginning of his career. In a letter to Edwin Chadwick of February 13, 1837, which has received some historical attention recently, Farr made it very clear he disapproved of the latter's plans for the use of registration material. He thought little of Chadwick's grasp of statistical methods, and had no intention of letting the Poor Law commissioners manage registration or medical statistics.[78] He enclosed "a scurrilous publication— the *British Annals of Medicine*," perhaps the editorial of February 10 which had attacked the government's implementation of the Registration Act.[79] Had Chadwick known more about the man he had recommended to Lister, he would not have been surprised at the response he received. The two men, as we shall see, were headed for some serious disagreements while Chadwick remained in public office.

Farr was influential in a variety of ways. He was probably not well-known to the general reader, although London newspapers gave some attention to his work, but he was read by an important group of administrators and professional men. Indeed, he became one of the main suppliers of facts for the sanitarians' arsenal. Farr also served as an expert witness for parliamentary committees and commissions. He was, for example, a member of the Royal Commission on the Sanitary State of the Army in India.[80] He gave testimony before the Select Committee on the Public Health Bill of 1854–1855,[81] before the Army Sanitary Commission,[82] and before the Royal Sanitary Commission.[83] He provided unique evidence consisting of life table calculations for miners for the Royal Commission of Mines in 1865.[84] He also spoke as an expert on actuary principles before the Select Committee on Assurance Associations,[85] before the Select Committee on Income and Property Tax,[86] and before the Select Committee on Police Superannuation Funds.[87] Farr also testified before the Royal Commission on the Water Supply of 1868–1869.[88]

Farr used his official statistics in advocating specific reforms outside government as well. The Statistical Society of London, the International Statistical Congresses, and the Social Science Association all provided places, as did the B.M.A. and the pages of the *Lancet*. He also collaborated with individual reformers. His most important collaboration was that with Florence Nightingale, most intense in the 1850s. We will discuss this work in Chapter Seven. In these private studies Farr exhibited the same breadth of knowledge and independence of judgment and used the same statistical techniques that appeared in his official publications.

Farr was also in large measure responsible for the evolution of techniques and procedures for gathering and analyzing the official mortality statistics. The Registration Act of 1836 had merely created the broad outlines of civil registration, leaving the details to be worked out later. There was no fundamental statutory change until 1874 when another Registration Act[89] was passed. In the meantime the G.R.O. staff created many of the distinctive features of the registration system. From the very beginning the office recognized that in order for the registration of deaths and their causes to be a success, the cooperation of the medical profession was essential. Even before registration began, Lister had secured support from the leadership of the three London medical corporations.[90] Lister asked doctors to provide a written statement of the cause of any death that occurred in their practices. Such a statement could be used by the person who would have to report the death to the registrar. Farr tried to encourage this practice, and in 1842 wrote letters to the profession that were published in the medical press, urging practitioners to cooperate in certifying the cause of death, and to note explicitly cases in which *post mortem* examinations had been performed.[91] A few years later George Graham simplified this procedure. In 1845 he provided every qualified medical practitioner in England and Wales with tablets of printed forms for this purpose.[92] Space was allotted for primary and secondary causes of death and the duration of illness. Hereafter any death not registered with the aid of this medical certificate was recorded as "not certified." The profession quite readily adopted the use of these forms. By 1870, 92 percent of all English deaths and 98 percent of London deaths were medically certified.[93] The medical certificates may have encouraged greater care and accuracy in reporting. Farr believed this to have been the case and felt justified in bringing out a new series of abstracts of the causes of death in 1847.[94] The certificate became an established part of the registration process, and its form suffered almost no change until 1902.[95]

The ready acceptance of these forms is a good indication that civil registration had the support of the medical profession. There was some criticism of the system in the forties, and proposals were made by physicians to collect more information at registration, to register still births, and to medically certify all deaths.[96] But the relationship of the G.R.O. to the profession was fairly cordial in the 1840s and 1850s. The *Lancet*, for example, welcomed the G.R.O.'s efforts to secure medical certification for the causes of death, although it carped repeatedly about the government's stinginess in expecting practitioners to provide the service *gratis*.[97] The editor, however, recognized the certification procedure would benefit the profession even without pay. Since only qualified practitioners would receive the forms, their use would provide some official recognition for these doctors denied to irregular or quack practitioners.[98]

The profession seemed proud of the official vital statistics and appreciative of the G.R.O.'s fairness and open-mindedness. As a *Lancet* editorial of 1855 explained: "So excellent has been the scientific basis, and so admirable the administrative efficiency of the General Register Office, that the English system of registration is deservedly looked upon by foreign governments and men of science as a model worthy of general adoption. Still it is not perfect; and it is not the least proof of Dr. Farr's great candour and ability, that he is ever found ready to listen to objections and to adopt well-founded and expedient improvements."[99]

With one exception, this happy relationship continued until the 1860s. That exception concerned the G.R.O.'s solution to an equally pressing demand, a scheme for arranging and analyzing the returns of death and their cause. Farr believed one of the most pressing needs of the new office was a statistical nosology, a classification of diseases. A nosology would help establish order in the mortuary records. An official scheme of nomenclature and classification was absolutely basic, he announced, and was as important to vital statistics as a system of weights and measures was to the physical sciences.[100] He made this one of his first projects at the G.R.O. and returned to revise and modify it at various times during his career.

Farr was familiar with existing nosologies. In the introduction to this first scheme, he cited about fifteen previous classifications.[101] He began by trying to adopt the one most commonly employed, William Cullen's, and he also tried Mason Good's. He found neither suited his needs, and so decided to draw up his own system.[102] Even before joining the G.R.O. he had made preliminary efforts in this direction. In his chapter "Vital Statistics" in McCulloch's *Statistical Account of the British Empire,* Farr analyzed the death records Heysham had collected for Carlisle, as well as those of the Equitable Society.[103] He arranged these returns by age group and according to the reported cause of death. In each case the data were classified twice by cause: first, according to the anatomical seat of disease, and second, according to the nature or the cause of illness. This rudimentary scheme was soon superseded by the more systematic nosology he devised for registration purposes. Farr's aim was to create a simple and practical classification based on sources and authorities familiar to practicing medical men.[104] The nosology also had to serve the administrative needs of the office. This meant, for example, that accidental deaths had to be included as well as those caused by disease. In spite of these practical aims, it is also clear that Farr became interested in the general principles of nosology and in the possible use of his scheme for other purposes. In his revised nosology he included nonfatal diseases, diseases which would not appear in the death register, in order, as he explained, to show where they should be placed if the nosology were used for classifying sickness.[105]

Farr's statistical nosology appeared initially in his first letter to the registrar general.[106] As he explained, the nosology was based upon "the mode in which diseases affect the population: whether they are generated and prevail only in particular localities (endemics), extend like cholera over nations (epidemics), or are propagated by contagion; whether they arise in an isolated manner (sporadically) from ordinary causes, and sources existing in the organization itself; or whether they are caused by violent means."[107] This nosology had three divisions. The first consisted of the epidemic, endemic, and contagious diseases. Smallpox, plague, mumps, cholera, puerperal fever, syphilis, and hydrophobia were all included. The second was labeled "Sporadic Diseases" and consisted of localized ailments arranged under eight organ systems plus subdivisions for diseases of uncertain seat and for old age. The third major division was for deaths by violence. No further indication was given for classifying violent deaths. The common English name for the disease was used, although Latin and English synonyms were also listed.

From a twentieth-century perspective the strangest feature of the nosology is the first division. This part also attracted the greatest amount of Victorian medical criticism. As we will see in discussing Farr's understanding of the causes of disease, he believed the members of this division were created by similar morbid processes. He eventually called them all "zymotic" diseases. But most important is the fact that Farr regarded this class of diseases as an index of public health and well-being.

This great class of maladies is the index of salubrity; it is this class which varies to the greatest extent in different climates and seasons; it is this class that has latterly been so much diminished in England, and that constitutes the principal difference between the health of different populations and different periods; for fearful and destructive as epidemics are in their strength, sweeping mankind of every age before them, like an irresistible conflagration, they can be controlled and almost always admit of prevention or mitigation. Of the utility of keeping this class of diseases distinct in a practical sanatory report there can be no question.[108]

The first version of Farr's nosology received some favorable comment in the medical press. The *British and Foreign Medical Review* urged practitioners to familiarize themselves with it in order to supply the registrars with accurate and statistically useful information.[109] The reviewer was especially pleased to see that Farr had taken cognizance of the latest advances in pathology, seeking, for example, entries for enteritis or peritonitis rather than merely for "inflammation of the bowels." In other circles, however, the nosology provoked criticism. A subcommittee of the Royal College of Physicians of Edinburgh headed by W. P. Alison reported critically and so did Marc D'Espine of Geneva.[110] Both of these physicians were keenly interested in the subject. Alison had led the British Association's subcommittee on the registration of deaths that reported in 1835.[111] D'Espine was already an experienced medical statistician and would in the future devise a rival statistical nosology. Alison and D'Espine voiced several of the same objections, objections that would be raised later in the century by other medical critics of the G.R.O.'s statistics. They were uneasy about Farr's first division: the epidemic, endemic, and contagious diseases. Some diseases, they pointed out, such as croup, diarrhea, and even cholera, might at one time be epidemic and at another be merely sporadic. Therefore it was, they claimed, very misleading to list these diseases under the epidemic class. Unlike Farr, Alison and D'Espine did not assume a similar mechanism of disease was at work in these cases. Alison could not see that cases of these diseases had much in common. Even deaths from the same disease Alison claimed, should be treated differently in the registers according to whether they occurred sporadically or in an epidemic.

Both critics believed a nosology should maintain a distinction between acute and chronic diseases. Alison wanted to see fatal cases entered by major anatomical seat in one of two columns labeled "acute" and "chronic." According to this scheme, deaths from croup, laryngitis, and quinsey would all be entered simply as acute diseases of the windpipe. Fatal cases of consumption would be entered under chronic diseases of the chest. In all instances except those in which the cause of death had been carefully determined by a competent medical authority, the disease would not be given a name. The English practice of assigning specific disease labels to all deaths was, in Alison's opinion, a great mistake. It gave a false impression of accuracy. His procedure would have abolished most of Farr's nosological entries.

For his part D'Espine insisted that it was more useful to distinguish the acute from the chronic than the epidemic from the sporadic. But true son of the Paris clinic that he was,[112] D'Espine favored a scheme that was based primarily on pathological distinctions. He wanted all tuberculous cases grouped together rather than listed separately by anatomical seat. D'Espine also questioned the practicality of Farr's scheme. Although he admitted it had value as a theoretical classification, he believed it was too complex and complete for its purposes. He would have preferred Farr's devising a nosology after registration was well under way, when he could see the types of returns the average informant was able to make.

Farr's response was a firm but polite defense.[113] He explained that the diseases in the first division were united in sharing a common means of causation. He also listed authorities to show that the members of that class were commonly considered epidemic, endemic, or contagious. While he agreed that the diseases Alison and D'Espine singled out might at one time cause few deaths, and at another, many, he argued the same was true of smallpox, which no one would deny belonged in the first division. Farr also claimed it was unreasonable to list deaths for the same disease sometimes under one heading and at others under another, depending on whether they were at the time epidemic. How common, he asked, must cases of a disease be for a compiler of abstracts to decide an epidemic was in progress? A similar arbitrary decision was also involved in deciding whether a fatal case was chronic or acute. The English practice of recording the duration of the final illness in common units of time was much to be preferred for statistical purposes. In response to D'Espine's suggestion that the nosology was too complete, rigid, and impractical, Farr reminded his critic that in registering a death the informant was under no obligation to follow the nosology or even to know of its existence. It was devised to aid the registration staff and medical practitioners, and it had to be comprehensive if it were to be of any use in systematizing the disease nomenclature used in the statistical returns.

Although Farr retained the basic features of this nosology, the critics had some effect. In the fourth *Annual Report*[114] he issued a revised nosology which in various ways reflected his attempts to answer earlier objections. In the first place, he explained more fully the rationale for his first division. He now explicitly named these diseases "zymotic," and gave one of the earliest and most complete explanations of his disease theory.[115]

He also listed several new entries to this division, such as rheumatic fever and diphtheria, and he subdivided the entry for smallpox into four groups in order to demonstrate the value of vaccination. Other entries were also subdivided. Syphilis, for example, was now entered separately for primary or secondary cases. The second division, sporadic diseases, now became two: sporadic diseases of uncertain or variable seat, and sporadic diseases of special systems and organs. The entries for the former were increased in number to include various forms of hemorrhage, dropsy, abscess, and tumors. D'Espine's suggestions were influential here because all forms of tuberculous disease, including pulmonary tuberculosis, were grouped together under this same heading. However, phthisis (pulmonary tuberculosis) also appeared in the third division under diseases of the lungs because, as Farr explained, there was not yet universal agreement that it belonged with the other tuberculous diseases. The old third division, now the fourth, external causes, was also expanded. Farr created subdivisions for such groups of causes as intemperance, starvation, poisoning, drowning, and mechanical injury. For the first time he also gave fairly specific instructions on reporting violent deaths. For many entries in the disease classes Farr listed standard medical authorities. In this way he helped practitioners in determining the cause of death. It was probably also a defense of the place he had assigned these diseases, another way of trying to silence criticism.

This revised edition seems to have been more favorably received. The *British and Foreign Medical Review* was again complimentary, and it welcomed in particular the use of the term zymotic to encompass the epidemic, endemic, and contagious diseases.[116] Another reviewer of the *Fourth Annual Report* offered guarded compliments and called Farr an "admirable conductor" for a reader "who shrinks from penetrating a forest of figures without aid."[117] Both reviewers, however, pointed to features of the nosology that must have bothered many doctors. In his passion for consistency Farr had been led to some bizarre creations. These are especially evident in the section for violent or accidental deaths. For many diseases Farr had adopted or coined a single Latinized term and offered this along with the more common disease names. He seems to have believed the violent deaths should, for consistency's sake, be entered as diseases. Since he had established for the zymotic diseases a consistent pattern between the Latin name of the disease and the name of the poisonous material he believed caused it, he applied a similar system to the naming of deaths by accident or violence. These names were derived from the causal agent. Farr's terms *arsenicia, nicotinia, psychria,* and *pinia* for example were the labels offered for deaths caused by arsenic poisoning, tobacco, cold, and starvation. Neither of these two reviewers welcomed such innovations in nomenclature nor thought the profession would adopt them. Here and in other places Farr was quite willing to use novel terms. This propensity lay behind some of the disagreements he had with at least two professional groups: medical men and, as we shall see, actuaries.

The G.R.O. used this revised nosology with slight modifications for twenty years.[118] Within ten years, however, Farr was at work on another nosology. This one had been requested by the first International Statistical Congress in 1853 and was presented to the next Congress in 1855.[119] Its purpose was to provide a classification of the causes of death which all member nations could adopt. Both Farr and his earlier critic D'Espine were engaged on the project. This time Farr wisely sought the counsel of the most prominent living British physicians and surgeons by eliciting their responses to a draft of his proposed nosology. He published the names and titles of about thirty of his respondents in the preface to his English summary of this nosology. The new system was both more complete and more formally arranged than its predecessors. Diseases were now grouped into classes and orders. There were five classes: zymotic, constitutional, local, developmental, and violent, and a total of twenty-three orders. The Zymotic class was the old division of epidemic, endemic, and contagious diseases. It now had five orders: miasmatic diseases, those diffusable through air or water such as smallpox, ague, or cholera; enthetic diseases, those in which a venom or contagious material passes through the skin, such as syphilis or glanders; dietic (dietetic) diseases including scurvy and ergotism; and parasitic diseases such as scabies and tapeworm. The second class in this international nosology was labeled constitutional diseases. Farr recognized that these diseases might affect several organs, that they were sometimes hereditary, and that they often left morbid deposits in diseased tissue. The class had two orders: diathetic diseases such as gout, dropsy, or cancer; and tubercular diseases. Phthisis (pulmonary tuberculosis) appeared now exclusively with the other tubercular diseases. The third class, the local diseases, had eight orders. These organ systems Farr had used in his first two versions. Developmental diseases, the fourth class, contained four orders. Two of these were defined by age: diseases of childhood and diseases of old age. One was for diseases of women. And the fourth was for diseases of nutrition. The final class listed violent deaths under five orders: accident, battle, homicide, suicide, and execution.

Farr spoke, quite correctly, of this scheme as a revision of the one then in use in England and Wales.[120] He recommended a procedure for registering individual deaths that was also borrowed from the G.R.O. practice. The nosology itself was his most elaborate. It was both larger and more thorough than his earlier versions. The change is best seen in the fate of the sporadic disease category of the first nosology. In the first major revision this category had been divided in two. By the time he devised his international nosology, Farr was considering these diseases under three classes: constitutional diseases, local diseases, and developmental diseases. The entries were identified and classified with greater care and in closer harmony with recent pathological findings. Farr freely admitted the benefit he had derived from the comments his consultants offered.[121]

He was also much less dogmatic in this third version about disease theory. His comments on the zymotic diseases were now very short. He merely noticed the differences in their prevalence with time and place and pointed to the facts that they could be diminished by public action, and that they were accompanied by specific transformations in the body.[122] Here was a major change from the version in the *Fourth Annual Report* where he gave a long and positive statement of his theory of zymotic disease.[123]

Farr hoped the member nations of the International Statistical Congress would adopt this nosology, and he tried to make it attractive by providing multilingual entries. Initially he listed English, Latin, French, and German synonyms. He apparently planned to include Italian, Swedish, Spanish, and Russian equivalents at a later time.[124] But European nations did not adopt his scheme. To the same meeting of the International Statistical Congress, D'Espine presented a rival nosology.[125] Faced with two conflicting nosologies, the Congress attempted a compromise. But even the compromise version failed to win general approval. Until 1893 no two continental nations used precisely the same methods of recording and registering the causes of death. In that year, however, Jacques Bertillon, the Parisian statistician, drew up the system that became the International List of the Causes of Death.[126]

This third version of Farr's nosology fared somewhat better at home, but even here there were critics. James Stark, M.D., Farr's statistical counterpart in Scotland, objected to the change.[127] He regarded Farr's older nosology, the one then used in Scotland, as the most suitable for statistical purposes—the new classification needlessly multiplied headings and broke the continuity of statistical records. It also, in Stark's view, pandered to fashions in medical theory such as the growing sympathy for the doctrine of contagion. Other conservative objections were raised as well, some of these from the civil service and the military. In the face of this criticism Farr turned to the Epidemiological Society of London for advice. The society circulated his questions to experts and published the responses. It appears from those responses that medical doubts continued about the disease theory on which the zymotic class had been formed, and that, in contrast to Alison and Stark, some physicians wanted information on such minute headings as to make almost any system of classification seem an arbitrary hindrance.[128]

In spite of the opposition, the G.R.O. began to use Farr's third nosology by 1860,[129] and it remained in use for the last twenty years of Farr's career. On succeeding Farr in 1881, William Ogle made some revisions in his predecessor's system, and this revised edition in turn was used for another fifteen years. Finally in 1896 the G.R.O. modified its nosology again by adopting the revised nomenclature published by the Royal College of Physicians.

Although the office eventually modified his system, Farr's nosology had a lasting influence. His schemes were adopted by statisticians in various English-speaking countries. In America, for example, the statistical pioneer Lemuel Shattuck urged Farr's nosology on the National Medical Convention of 1847. Within the next two decades several states and the United States Army had adopted the English scheme.[130] Even the present International List of the Causes of Death evinces Farr's hand with its opening division for epidemic, endemic and contagious diseases, its final division for deaths by external causes, and its divisions for diseases of organ systems.[131]

The Medical Profession and the Reform of Registration

It is easy to point out the deficiencies in Victorian vital statistics. Modern demographers have done so; Victorian doctors did so; William Farr himself did so. But in view of the circumstances we may marvel that these statistics were as good as they were. Almost all adult deaths were recorded after registration had been in operation several years. Although the registration of births was much more deficient, it was greatly improved as the century wore on. In order to appreciate the quality of the English vital statistics, we have only to compare them to the rudimentary vital statistics of the United States or even of France.[132] The real problems with the English statistics arose with their use of special purposes, including medicine. Since many Victorian doctors were interested in such specialized uses, it comes as no surprise to find these men prominent among the critics of the national registration system. By the 1860s some of medicine's enchantment with the official statistics had worn off, and the profession was becoming critical of things besides Farr's nosology. The reasons for these changes seem to lie both in the increasing sophistication and higher critical standards among the leaders of the public health movement and in the backlash, lay and medical, against the ways these statistics had sometimes been used by the proponents of state medicine.[133]

Some defects in the registration system were obvious to medical sanitarians. The Registration Act of 1836 had serious omissions. As we have seen, Farr recognized this fact even before he joined the G.R.O. The registration of births was not compulsory, nor was the registration of the deaths of stillborn infants. The Act did nothing to encourage accuracy in recording the cause of death, and it permitted informants to sign the register with their mark. Farr pointed out in 1866 that such defects had legal as well as statistical consequences.[134] They opened the door to fraud and made it comparatively easy to conceal infanticide and other forms of murder. In addition, the local registration procedure itself might be corrupted. Some local registrars were unqualified or irresponsible.[135] A tiny number had been known to add bogus entries to their registers to enlarge their fees.[136] Such deliberate falsification was probably too rare to exercise much influence on the overall statistical rates, although it could ruin local returns.

But there were other, more fundamental problems. Diagnosis was difficult. It was also difficult to select from several diagnosed conditions the primary cause of death, yet only the primary cause would appear in the G.R.O. abstract. Farr was acutely aware of these problems, especially in his mature years.[137] They were not easily solved and they remained to earn the serious attention of later statisticians.[138]

During Farr's lifetime the most thorough medical critic of registration was Henry Wyldbore Rumsey, physician from Cheltenham and one of the outstanding Victorian spokesmen of a coherent, comprehensive, and centralized system of state medicine.[139] Rumsey fully believed in the importance of vital statistics. In fact, he had made their collection and interpretation one of the pillars of his plan for state medicine.[140] He recognized, however, that the official statistics of his age contained serious errors and defects, and that they had sometimes been seriously abused. His book on the fallacies of statistics is dedicated to Farr. Rumsey did this not with a sense of malicious irony but as a mark of respect. Farr, he claimed, was "unanimously and most deservedly recognized as our highest European authority" on vital statistics, the "earliest guide" in his own study, and one of his "oldest allies in the warfare of sanitary science against indifference, ignorance, and prejudice."[141] The two men and their families had been on friendly terms for several decades, and remained so until Rumsey's death.[142] Rumsey began his criticism with two papers before the Social Science Association's Public Health Section in 1859.[143] In 1865 and 1866 he wrote a series of articles on the subject for the *Social Science Review*,[144] and slightly later read papers to the Manchester Statistical Society.[145] In 1875 these papers were collected and republished as his *Essays and Papers on Some Fallacies of Statistics Concerning Life and Death . . .*[146]

Although sympathetic with Farr's purposes, Rumsey was extremely critical of the flaws in the registration system. He pointed to the now familiar limitations in the Registration Act. He dealt very harshly with the system for reporting cause of death.[147] Despite the G.R.O.'s encouragement, these returns were still not carefully made. According to the registrar general's own figures, by 1860 nearly 20 percent of registered deaths were still recorded without the use of the medical certificate. For 2 percent of these no return whatsoever was made of the cause of death. In the remaining 18 percent the causes of death, usually returned by lay informants, were often "utterly worthless." But even when a medical man filled out a certificate for the cause of death, Rumsey was not certain that accuracy was always better served. Physicians might see a dying patient only in his last moments or might make out the certificate with information supplied by the family. More sinister was the temptation for practitioners to obscure or falsify the cause of death to save respectable families embarrassment in certain sorts of deaths.[148]

Rumsey also explained the difficulty of selecting the particular process, structural change, or derangement of function that would be formally recorded as the cause of death. There was no guarantee that uniform principles were used by various practitioners. The problem was compounded by the fact that the certificate limited the practitioner to ten descriptive words for recording the primary and secondary causes of death.

Rumsey provided a "registration puzzle" to illustrate his point, a certificate submitted by a medical officer of health in Gloucestershire in 1874 for a male, age 74.

Causes of Death—(1) alcoholism (2) fracture of the jaw (3) bronchitis (4) morbus
     brightii (5) inguinal hernia (6) cerebral haemorrhage
Duration of Disease—(a) Two months and 14 days (b) Two Days[149]

What meaning did the "cause of death" have in such a return? Furthermore, what was the compiler of abstracts, who sat in London, to do with such returns? His decision on entering such deaths by cause must be arbitrary, and a slight change in the G.R.O.'s selection process in such matters could profoundly affect the profile of the mortuary abstracts.

Rumsey was also critical of the official nosology, claiming it served in some cases to create rather than to eliminate confusion. He showed, for instance, how the same cause of death could appear in several places. A death returned as due to mortification or gangrene should be entered under class II, constitutional diseases. But if it resulted from frostbite or an accidental injury, it might also be entered in one of two places in class V, violent deaths. On the other hand it could also appear under class III, local diseases, if it were preceded by ossification of the heart, or under class IV, developmental diseases, if it followed a bed sore.[150] The medical needs of registering the cause of death would be best served by abandoning the use of nosology altogether and by simply listing the immediate cause of each death under its scientific name. In making his point he used the analogy of classifying books in a library. Just as a knowledgeable reader knew the proper title entry, so the person using the abstracts of deaths should be expected to know the proper scientific names for the diseases or modes of death in which he was interested. This was the extreme solution to the debates over the official nosology. It might have eliminated formal difficulties, but it would have severely hampered the G.R.O.'s operation.

Rumsey could have been faulted for overestimating the logical flaws and for underestimating the practical difficulties of registration. But he did find some vulnerable spots in the system, and he generated interest within the medical profession for seeking further improvements in the official statistics. By the time Rumsey wrote, critics had begun to point out another omission: national statistics of sickness. In the first half of the century statisticians like Farr had argued that a rather constant relation between morbidity and mortality permitted the cases of a given illness to be inferred from deaths by that disease.[151] This method of inferring morbidity from mortality, of course, ignored nonfatal illness. Rumsey pointed out a variety of objections to assuming a relationship between mortality and morbidity.[152]

By 1860 leaders in preventive medicine began to advocate the keeping of morbidity statistics. Their initial schemes called for using the Poor Law medical services to generate sickness statistics to supplement the registrar general's reports. Benjamin Ward Richardson and Galvin Milroy proposed such ideas, and John Simon, as the Privy Council's medical officer, attempted unsuccessfully to get the cooperation of the Poor Law commissioners.[153] Rumsey, in typical form, made more sweeping proposals. He thought public opinion would accept a national sickness register for certain classes of patients: those attended at public expense or relieved by a medical charity.[154] In the 1860s and 1870s several institutions added the registration of infectious diseases to their list of reform demands. As we shall see, the B.M.A. and the Social Science Association were probably the most important, although the Epidemiological Society of London, the Poor Law Medical Officer's Association, and the International Statistical Congress also offered support. Although notification of infectious diseases was not made compulsory for the nation until 1899, it had been put in force in many places by local initiative during the nineties.[155]

Elsewhere reforms in the nation's system of vital statistics had begun somewhat earlier. Farr himself had repeatedly suggested ways registration could be improved by instituting stricter local supervision of the registration process. The coroner's office was important to this end, and Farr gave it attention in the *Third* and *Nineteenth Annual Reports.*[156] The coroner's inquests served legal ends: to deter crime, to assist the courts, to protect the innocent from false accusation and from fear of violence. They might serve preventive means in other ways as well by discovering the causes for accidental injury and deaths. The coroner's duties also made him party to the registration system, since the Registration Act of 1836 required the verdict of the coroner's jury to be reported to the registrar of births and deaths as the cause of death. Such returns were sometimes highly defective. Farr discovered that in the early years of registration juries often gave perfunctory returns for the cause of death such as "natural," or "visitation of God." In other cases they did not determine a cause at all. Farr listed both sorts in the abstracts as "Sudden Deaths," the nosological miscellany that in 1839 had no fewer than 3,696 entries, about 1 percent of all registered deaths.[157] He made a variety of suggestions for how the coroner's returns might be improved. The most important of these was that coroners should be given greater independence from the magistrates. He suggested they be paid fixed salaries and an effort be made to raise their status in the public eye to a level commensurate with the importance of their duties. Finally, they should possess special skill. Since in many cases the cause of death could not be accurately determined without an autopsy, Farr declared coroners must be trained in medical jurisprudence and might be required to give evidence of such training before standing for election.[158]

Rumsey's criticism may have sharpened Farr's awareness of the deficiencies in the registration of deaths and elicited another of Farr's suggestions that was more influential. This was Farr's proposal for the creation of a new public medical office, the registration medical officer, whose duties would include investigating all deaths that were not medically certified, determining the cause of death when possible, and calling for a coroner's inquest in other cases. The plan is most fully outlined in his twenty-seventh annual letter to the registrar general of 1866.[159] But he had suggested the basic feature of the plan twenty-three years earlier, and called attention to it again in 1869 and 1870.[160] The new office would in fact perform many of the duties that could have been performed by an enlightened medical coroner. Farr maintained that besides improving the returns for the cause of death, the new officer would, like a good coroner, help detect and deter crime. He would also serve to guard the registration system against the entering of fictitious deaths. In addition, because he would frequently be called upon to enter the homes of the poor, he would obtain much knowledge of their condition and illnesses and could offer local authorities good advice on sanitary matters. The registration medical officer might therefore also hold the offices of coroner or of medical officer of health. He would, of course, be expected to be a medical man of good education who had knowledge and experience with *post mortem* examination. In addition, Farr urged the registrar general to appoint a medical inspector to oversee the work of the registration medical officers, just as the

G.R.O.'s existing inspectors supervised the work of the registrars and superintendent registrars.

The object of both these proposals, for the Coroner and for the registration medical officer, was to insure that the causes of all deaths would be determined by medically competent men. The proposals would enlarge the role of the medical profession in the registration system. By the 1860s leadership in public health and social medicine had changed from lay reformers to the medical profession.[161] Initiative for new health legislation now came from John Simon's Privy Council health office and outside government from the B.M.A. and the medical members of the Social Science Association. Rumsey was a leading spokesman for both of these private associations. He introduced Farr's plan for the registration medical officer into the deliberations of the B.M.A.'s committee on the registration of disease in 1866.[162] The committee endorsed the plan the following year and added to the proposed officer's duties the task of registering disease in his district. In 1872 the Social Science Association also gave Farr's proposal its support.

Rumsey's speech of 1867 to the B.M.A. contained the core of his observations on registration and state medicine, and it urged the adoption of Farr's plan to create registration medical officers.[163] This speech also seems to have focused the profession's concern for legislative reform, a concern embodied in the deliberations of the Joint Committee of the B.M.A. and the Social Science Association and the Royal Sanitary Commission.[164] Although registration was excluded from the commission's deliberation, it did benefit from the reforms that followed in the 1870s. The Registration Act of 1874[165] removed some of the most glaring defects in the registration system, but without giving the doctors their more novel demands. The act made the registration of births compulsory and imposed penalties for noncompliance. It also required the use of the medical certificate for registering the cause of death except in cases where a coroner's inquest was held. Other loopholes in the regulations were closed, and the superintendent registrar was given authority to prosecute offenders in his district. The act did not require the registration of sickness nor authorize the appointment of registration medical officers. In effect, it completed but did not extend the original vision of a medically useful system of registration which professional spokesmen had advocated in the 1830s. By the time the legislative changes were passed, much of the work in improving the system had already been done in piecemeal fashion. As we have seen, the use of the medical certificate for the cause of death was almost universal by 1870.[166] Although they could not satisfy the most expansive minds, the G.R.O.'s leaders had done a remarkably successful job exploiting an incomplete system.

FOUR

FARR'S BIOMETER

THE LIFE TABLE AND ITS APPLICATIONS
IN MEDICINE AND ECONOMICS

*Farr's Basic Statistical Tools: The Rate of Mortality
and the Life Table*

When William Farr began working for the registrar general, he faced not only the problem of helping devise a system for collecting and abstracting the registration materials but also the more mundane problems of tabulating and computing results. This work was tedious and exacting, and it occupied a great deal of Farr's time in his early career. He explained that he alone prepared the abstract for the 148,701 deaths reported in the first six months of registration.[1] In each case he had to decide under which cause the death would be entered.

The routine calculations of the office were laborious scribal exercises which were usually performed by pairs of clerks who worked on the same problem independently and then compared results.[2] Babbage's calculating machine promised some reprieve from the computational tedium. The G.R.O. bought a working model and employed it in calculating Farr's later life tables,[3] but the machine required constant attention and its results were disappointing.[4] Painstaking calculations employing logarithms remained the standard office procedure during Farr's lifetime. In fact, the G.R.O. did not employ mechanical means of tabulating its census material until 1911.[5]

Although he might call mathematics "the soul of statistics,"[6] Farr never became expert in mathematical theory. He had taught himself the elements of calculus, and was familiar with the work of Laplace and Quetelet. But he made little attempt to use the most sophisticated mathematical methods. He rarely used calculus in his published works, and with the exception of his life tables he seldom treated phenomena as continuous functions.[7] Farr never spoke explicitly of the distribution of data in the sense Quetelet did, nor did he use Quetelet's law of error.

There were undoubtedly practical reasons for this neglect. The problems of obtaining the most accurate data possible and of using basic statistical indices were the issues demanding immediate attention. Probably Farr recognized that most of his audience had less mathematical ability than he. We have noticed already how few members of the statistical societies knew more than shop arithmetic. Medical readers were scarcely any better prepared. In one of his early articles in the *British Annals of Medicine,* Farr encouraged medical students to acquire skill in numerical methods, but what he urged them to study was only the use of logarithms.[8] He did not change his mind very much during his career. The questions he submitted on vital statistics for the examination on public health at London University in December 1875 required mathematical knowledge no more advanced than basic algebra.[9] He asked the candidates how birth and death rates were computed, what were the present rates for various sorts of districts, what factors affected the rates, and how such rates should be interpreted.

Other indications suggest that despite the limitations of his audience and the practical nature of his responsibilities, Farr was not alert to the importance of mathematical theory. In a set of his notes,[10] presumably the draft of an article on permutations, Farr sought to prove the number of ways that $1, 2, 3, \ldots , n$ integers can be arranged in a row. In doing so he did not attempt a general proof but only calculated the solution for enough real examples to convince himself of the answer. More revealing still is the fact that Farr apparently failed to realize that his mortality figures for a smallpox epidemic he reported in the *Second Annual Report* produce a normal curve.[11]

One can easily make too much of Farr's mathematical limitations. Had he been more of a mathematician it is questionable whether the results of his work or his impact on contemporaries and immediate successors would have been much greater. Farr was a practical, working statistician. His duties called for someone who could make the best of imperfect data and put available information to good use. Farr was eminently successful in these matters. He established standards and techniques which became fundamental to demography and social medicine. These derived from experience, sound judgment, and the commitment to utility more than from high mathematical skill. Major Greenwood believed Farr's amateur status as a mathematician may have been a blessing in disguise, because it kept him from trying to squeeze good results from bad data under the cover of sophisticated manipulations.[12] Had he lived long enough, Farr probably would have become as suspicious as Sir Arthur Newsholme of the excessive mathematical manipulation of raw data by the Galton-Pearson school.[13]

The question of Farr's mathematical competence ought to be looked at from another point of view. Compared to the expectations of the age and to the performance of other statisticians, Farr clearly deserved the international reputation he acquired. At a time when statisticians, especially medical statisticians, were markedly uncritical of their data and showed little uneasiness about basing results on a handful of observations,[14] Farr worked to establish his conclusions on more critical standards. Thanks to the national data he inherited, a paucity of observations was seldom a problem. In addition, he was aware of the importance of choosing wisely the units to be used in statistical investigations.[15] These, he explained, should be both appropriate to the problem and consistent with existing studies. Farr also recognized many of the defects in the registration materials. He not only worked to improve the quality of future data, but he also tried whenever possible to account for and to correct probable inaccuracies in existing records.[16] Much of the latter was educated guesswork which depended on his experience and knowledge of the problem at hand. Perhaps most important, unlike the "careless or uninstructed retailers of official figures" Rumsey castigated,[17] Farr was aware of the effect the age composition of the population had on its morbidity and mortality rates. Farr had some appreciation of the importance of age differences for the evaluation of these rates even in his earliest publications.[18] But it was his later work, especially his decennial supplements, that developed the implications of this problem most fully. By that time, for example, he had developed a rather thorough appreciation of the effect population growth had on the age composition of a locality and hence of its importance to any study that attempted to compare sickness and mortality statistics from different areas.[19]

Turning now to Farr's statistical methods, we find that his most basic tools were simple ratios: birth rates, fertility rates, and especially death rates. Mervyn Susser and Abraham Adelstein have recently put the matter rather well in explaining that Farr took his numerators from the registration materials and his denominators from the census.[20] The combining of these two sets of data proved very fruitful. The two sets of figures were reasonably compatible, since both were gathered in the same geographical districts. In addition, Farr came to have statistical supervision over both sources during the middle decades of the century.

One can also describe Farr's approach another way by saying he applied some of the actuary's basic techniques to problems in medicine, public health, and economics. Farr chose in particular the life table and the rate of mortality, and he used several analogies to illustrate their importance. He once claimed the rate of mortality was as essential to the social sciences concerned with health as the concept of value was to economics.[21] The thermometer was a favorite analogy. On one occasion he described the mortality rate as a scale which "serves to measure the life-force, or the complementary death-force, in the same way as the centigrade scale of the thermometer serves to measure heat."[22] The life table was even more fundamental. Although it may have developed in the insurance office, it was really more than an actuary's tool. Farr called it a "biometer,"[23] and regarded it as a basic technique for the study of man.

Farr's use of the rates of mortality and the life table depended on the belief that life processes were law-abiding and subject to several forces whose effects could be measured. At each age and for each set of circumstances, he explained, the human frame is acted upon by two influences, one towards life and another towards death.[24] In sickness another set of opposing forces determines at every instant the chances of recovery or of death.[25] Over the course of a lifetime the balance of forces changes even during good health so that "a unit of life loses a certain fractional part by death every moment."[26] The proper measure of that loss of life with time is the rate of mortality. From the context of Farr's statements on this subject, it is obvious he was thinking of the example of the life table, which demonstrated a regular change in mortality with age. Seen this way, the rate of mortality was an accurate numerical measure of "the forces of the causes that induce death, of the death-force, *vis mortalis*," and its reciprocal became the measure of the *vis vitalis*.[27] The force of mortality itself had two components: the natural, due to ordinary physiological change, and the external, due to the influence of the environment.[28] This last distinction was very important to Farr's approach, because it was the latter component that made mortality rates potent weapons in the public health campaign.

The rate of mortality was Farr's primary statistical index. It had been used by his predecessors, but they had been neither consistent in the expression of the rate nor careful in its calculation. In the 1830s Farr's contemporaries recorded mortality either as a percentage of deaths to living or by the phrase, one death in so many lives.[29] Farr helped make the standard expression of mortality "deaths per thousand." In addition he was careful, especially in his mature writings, in defining the rate of mortality. It was not sufficient, he explained, to calculate mortality as simply the ratio of deaths to population. Three factors were involved: deaths, lives at risk, and time. The correct formula, Farr insisted, was the ratio of deaths to years of life. Returning to his favorite analogy, Farr explained that just as a thermometer was a useful instrument only when the amount of mercury remained constant or when the observer knew how much had been added or lost between readings, so the calculation of mortality depended on a knowledge of human lives being considered.[30] In order to calculate the rate of mortality one had to know the years of life at risk. In most real calculations this figure was not simply the enumerated population because population changes occurred during the period of observation. Farr explained how years of life could be determined for a variety of demographic circumstances.[31] In a stationary population the years of life were simply the constant population multiplied by the years involved. If the population were not stationary, the question became more complex. In an irregularly fluctuating population or in one increasing in arithmetic progression, the years of life were found by multiplying the mean population by the number of years, understanding of course that to determine the mean for the fluctuating population, very frequent enumerations had to be taken. In the case of a population's increasing as a geometrical progression, a special formula was deduced.[32] Farr explained how this formula gave the true mean for a population increasing in geometrical fashion, and he showed how its application avoided the understatement of the mortality resulting from the use of the arithmetical mean of the extremes or of the population at the midpoint in time.

Strictly speaking, Farr's strategy here was correct. This method of computing mortality would give accurate results for a rapidly increasing population. But with the benefit of hindsight, we can see that it was often impossible to calculate mortality in this way. In many of the routine calculations Farr could use only the population at the last census as his denominator. In better studies he used the census figures as the population at the midpoint of a series of registration years. Although not strictly correct, these latter methods probably gave relatively accurate results. It was only when he applied his mode of computation far afield, to the calculation of hospital mortality, that, as we shall see, his methods were successfully challenged.

Farr and his contemporaries used the rate of mortality for a variety of purposes, especially as an index of the health or vitality of a population. This use was widespread but by no means uncontroversial.[33] The mean age of death had already been used for this purpose, and at a time when civil registration was just getting under way it found a very powerful champion. In his famous 1842 *Report on the Sanitary Condition of the Labouring Population,* Edwin Chadwick used the mean age at death as a measure of the healthiness of a locality, and in a paper to the Statistical Society of London two years later he proposed the general use of this method.[34] Farr joined other statisticians and actuaries, William Guy and F. G. P. Neison in particular, in condemning this statistical heresy.[35] As Farr pointed out, the fallacy of this method had already been demonstrated by the actuary Joshua Milne and was no different from the error committed by those who constructed life tables from deaths alone without a knowledge of the number living at each age. Although Farr accepted Chadwick's underlying goal of showing how much an individual's manner of living shortened his lifetime, he agreed with Guy and Neison that the mean age at death was a deceptive way of determining that influence. The mean age at death was dependent on the age distribution of the population. In a population that had been growing for some time from an excess of births over deaths, the mean age at death and the annual mortality would both be less than the same figures for a stationary population that had the same expectation of life. The statisticians maintained that only a life table gave the proper average length of life, and in the absence of a local life table, the rate of mortality was the best measure of comparative health. In a section of George Graham's letter in the *Fifth Annual Report* that most certainly was written by Farr, the principles of a life table were set out in a popular style, and the fallacy of employing the mean age at death as a measure of a community's health was explained in general terms and by several clever examples.[36] This explanation appeared in 1843, the year following the publication of Chadwick's *Sanitary Report* and the year before the latter's paper to the statistical society. This incident shows very clearly that Farr and other professional statisticians recognized even in the opening phases of the sanitary campaign both the dangers of overlooking demographic factors and the fact that mortality rates were second-best indices of health.

Although life tables were to be preferred for comparative studies, mortality rates were easier to obtain and proved immensely useful. Farr employed a number of them. The backbone of the registrar general's reports was the general or crude mortality rate. This rate was based upon all registered deaths regardless of person or cause. It was the most easily obtained and most widely employed death rate. Farr used the general mortality rates for a variety of purposes: to monitor changes in health over time; to compare the salubrity of various geographical areas; and, by adding other socio-economic or geographical information, to explore the causes of high mortality. He used the general mortality rate throughout his career, although, in part because of criticism, he used it more cautiously as an index of health and well-being in his later career. He also calculated mortality rates for each sex, for various age groups, and for a number of causes of death. These more specialized rates were the basis of his most sophisticated studies of mortality and morbidity. We will consider specific examples of their use in later chapters.

There is one special mortality rate that should be mentioned here. That is the rate of 17 per 1,000, which was known as the "healthy district" mortality rate. Farr proposed using this rate as an index of health in the mid-1850s, and John Simon soon accepted it for this purpose.[37] In proposing this standard, Farr was making use of the differences in the two components he had identified in the force of mortality: the internal and the external. He recognized that it was impossible to observe the effects of the internal or physiological force working alone, since no known population lived in an ideal hygienic state. Still he knew that for the decade 1841–1850, one-tenth of the registration districts, the so-called health districts, had annual rates below 17 per 1,000. This fact convinced him that the natural rate of mortality was at least as low as 17 per 1,000, and he suggested that deaths above that rate could be considered due to preventible causes. The healthy districts not only offered one of the first standard populations for the computation of standarized death rates, but they also served as a sanitary yardstick. Farr used the rate explicitly as a standard of health by calculating "degrees of insalubrity" for town districts, each degree representing 1 death per 1,000 above the healthy district rate.[38]

These various mortality rates were Farr's common tools, but he recognized that they did not give as accurate a picture of the relative health of a population as a life table. The life table was for him the ultimate demographic tool. In its most rudimentary form a life table follows through life a certain large number of infants, born simultaneously, and it records at convenient intervals, usually on each successive birthday, the numbers still alive until all have died. In the popular account on life tables which Farr wrote for Graham in the *Fifth Annual Report,* there is a very clear description of the life table and its meaning. This section might still serve as an introduction to life tables and mortality statistics for a general reader. It also conveys something of Farr's enthusiasm for the life table approach. The life table, Farr explained, describes "the march of a generation through life," and he employed the analogy Addison used in "The Vision of Mirza": a column of pedestrians crossing a bridge whose consecutive arches concealed trap doors, numerous at the beginning, more sparse in the middle of the bridge, and frequent again at the end.[39] Although no one could say who among the walkers would vanish into the torrential stream below during the crossing of any arch, one could predict the relative numbers to disappear in the crossing of the various spans. Farr continued in a speculative vein:

In the law which regulates the waste of life, two things have been reconciled: the uncertainty of the hour of death, and the constancy in the same circumstances of the mean duration of man's existence. The days of successive generations are numbered, yet a child born today may die in any day, hour, or minute, of the next *hundred years;* and until a very advanced age the chances always are that the time of death will be several years distant: the danger of death we know varies at different ages, and in different states of health; but if the limit of life be 100 years, it is on an average 36,525 to one that a person will not die on a given day; 876,600 to one that he will not die on a given hour, and 52,596,200 to one that he will not die at a given minute. These chances—doubled or trebled as life advances—are so low that practically they have little or no influence in ordinary affairs; and as a general rule men have indeed no fear of dying upon any *day;* yet the knowledge that they *may* die at any instant, exercises a salutary check upon their conduct; and, notwithstanding its sometimes appalling effects, the changing certainty or uncertainty of life, according to the different aspects and points of view, is in harmony with the feelings, hopes, moral constitution, and destinies of mankind.[40]

Farr traced in this account the fate of the 100,000 infants of his table. His treatment of the final ages is entirely characteristic of both his enthusiasm and his faith in the laws of human life.

The mental faculties, ripened and developed by experiences, will not protect the frame from the accelerated and insidious progress of decay; the toil of the labourer, the wear and tear of the artisan, the exhausting passions, the struggles and strains of intellect, and more than all these, the natural falling off of vitality, will reduce the numbers to 9,398 by the age of eighty. Here we may pause for a moment. It would formerly have been considered a rash prediction in a matter so uncertain as human life to pretend to assert that 9000 of the children born in 1841 would be alive in 1921; such an announcement would have been received with as much incredulity as Halley's prediction of the return of a comet, after the lapse of 77 years. What knew Halley of the vast realms of aether in which that comet disappeared? Upon what grounds did he dare to expect its re-appearance from the distant regions of the heavens? Halley believed in the constancy of the laws of nature; hence he ventured from an observation of parts of the comet's course to calculate the time in which the whole would be described; and it will shortly be proved that the experience of a century has verified quite as remarkable predictions of the duration of human generations, so that, although we little know the labours, the privations, the happiness or misery, the calms or tempests, which are prepared for the next generation of Englishmen, we entertain little doubt that about 9000 of 100,000 of them will be found alive at the distant Census in 1921. After the age of 80 the observations grow uncertain; but if we admit their accuracy, 1140 will attain the age of 90; 16 will be centenarians; and of the 100,000, one man and one woman—like the lingering barks of an innumerable convoy—will reach their distant haven in 105 years and die in 1945.[41]

As Farr realized, life tables were nothing new when he began his career.[42] Edmond Halley, the astronomer, had calculated one as early as 1693 from records of 5,869 deaths that occurred during 1687–1691 in Breslau.[43] Of greater practical use was the Northampton table that Richard Price computed in 1783 at the request of the Equitable Society from information taken from the parish registers.[44] Such early tables were as defective as the data from which they were derived. Accurate tables could not be composed, as these had been, from deaths alone. Halley had been forced to assume the population of Breslau was stationary.[45] Price had even greater difficulties. The parish registers he used seriously underestimated the number of births because of the prevalence of religious dissent in the area. Price compounded the error by estimating the total population from the number of births. As a result, he seriously overestimated the death rate and gave the average life expectancy as twenty-four years, when it was probably around thirty. The results were unhappy. The Northampton table was widely adopted by insurance companies and by the annuity scheme the government introduced as a revenue measure in 1808. Because Price's table overestimated mortality, premiums were artificially high, and because it underestimated expectation of life, the government lost enormous sums on its annuities.

By the early nineteenth century better life tables appeared. Not only had commercial insurance offices been in business long enough to begin relying on their own experience, but also the first reasonably accurate life table for an English community was produced. This was the Carlisle table, published in 1815 by Joshua Milne, actuary to the Sun Life Assurance Company. Unlike Price, Milne had the results of two censuses for information on the living. The enumerations had been taken by Dr. John Heysham in 1780 and 1788. Milne also used Heysham's summary of the Carlisle Bills of Mortality for the years 1779 to 1787. Milne provided a table that gradually replaced the Northampton Table in practice, and in addition his *Treatise on Annuities*[46] became a standard actuarial authority.

Farr, of course, studied the works of Price and Milne as well as those of other nineteenth-century actuaries.[47] But he seems to have been particularly indebted to the works of Thomas Rowe Edmonds that appeared in the 1830s.[48] Edmonds (1803–1889) had studied mathematics at Trinity College, Cambridge, had absorbed the principles of Owenite socialism, and had published an original work on political theory before taking the post of actuary of the Legal and General Life Assurance Society.[49] What distinguished his actuary publications was his use of the national census materials, in particular the voluntary census of ages for the 1821 census, and the search of the parish registers for the ages of the dying from 1813 to 1830 for the 1831 census. This information allowed Edmonds to compile life tables for the entire nation or for such large areas as counties. He had information on the number and ages of the living at one point in time and information on the number and ages of the dying for a period spanning that census year. His data could have been more complete, but it was the right sort of data for computing life tables correctly. In addition, he used recent information for special groups: burial records kept by the Glasgow Committee on Churchyards and Southwood Smith's sickness statistics for the London Fever Hospital.

Edmonds claimed above all to have discovered a fundamental law of mortality from his tables. He established that the rate of mortality for each human age changes regularly year by year for three intervals of life: before, during, and after the years of procreative power. The precise limits of these periods depended on the population being considered. In the first period mortality dropped very rapidly, at an annual rate of 32.4 percent from about six weeks of age to the ages of six to nine, and from then to about fifteen years of age mortality was at a minimum. In the second period mortality increased annually at a rate of 2.99 percent from fifteen to fifty-five or sixty years. In the final period the annual increase in the rate of mortality was 7.97 percent for each year of life.[50] He believed that this was a fundamental law regulating human existence. The relative rate of change with age was universal although the absolute value of the mortality and the precise limits of the three periods of life might differ for various populations.

Between Ages.	Six Towns of England.	Glasgow.	London.	Theoretical Tables.			Sweden, 21 years, 1755-75.	England and Wales.	Carlisle, 9 Years, 1779-87.
				City Mortality.	Mean Mortality.	Village Mortality.			
0— 5	8.63	8.10	8.27	8.46	6.73	7.48	9.01	4.98	8.23
5—10	1.03	1.24	1.08	1.24	.99	1.02	1.42	.70	1.02
10—20	.73	.76	.60	.88	.70	.58	.71	.63	.59
20—30	1.39	1.17	1.07	1.17	.93	.78	.92	1.02	.75
30—40	1.56	1.57	1.52	1.57	1.25	1.05	1.22	1.19	1.06
40—50	1.96	2.31	2.29	2.10	1.68	1.40	1.74	1.49	1.43
50—60	3.00	3.50	3.61	2.99	2.40	2.01	2.64	2.25	1.83
60—70	5.83	6.04	7.34	5.99	4.83	4.05	4.81	4.33	4.12
70—80	12.10	13.57	15.23	12.36	10.04	8.46	10.23	9.90	8.30
80—90	24.62	23.81	29.91	24.53	20.18	17.16	20.78	22.08	17.56
Above 90	42.72	42.55	33.55	47.20	39.85	33.45	39.41	37.10	28.44
All ages	2.95	2.83	2.84	—	—	—	2.89	2.12	2.50

Figure 1. Three theoretical life tables by Thomas Rowe Edmonds. T. R. Edmonds, "On the Mortality at Glasgow, and on the Increasing Mortality in England," *Lancet*, 1835-36, ii, 358.

Edmonds suggested his discovery made it possible to construct more accurate life tables because by using his law and the technique of interpolation one could eliminate the yearly fluctuations that appeared in tables constructed from observation alone. To prove his point he constructed three theoretical tables.[51] (See fig. 1.) In each case he assumed a minimum mortality rate at age ten, and constructed the rest of the table by generating mortality rates for other ages using his law of mortality. For his village mortality table he assumed a rate of 5 per 1,000. For the mean mortality table he assumed the minimum rate was 6 per 1,000. For his city mortality table he assumed 7.5 per 1,000 as the base. These tables, he asserted, agreed very well with the best available tables constructed from observation. The village mortality table was much like the Carlisle table. The mean mortality table agreed with the table Milne had constructed from the national mortality figures from Sweden. And the city mortality table agreed with the figures available for Glasgow and other large cities. His commitment to this discovery was tarnished only slightly by the fact that the available data for all of England and Wales did not seem to agree. He held firm to his discovery, however, and criticized the national data for England as well as Richman's incompetence.[52]

In effect, what Edmonds seems to have done was to have discovered independently the same regularities in life tables that Benjamin Gompertz had pointed out more elegantly a few years before.[53] Some two decades later Edmonds became involved in a priority dispute over this matter that was thrashed out in the pages of the *Journal of the Institute of Actuaries*.[54] Posterity has decided in Gompertz's favor.[55]

Edmonds's work was a revelation to young Farr. It seems to have profoundly influenced his notions about the nature of vital statistics and to have offered him important suggestions about methodology. Most important was the concept of a statistical law. It was Edmonds's law of mortality which seems to have been Farr's paradigm. In his own statistical studies he hoped ultimately to discover laws analogous to the one Edmonds found in life tables.

Edmonds's work also pointed out to Farr the ways life tables might be computed and put to use in medical and social analysis. In Edmonds's *Lancet* articles we can find clear anticipations of approaches Farr would develop much more fully. First, Edmonds constructed life tables for entire communities, using data from the national census and from death records. Second, he showed an interest in using those tables and mortality rates derived from the same sources to compare the health of various places. In an article on the mortality of English counties, Edmonds reported finding a geographical pattern in the incidence of high death rates. The counties with the highest rates fell on a line running northwest from Brighton to Liverpool.[56] The lowest mortality occurred farthest away from this line, particularly in Northumberland, Cornwall, Devon, and Wales. Edmonds was aware that differences in the age composition of districts made the comparison of their crude mortality rates hazardous. He suggested that age-specific rates might be used to overcome such risks. He recommended in particular the use of the mortality rate for ages 15 to 60, especially the rate for women, as the best index of comparative health.[57] Third, Edmonds, like Farr, believed life tables would help advance medical knowledge and improve medical practice. In his articles in the *Lancet* Edmonds recommended the study of life tables as a means of assessing medical progress, because, as he said, the "only sure index of the practical success of the science of medicine is in the increase of collective vitality, or in the diminution of collective mortality."[58] As Farr was to do two years later, Edmonds also suggested that it was through the study of the laws of collective vitality and mortality that the laws of individual vitality and the chief causes affecting the length of human life would be discovered.[59]

Farr's early works show Edmonds's influence. In his article "Vital Statistics" in McCulloch's *Statistical Account of the British Empire* of 1837 Farr relied on both data and approaches he found in Edmonds.[60] For his part, Edmonds on at least one occasion used material from one of Farr's early articles.[61] By mid-century, however, circumstances had changed. Now Farr was the more eminent authority. Edmonds wrote to him asking for help during the dispute in the Institute of Actuaries in April 1859 and May 1869.[62] Farr defended the importance of his correspondent's work, but he saw that Edmonds's law was simply an independent discovery of the phenomenon described by Gompertz, which had been recognized in less complete form even earlier by Milne and Price.[63]

The construction and application of life tables were Farr's most serious statistical enterprise. Over the course of his career he constructed three national tables from the registration and census returns, as well as several other tables for particular regions or occupational groups. His first English life table appeared in the registrar general's *Fifth* and *Sixth Annual Reports* and was based on vital records for the census year 1841.[64] English life table number two appeared for each sex separately in the *Twelfth* and the *Twentieth Annual Reports*.[65] It was based upon the census of 1841 and the death registration for the years 1838 to 1844. The third national life table was Farr's major effort, and it appeared as a separate volume entitled *English Life Table*.[66] For its calculation he used the censuses of 1841 and 1851 and the death registration for seventeen years, 1838–1854.

By the time Farr began constructing life tables, the rudimentary table Farr described in his popular accounts had grown to more elaborate proportions. Typically there were columns not only for the number of the living at each age, but for the dying in each year, and several other columns derived from the living and the dying of use in determining life expectancy, the probability of living one year, or other factors of use in insurance practice. Life table works usually contained tables of annuities and premiums at various rates of interest. Farr's life tables in this regard were quite typical. They were, in fact, collections of many tables, not only survival tables for single persons and joint lives, but also tables of probability of survivals, life expectancy, and values and annuities at various rates of interest. The entries in some tables were proportional parts of an original number while other tables were entirely logarithmic. Farr's life tables also included instructions, formulae, and examples of the application of the tables to practical purposes. Farr's description of the basic life table relations before the Royal Society contains, for example, seventeen such formulae,[67] while English life table number three devoted some fourteen pages to mere lists of algebraic formulae, primarily of actuary use, which he had explained in the earlier pages.[68]

Farr gave several descriptions of his life tables. For details the interested reader is referred to the most thorough of these, Farr's account in the *Philosophical Transactions* and the introduction to his third national life table.[69] We offer here as figure 2 a sample page from Farr's health district life table. For the following account it may be useful to refer to this figure. The columns are labeled using the notation Farr employed in his later tables, and the headings above the columns give formulae for computing the entries and concise descriptions of the meaning of the entries.[70] Farr's tables were based on either 100,000 or 1,000,000 births. The initial

Table E.—Healthy Districts. Males.

Age.	Dying in each year of age x, 1 to x, x+1.	Born and living at each age.	Sum of the numbers born and living at each age x from x to the last age in the Table.	Population, or the living in each year of age 0, 1 to 2, &c.	Sum of the living, and of the living of every age x and upwards to the last age in the Table; also the years which the male, l_x, will live.	The years which the males at the age x and upward will live; also the years which they have lived over x.	Age.
x	d_x	Σd_x, l_x	Σl_x, L_x	$\tfrac12(l_x + l_{x+1}) = L_{x+1} + M_x$, P_x	ΣP_x, Q_x	$\tfrac12\{Q_x + (x+1)\} = Y_{x+1} + (Q_{x+1} + \tfrac12 P_x)$, Y_x	x
0	5767	51125	2509515	46915*	2887245	84008231	0
1	1591	45358	2458390	44562	2841530	81519733	1
2	923	43767	2413132	43152	2791168	79061404	2
3	662	42844	2369385	43283	2747977	76648272	3
4	512	42153	2326571	42887	2705494	74278926	4
5	427	41621	2284418	44408	2665607	72155176	5
6	341	41294	2242797	42103	2223992	69712273	6
7	275	40953	2201797	40766	2181172	67726385	7
8	223	40678	2160750	40266	2140060	65549767	8
9	186	40355	2120172	40365	2099994	63417940	9
10	161	40169	2079817	40089	2059273	61319677	10
11	146	40008	2039648	39935	2019943	59309990	11
12	141	39862	1999640	39791	1979708	57310314	12
13	144	39720	1959778	39648	1939917	55350502	13
14	154	39576	1920058	39499	1900226	53430409	14
15	168	39422	1880482	39338	1860770	51565889	15
16	186	39254	1841060	39161	1821432	49708782	16
17	205	39068	1801806	38965	1782271	47906937	17
18	227	38863	1762738	38750	1743306	46144418	18
19	248	38636	1723875	38512	1704556	44420217	19
20	267	38388	1685239	38254	1666044	42734917	20
21	272	38121	1646851	37985	1627790	41082000	21
22	277	37849	1608730	37711	1589805	39475203	22
23	281	37572	1570881	37431	1552094	37908233	23
24	284	37291	1533109	37149	1514663	36417875	24
25	287	37007	1496018	36864	1477514	34878786	25
26	288	36720	1459011	36576	1440650	33419704	26
27	289	36431	1422291	36287	1404074	31997341	27
28	290	36143	1385859	35998	1367787	30611412	28
29	291	35853	1349716	35708	1331789	29261644	29
30	292	35562	1313863	35416	1296081	27927683	30
31	292	35270	1278301	35124	1260665	26694316	31
32	292	34978	1243031	34832	1225541	25452213	32
33	293	34686	1208053	34539	1190709	24218088	33
34	293	34393	1173367	34247	1156170	23044648	34
35	293	34100	1139074	33957	1121923	21903602	35
36	298	33805	1104874	33667	1087977	20806055	36
37	298	33509	1071069	33360	1054314	19729311	37
38	300	33211	1037560	33061	1020954	18693858	38
39	302	32911	1004349	33760	987893	17682455	39
40	306	32609	971458	32456	955133	16715942	40
41	310	32303	938209	32248	922677	15777037	41
42	315	31993	905029	31826	890429	14870434	42
43	320	31678	874531	31518	858603	13995813	43
44	326	31358	843855	31260	827775	13158889	44

Figure 2. Sample page of Farr's healthy district table. William Farr, "On the Constructions of Life-Tables, Illustrated by a New Life-Table of the Healthy Districts of England," *Phil. Trans.* 149 (1859): 874.

entries for males and females were proportional to the relative number of male and female live births. His tables showed therefore the proportional numbers of the two sexes alive at any age.

There were seven basic columns in Farr's life tables. The first, the "x" column, gave the year of life. Actually it represented the precise moment of consecutive birthdays, beginning with the moment of birth equal to zero. The "l" column was for the living. It represented the number of the original life table population to reach each birthday. The dying were represented in column "d." Thus "d" represented the number to die after celebrating their x birthday but before reaching their $x + 1$ birthday.

These were the fundamental columns from which, as figure 2 shows, four other columns "L," "P," "Q," and "Y," were computed by summation processes. A good deal of basic demographic information could be obtained from these columns by simple arithmetic. For example the ratio of "d_x" to "P_x" gave the mortality at age x, and the reciprocal of this ratio was the number living out of which one death occurred in the year following moment x. Similarly, life expectancy at any age, or "mean afterlifetime" as Farr preferred to call it, was found by dividing the entry in the "Q" column by its counterpart in the "l" column at the age in question.[71] The seven basic columns also served as the basis for computing monetary tables of interest to practicing actuaries.[72]

The key to constructing the table was a complete set of figures for either the "d" or the "l" column. Once either of these columns was complete the remaining five could be found by summations. Farr chose to make the "l" column the basis for construction. It was no simple task to calculate these entries from vital data. Farr simplified his labor by making two assumptions. First he assumed that although human mortality varied with age, that, at least after the first five years of life, the rate of mortality at a given age was constant during the year and that those who died during that year did so at equal intervals of time. This assumption permitted Farr to ignore instantaneous change and consequently the need for using calculus. Farr recognized that, strictly speaking, his assumption was inaccurate, but he argued it was both necessary (because of manpower limitations in his office) and reasonable since it introduced no errors of significance in comparison to errors in registration and the census.[73] Even his formula for living one year derived from this assumption was not much different from the formula Edmonds derived using calculus and assuming instantaneous change.[74]

Farr's second assumption was that human mortality varied with age in a manner described by the law of mortality Edmonds had first brought to his attention. The law of mortality allowed him to use extensive interpolation techniques which both saved tedious labor and also helped smooth out irregularities in the census and registration records. Farr explained how life tables could be computed directly from observations on the numbers living and dying at each age, but he pointed out that ambiguities in the age returns of the census and the yearly fluctuations in vital events made this a risky procedure.[75] Tables constructed by this method would be especially inaccurate in the early years of life where the census enumeration of ages was most defective. Farr hoped to overcome some of the defects of this data by averaging and interpolating.

In broad outline what he did was to compute first the mortality at select ages using census and registration records. He ordinarily used mortality records for a period of years and for a series of ages, making the age in question the midpoint of the series. From the mortality at these ages he could next compute, using a formula he had devised, the probability of living one more year.[76] At this point he found by interpolation the probability of living one more year at every age in the table. Since he now knew both these probabilities and the number living at key ages, he could compute the entire "l" column by multiplication.

In his first tables, his choice of ages to serve as starting points was dictated by a simple application of Edmonds's law of mortality.[77] By the time he computed his third national life table his interpolation techniques had become much more complex.[78] The major exception to Farr's basic computation technique was the computation of entries for infants. Farr believed the census returns of age at early ages to be quite defective, while he thought the registration of births and deaths was more accurate. For this reason he computed the mortality for ages under five years directly from registration records, ignoring the census entirely.

The Applications of the Life Table: Health, Economics, and Insurance

A life table for Farr was much more than an actuary's tool. It was a general statistical device for studying human life and society. He explained: "The applications and uses of National Life Tables are almost innumerable: without an intimate knowledge of their properties it is impossible to determine the laws of population, which are the basis of statistics, or to reason upon such matters without falling into great errors, of which, if it were not invidious, too many instances might be cited from current works on population and public health."[79] Farr most often used the life table to describe vital phenomena, in particular, mortality. But this was not all. He also constructed for the Royal Society of London a fertility table for English women ages 15 to 55.[80] The table was like a life table except that it showed for each age of life the total number of children and the number of legitimate and illegitimate children separately born to mothers at each age. In this case it was fertility, not mortality, that was shown to change regularly with age. As we shall see in Chapter Five, Farr also adopted the life table to study morbidity by producing for certain diseases sickness tables that represented the living and dying in various periods of a disease. The life table described in the most general terms the vital structure of a "normal" population and showed there was an "indissoluble connexion between (1) the numbers living, (2) the mean after-lifetime, (3) the births, (4) the deaths, (5) the rate of mortality, (6) the probable duration of life."[81] The life table thus confirmed Farr's belief that vital phenomena are governed by natural laws. Statisticians of the early twentieth century showed some interest in a suggestion by Farr that a positive relationship existed among the rate of mortality, the birth rate, and the expectancy of life in a population.[82]

He found other uses for the life table as well. Using historical records dating back to 1689, he constructed a table for the lifetime of government ministries. This table resembled a life table and showed for each year of their tenure the number of ministries that were terminated. Such a table could therefore be used to calculate the probability that any ministry would remain in office one more year.[83] He also indicated how life table methods could be used to describe promotions in the army and in the civil service, assuming that retirements were few and advancement depended primarily on years of service.[84] The tables of annuities and insurance published with life tables suggested that the life table could be used to describe economic change. Farr demonstrated, for example, how to calculate the value which had been added to taxable property in England by the reduction of the poor rates in 1834.[85]

These exotic applications were the exception. More commonly, Farr used life tables to assess the health of the people. A life table, he and other actuaries had argued, was the only correct measure of average length of life. As we have seen, early Victorians were prepared to accept length of life as the measure of health and vitality. A national life table represented in numerical form national health and vitality. Farr hoped international actuarial comparisons would stimulate reform.

Since an English Life Table has now been framed from the necessary data, I venture to express a hope that the facts may be collected and abstracted, from which Life Tables for other nations can be constructed. A comparison of the duration of successive generations in England, France, Prussia, Austria, Russia, America, and other States, would throw much light on the physical condition of the respective populations, and suggest to scientific and benevolent individuals in every country—and to the Governments—many ways of diminishing the sufferings, and ameliorating the health and condition of the people; for the longer life of a nation denotes more than it does in an individual—a happier life—a life more exempt from sickness and infirmity—a life of greater energy and industry, of greater experience and wisdom. By these comparisons a noble national emulation might be excited and rival nations would read of sickness diminished, deformity banished, life saved—of victories over death and the grave,—with as much enthusiasm as of victories over each other's armies in the field; and the triumph of one would not be the humiliation of the other; for in this contention none could lose territory, or honour, or blood, but all would gain strength.[86]

Farr played an important part in making the life table the criterion of collective health in Victorian England. Writing in the 1860s, Henry Rumsey claimed "almost all recent writers on the subject seem to agree in the opinion that a Life Table . . . is the surest and safest test of its [the nation's, district's, group's, or class's] healthiness and vitality."[87] The census of 1841 and the first years of registration provided Farr the data he needed to construct national and local life tables, and he announced in the *Fifth Annual Report* his plan to publish a series of life tables which would "furnish a standard; any deviation from which will denote an improvement or deterioration in the national health."[88] The same volume contained his first contributions: his first national life table and local tables for three carefully selected areas: Surrey (excluding the metropolitan portions), the metropolis, and Liverpool.[89] These districts provided representative extremes in salubrity. He published a life table for Manchester in the *Seventh Annual Report*.[90] The *Eighth Annual Report* contains very interesting life tables for Northampton.[91] Using the city population according to the 1841 census and the registered deaths 1838–1841, Farr first constructed a life table for the city using his methods. He then constructed a second table using the procedure Richard Price had used for his Northampton table using the death registers alone. A comparison of these two new Northampton tables provided Farr with an excellent opportunity to discuss the principles of the life table and to illustrate the fallacies of working, as Price did, from deaths alone. In a section that was not at all atypical he also offered a historical account of the town and its vital statistics.[92]

This work was the beginning of one of Farr's major programs, the statistical analysis of the health of towns. It is the subject of extended discussion in Chapter Six. Farr's interest in the subject was keenest in the early forties and then seems to have waned a bit until the sixties. By the latter period his approach had changed, and he began to use the experience of standard populations to measure the health of populations. The most important of his standards were all of England and Wales, whose health was reflected in the national life tables, and the healthy districts, for whom he computed a life table in 1859.[93] The healthy districts, it should be recalled, were districts having average crude mortality rates below 17 per 1,000. The healthy district life table was based upon the experience of sixty-three registration districts—on the deaths registered during the years 1849–1853, and on the population according to the census of

1851, the midpoint in the interval. This table and the national life tables became for Farr standards of health against which the mortality of localities or occupational groups might be compared. Such a comparison was a marked improvement over the comparison of crude mortality rates which overlooked differences in age composition or other demographic differences. In his late career, Farr began to make allowances for the differences in age composition by a technique his successors would call the indirect method of computing standardized death rates.[94] Farr did not use the term, but he introduced the essence of the procedure by computing how many deaths would have occurred in each age group of the population in question, had that population experienced the same law of mortality which prevailed in his standard population (the entire nation or the healthy districts). (See Fig. 3.) Farr employed this technique in his decennial supplement for the years 1851-1860 in discussing the death rates of large towns, and he used it again for the mining population in evidence he presented to the Royal Commission on Mines in 1864.[95] In the latter case he constructed life tables for miners and compared mortality, mean afterlifetimes, life insurance premiums, and other figures from this table and from the healthy district and the English life tables.

The life table in Farr's hands was a general statistical tool, but of course it had developed to meet the needs of the insurance business. Farr was keenly aware of this fact, and like other early Victorian statisticians was interested in the financial uses of such tables and in economic ques-

TABLE XVIII.—**Deaths in 30 Large Town Districts** in the 10 Years 1851-60 ; and also the DEATHS which would have occurred in the 10 Years if the MORTALITY had been at the same Rate as prevailed in the 63 HEALTHY DISTRICTS (1849-53).

AGES.	DEATHS in 10 Years 1851-60.	DEATHS which would have occurred in the 10 Years at HEALTHY DISTRICT RATES.	EXCESS of ACTUAL DEATHS in 10 Years over DEATHS at HEALTHY DISTRICT RATES.
ALL AGES -	711,944	384,590	327,354
0— - -	338,990	135,470	203,520
5— - -	31,319	19,290	12,029
10— - -	14,240	11,020	3,220
15— - -	43,807	37,550	6,257
25— - -	48,625	36,150	12,475
35— - -	50,071	30,320	19,751
45— - -	49,638	26,680	22,958
55— - -	49,763	27,020	22,743
65— - -	47,445	31,510	15,935
75— - -	30,583	22,620	7,963
85 & upwards -	7,463	6,660	803

Figure 3. Farr's method of correcting for differences in the age composition of populations whose mortality rates were being compared. Farr, "Letter," *Suppl. 25th A.R.R.G.*, p. xxvi [PP, 1865, XIII].

tions in general. Farr apparently had hoped to see his national life tables adopted by private life insurance offices, because he published with each of his national tables a full set of actuary tables and instructions for their use. Some offices adopted his tables. The Scottish Amicable and the Standard companies used his first national table; the British Equitable Company used the second table; and the Positive Company used English life table number three.[96] As a general rule, however, life offices did not adopt the national tables. This fact, in retrospect, is not too surprising. Although Farr's tables were the best for the English population at large, they were not the sort of table commercial offices felt they needed. These offices were not interested in the mortality and life expectancy for the general population but rather in these phenomena for the classes of the population that purchased insurance. Also by mid-century life insurance companies had sufficient experience of their own to serve as a basis for estimations of risks and costs.

Actuaries ignored Farr's national tables for other reasons as well. He was, after all, an outsider despite his reputation as a statistician and the interest some actuaries had shown in his plan for a government-sponsored, working-class insurance.[97] He adopted a novel perspective on actuary problems, and he made annoying changes in notation and in the details of tables of premiums and annuities.[98] Furthermore, by the time of his death certain actuaries had grown suspicious of theoretical life tables.[99] By that time at least one actuary had even called into question the law of mortality.[100]

For his part Farr was critical of actuary practice. In articles on life insurance which he wrote for medical journals or for the registrar general's *Annual Reports,* he not only recommended life insurance as an investment and as a protection against financial losses, but he also criticized the management of commercial firms.[101] There was good reason for concern, for not only were known actuary principles imperfectly applied, but speculation, fraud, and financial failure were rampant in the insurance industry from the 1820s through the 1860s.[102] Farr objected to the use of defective life tables, such as the Northampton table, which overestimated mortality and hence justified high premiums. But he also pointed out that by the selection of lives and by calculating premiums on lower rates of interest than could be obtained, life insurance offices inflated premiums still further. Surplus funds, moreover, usually were not divided equitably.

Farr testified before a House of Commons select committee that investigated the insurance business, and he published a lengthy statement of his views on the subject about the same time.[103] Four principles, he maintained, should be observed in equitable insurance schemes: a true life table should be the basis of operations; public accounts and public audit should be undertaken to gain public confidence; access to deposited money should be guaranteed; and, finally, a reserve fund should be created by an addition to the premiums to guard against fluctuations in interest rates or mortality and other uncertainties.[104]

He proposed several insurance schemes of his own. One of these was a publicly regulated plan for the professional and commercial classes.[105] This plan would use his English life table number two, calculate premiums at 3 percent interest, and then add a surcharge of 20 percent of the premium for the reserve fund. An annual report would describe the financial status of the company in detail. The insured could withdraw his sum in deposit, less any bonuses, after three months' notice, while the company reserved the right to refuse coverage to the unhealthy and to cancel during its first year any policy, should fraud or deception be discovered. The company would offer three types of life policies, differing in their term of coverage, the amount insured, and the amount left in deposit.

Farr was not content merely to see life insurance offered to the middle classes on equitable principles. He also proposed a scheme for offering it to the wage-earning population through the savings banks.[106] These banks were unique British combinations of private enterprise and government regulation in investment. They had developed in Britain during the eighteenth century to cater to very small investors. By 1817 they were under some governmental control and, while managed by private trustees, were obliged to invest their deposited capital with the national debt commissioners, who paid a bonus interest rate. In 1861 Post Office savings banks were authorized and rather quickly absorbed most of the semi-private savings banks.[107] Life insurance for the masses, Farr claimed, could be managed much as banking for the masses was managed and through the same institutions. His scheme would allow a wage earner in good health, once admitted to the program, to buy as many separate annual policies at £1 plus 4s for expenses as he could afford. If he were unable to purchase any policies a given year, he sacrificed nothing other than the increased coverage he might have obtained. The amount of coverage depended upon the amount invested and the time it had accumulated interest. The deposit remained subject to withdrawal by the insured in the event of financial need, and surplus profits were to be distributed among the insured at five-year intervals. The investor could also specify that a certain amount of his deposit go for life insurance and the rest for an extended annuity, payable to him when he reached a given age.

This was one of Farr's insurance schemes that was enacted. It ultimately served as the basis of the Post Office insurance system, which the government authorized in 1864.[108] The Post Office savings banks received, invested, and managed the funds. The plan used Farr's English life table number three and retained Farr as a consulting actuary. Life insurance was thus placed within the reach of almost every man with an appreciable, even if irregular, income; the government served as the ultimate guarantor of the coverage.

At the same time that he was planning a government-sponsored life insurance program for the working class, Farr proposed the government underwrite a health insurance scheme for the same population.[109] He considered his plan a supplement to the Poor Law and a remedy to one of its major defects: the fact that the same relief was offered to all, regardless of previous status or contribution to society. He hoped to provide health insurance for low and moderate income groups through a plan which would function like a national friendly society. In answering *laissez faire* objections he made it clear that part of his motive was to protect private property.

Society without a legal system of relief for destitution can be scarcely said to exist . . . . Anarchy, riot, insecurity of life, communism, are common and ever recurring symptoms of this constitutional evil in countries where the owners of property have not yet discovered that the appropriation of a small part of the profits, as a premium for the insurance of the life of the population, is at the same time a cheap insurance of their titles and possessions,—that the insurance of the life of all, is the insurance of the property of all.[110]

As he called upon the property-holding classes for assistance in this program, he reminded them that their cooperation would insure better relations with their employees and more control over the labor market, and that the industrialist could not afford, any more than a general, to abandon wounded troops.

Farr wished to take health insurance for working men out of the hands of the friendly society, the workingmen's clubs, and the trade unions, which were under the control of working-class leaders. Such goals as organizing to seek wage increases should, he believed, be "entirely dissociated from the serious business of making a provision against sickness, infirmity, old age, and untimely death, as they are among the higher and professional classes."[111] His plan, therefore, placed the national health insurance system in the hands of employers who would make payroll deductions from the weekly wages of their employees, manage the insurance fund, and perhaps contribute to it. As in the case of working-class life insurance, policies would be of short term and capable of being closed by mutual consent of employer and employee, and the premium would be small and variable. The weekly premium necessary to insure a fixed, guaranteed, weekly sick wage would be determined by occupational morbidity statistics. Farr anticipated this scheme would result in a profit, which he hoped would be distributed among the employees either as deposits in a savings bank or saved as a sum to be paid to the widow or children in the event of the employee's death. He believed it was desirable that the plan operate as nearly as possible within the confines of the industry or business to bind employer and employee together in common interest. He recognized, however, that the government alone had the necessary knowledge and resources to guarantee pensions and life insurance. He called on the government to encourage employers by defraying the administrative costs of the program or by permitting such costs to be deducted from profits in figuring taxes. Unlike his plans for working-class life insurance, this scheme for health insurance apparently found no immediate application.

These suggestions reveal a creative, expansive mind at work. They also show Farr's continued anxiety about social welfare and security and his notion that insurance could help offset some of the insecurities in the present economic system. He considered, too, other forms of insurance, some rather unconventional in his age. He pointed out in the late 1830s that the lawful behavior of disease mortality made it feasible to write life insurance for unhealthy persons who otherwise could not obtain policies.[112] All that was necessary was the collection of data permitting sickness tables to be compiled for the major diseases, giving mean afterlifetimes by age, sex, and duration of illness. Premiums could be figured accordingly. The principle was simple even if the application was not. In his later career Farr proposed insurance programs to cover certain unusual financial losses. Following the 1866 cattle plague, he suggested that such heavy agricultural losses might be covered by a national agricultural insurance scheme which promised protection no local insurance could offer.[113] The insurance was to be privately financed but to have government assistance in administration. Again, in discussing deaths and injuries caused by railway accidents, Farr proposed a scheme for railway insurance.[114] Its purpose was to provide protection for financial losses and to encourage companies to make the facilities safer. According to Farr's plan, passengers would purchase annual policies from the railway companies. These policies would provide varying amounts of coverage on a graduated scale of premiums. The policies insured the passenger against death or injury incurred on that railway and awarded damages without the necessity of determining liability by expensive litigation. Neither of these schemes was enacted in Farr's lifetime.

Farr also brought his experience with insurance and annuity schemes to a favorite reform issue, the financial plight of civil servants. His paper of 1849 on the "Statistics of the Civil Service"[115] should be seen as part of the campaign by civil servants to have the Superannuation Act amended. For that paper Farr circulated a questionnaire among civil servants, seeking information about their ages, years of service, salaries, number of dependents, etc. and received about 8,000 replies, heavily weighted in favor of men in lower grades. The questionnaire showed that civil servants were paid much less than men in the learned professions or the trades with whom the civil servants were fond of comparing themselves. But Farr claimed the greater injustice was found in the terms of the Superannuation Act, which he regarded as both unjust and actuarially unsound. The amount one could withdraw from the retirement fund was not proportional to the amount contributed. In fact, older men in higher grades and the holders of certain lucrative sinecures were not required to contribute at all, although they might withdraw funds on retirement. The burden of supporting the scheme therefore fell on younger men in the lowest paid positions. Furthermore, Farr claimed, the retirement fund was badly managed. It was not invested at compound interest nor was there a reserve or guarantee fund to protect the scheme from unexpected demands. He suggested that contributions be made compulsory and universal, and the amount collected be managed as a provident fund for the support of civil service widows and orphans. He went on to explain the actuarial principles on which it could operate.[116]

Farr not only recommended these changes, but he also sought to bring them about. He first had this 1849 article republished as a pamphlet.[117] When the issue finally was brought before Parliament in 1857, Farr was active again. In another paper to the Statistical Society he described the history of the financial rewards of public servants, crown ministers in particular, and argued that such ministers should be included in a revised superannuation scheme.[118] He also helped the General Committee of Civil Servants of the Crown marshall evidence and arguments for a reconsideration of the superannuation question.[119] After a reform measure had passed the House of Commons, Farr wrote to Lord Brougham offering a primer of facts and suggesting how Brougham might answer the objections raised by William Gladstone and others.[120] There is evidence that Farr remained active in the civil servants organization. We find him writing to the Second Earl Granville in May of 1871, asking the Earl to become Vice-President of the Committee of the Civil Service Cooperative Society.[121]

We can see therefore that by the fifties Farr was active as an actuary within official circles. He continued this practice in the sixties. In that decade he served as a paid actuary consultant to the Royal Commission on the Sanitary State of the Army in India.[122] He was also asked to prepare a memorandum for Gladstone to help institute the Post Office insurance scheme he had helped plan.[123] But Farr's activities in matters of insurance did not stop at the boundaries of officialdom. By the sixties he also had an actuary consultantship with private parties. It is difficult to obtain detailed information about these activities. Farr did not leave any accounts of these matters, nor did his friends who wrote biographical sketches describe his private insurance ventures. What we can learn about such matters comes from his surviving letters and papers and from some guarded references by younger contemporaries to his unfortunate financial associations. Letters in the Farr collection at the London School of Economics suggest that Farr was consulted by the National Mutual Life Association, the Royal Mail Steam Packet Company, W. I. Bain of the North American Life Insurance Company, and the "Captain" Relief Fund.[124] Joseph Whittall, in his notes for a biography of Farr, listed the dates of Farr's appointment as auditor of the Life Insurance Fund of the British Imperial Insurance Company and as auditor of the Positive Insurance Company.[125] Farr also served as director's actuary to the London and North Western Railway Company.[126] By the middle 1860s he had enough of an international reputation that New York State published in 1868 a pamphlet summarizing the symbols and formulae used in his English life table number three.[127] His active concern with the insurance business was retained throughout his career, and he published as late as 1880 a table of premiums for accident insurance.[128]

But all did not go well in these matters. Humphreys wrote: "These qualities [lack of jealousy and lack of suspicion of others' motives] made him a somewhat bad judge of character, and exposed him to imposition from scheming speculators, who were desirous of and too frequently obtained his name and support in the furtherance of disastrous financial ventures. For this want of worldly wisdom, and of due caution in putting his actuarial reputation and his money at the mercy of others, he paid dearly."[129] Hare expressed similar views. "Clever men of the world knew the doctor's weaknesses, and by praising his crochet and playing on his ambition, "used" him, his name, his official position, and his money, to answer their own ends, at the costs of his and other people's disaster."[130] This "crochet," which both Hare and Farr's obituary writer for *The Insurance Record* (who may have been Hare[131]) referred to, was Farr's insistence that the reserve of an insurance fund be invested in consols. Consols were British government stock which paid only 3 percent annual interest but which paid bonuses to the principal.[132] The price of consols was variable enough to allow speculation. Unfortunately, in 1854 additional consols were issued and the price dropped, not to rise again to par until 1887. It appears that in the opinion of certain actuary contemporaries of Farr his commitment to investment in consols had caused financial difficulties for several firms with which he was associated and the ruin of at least one of these, the Consols Insurance Association. *The Insurance Record* obituary claimed: "His great crochet related to the investment of a life assurance company's reserve in consols. This one thing must, if we mistake not, have cost him dear; for we have reason to believe he "was in" first with the company of that name, then with the British Imperial, and lastly with the Positive. He gave at least these proofs of his sincerity."[133] Although the actuary in charge of closing the Consols Insurance Association denied that Farr was responsible for the failure and claimed the only part of the association that did well was the Life Insurance Fund of which Farr was the auditor,[134] the suspicion of Farr's role lingered to reappear in his obituaries twenty years later. With characteristic overstatement, George Bernard Shaw put the matter rather bluntly: "Dr. Farr survived his wits and lost most of his means by senile speculations before his death . . . ."[135] Besides his insurance investments Farr apparently invested money in building societies and in buying mortgages.[136] He may also have lost money in these ventures. As we shall see, his financial losses left his children, especially his unmarried daughters, in some difficulty and caused concern among his friends in the civil service and in the medical profession.

Farr's Economic Ideas and the Monetary Value of Human Life

Like many other members of the statistical societies, Farr was interested in economics, both economic theory and practical economic affairs. His economic ideas and their application both illustrate the pervasiveness of his interest in actuary affairs and serve as further illustration of his place in the spectrum of Victorian opinion. We see in this instance, perhaps better than in any other, the expansive nature of Farr's mental processes. Having once outlined his position, he applied it to a wide range of problems, from capital investment to public health. Of particular interest is his application of economic analysis to human beings.

In matters of theory, Farr's position was based upon a rejection of the labor theory of value.[137] He pointed out that the value of an object depended not on the labor that went into its manufacture but on its market price, which was a measure of the degree to which the prospective buyer and present owner desired possession of it. There was, Farr believed, no intrinsic value in the object. Its value depended rather on human needs and whims. Without any change occurring in an object, its value might change with time or place or even with the psychological states of the individuals involved in transactions. Irrational as well as rational factors might come into play in determining value. Speaking of the stock exchange he wrote, "As value originates in a psychial affection, it may be expected to vary in every person not only with facts, knowledge, and opinions, but with the states of ebb and flow—of exaltation or depression—of men's minds."[138] His best illustration was his account of an auction.

Every article put up for sale has a different value in the minds of the spectators; for one article there is no bidding at all, for a second a few bid, for a third there is the keenest competition; scarcely two articles sell for the same price. Question the purchasers, and you will find that every one has in each case his own ideas of value. . . . It is possible that some might take into account the labour of making a lot; but as a general rule that does not influence a single bid; every bidding expresses the desire to acquire its possession. . . . Go to another auction, and you will find similar articles sell for very different prices; the things may be identical, but the minds of the people are different; their circumstances are not the same. . . . Take a sale at Christie and Manson's; there the picture fanciers and dealers meet; the price of no single picture depends upon the amount of labour the artists have expended upon its production, but chiefly on its beauty, on the reputations of the artist, on its rarity, on the rarity of similar works, and on the means of purchase.[139]

The labor theory of value, Farr asserted, owed its origin to fallacious reasoning upon sound observation. While it was true that labor expended on certain products was accompanied by an increase in their value, it did not follow that labor was the cause of value. While he admitted that there was a general relationship between the amount of capital, including labor, invested in a product and its value, the relationship was not constant. It was possible to invest labor without increasing value at all. Similarly, the weight of the object or the good it might do did not bear any necessary relation to its value, although each might exert an influence. Finally value depended on the ability to make the purchase. Men without money had no effect on value, regardless of how much they might desire the object in question.

In defining value as market price Farr gained several advantages, two of them major ones. First, he was permitted to discuss more easily than the physiocrats or classical economists the value of luxury goods and services whose price bore little relation to the amount of labor actually performed in producing them. Second, in using market price as a measure, he obtained convenient numerical units for economic statistics, monetary units. "Value for scientific purposes, however constituted, can only be dealt with like time when it is measured; and as time can be measured by the shadows on a sun-dial or by the revolutions of worlds, so value may be measured by paper money or by gold, or by any unit of value on which people agree. These units are money, in which all values can be reckoned. . . ."[140] In a business transaction money was exchanged for services tangible or intangible. Such services, Farr held, were products whose value was accurately given by their exchange price. The idea that any product or service was unproductive was repugnant to Farr. He took issue with Adam Smith's insistence that the army and navy were unproductive. These forces, Farr claimed, protected life and property, and the value of this service was properly measured by "the rate of insurance indispensable to maintain the security it affords."[141] Similar considerations applied to luxury goods.

A large quantity of the property of the country—such as furniture, jewels, the precious metals, cash, pictures, parks—is often called unproductive; but, I apprehend, erroneously. All these things have been purchased with money, and may again be converted into money, the representative of capital, which can always be invested productively; and if, instead of investing 10,000 l. in land, which would produce 300 l. a-year, you invest it in furniture, pictures, or jewels, it is evident that you select this investment because property in such a form yields services which you esteem at a higher value than 300 l. a-year. These services are products; and the property is, therefore, productive. When an object ceases to be serviceable, and ceases to be exchangeable for value, it ceases to be property, and at the same time ceases to be productive.[142]

One way Farr used his concept of value was in discussing the means of determining just compensations for utility companies the government was considering purchasing. Two of Farr's papers to the Statistical Society of London dealt with this topic in the 1870s.[143] Farr decided to do the valuation by calculating the present values of future dividends. This reduced the problem to a procedure familiar to actuaries: calculating the present value of future annuities. Variable profits or dividends could be considered as the sum of a fixed annuity plus an increment which was assumed to vary either as an arithmetic or a geometric progression.[144] In his first article he gave a general formula for the valuation in these terms.[145] His second article was much more detailed and included the results of an investigation of the financial history of several utility companies. In that article he gave valuation tables for interest rates of 3, 4, 5, 6, and 7 percent, tables of dividends and stock prices for several companies, and tables of valuation for specific companies.[146]

Farr applied his economic notions more fruitfully to human beings. As we shall see again in Chapter Six, he recognized the importance of differences among individuals. But although he was unsuccessful in finding precise physiological or psychological definitions for individual differences, he was more successful in giving economic meaning to the concept. Men clearly differed in skill and work capacity and hence in economic value, just as they did in physical appearance or in intelligence. In speaking of the proper statistical units for measuring national resources he wrote:

What are we to say to the human unit? Here also distinctions have to be drawn. As hectars [a measure of land] differ, so does the average man of different states. Besides the divisions incidental to sex and age, the work of different races of men varies in quantity. . . .

The mechanical force of a country is the sum of the working forces of its population, with its steam-engines, horses, winds, waters, which can all be measured by the engineer's unit of work. Adam Smith proposed to employ a unit of labour as the unit of value. The wages of men express the value of their labour in gold, and from the mean value of these earnings at different ages of life, the economic value of a man is calculated by taking the interest of money and the contingencies of his life into account. . . . The value of the mean worktime of artisans, artists, and professional men, varies indefinitely; and it is evident that the human units differ, so the difference can be appreciated by the value of their works.[147]

Consistent with his value theory, Farr believed that the market value of a man's services, his wages, accurately reflected his economic value. This definition brought Farr to consider what economists call human capital, investments in the quality of the work force, in such things as training, education, and health services. One approach to the problem has been to assign monetary value to human beings. B. F. Kiker, an economist who has written a history of the concept, assigns Farr an important place in its development.[148] Kiker traced the history of estimates of human capital to the seventeenth century and listed six major uses the concept has had since that time: first, to estimate the power and prestige of a nation; second, to estimate the economic effects of education, migration, or health investment; third, to propose tax reforms; fourth, to calculate the total cost of war; fifth, to point out the need of measures to protect health or life; and sixth, to assist courts in making fair financial settlements.[149] Basically there have been two methods of calculating human capital: by estimating the cost of production or by taking the capital value of probable future earnings. Farr used the second method, and his treatment, which modern economists regard as the "first truly scientific procedure," was followed by later economists.[150]

Farr's most thorough treatment of the subject and the only one known to Kiker, apparently, was occasioned by his study of tax reform proposals.[151] He maintained that property, not profits, should be the basis of taxation, and he proposed to treat earning capacity as a kind of taxable property.

The characteristic of this property is that it is inherent in man, and is the value of his services—of the direct produce of his skill and industry. In slaves it is vendible and transferable; in freemen it is inalienable; but is not the less on that account property, which in the early states of society is assessed and taxed in the form of personal services.[152]

Produce then is expressed by the value in money which the property yields during the year, either in separate products, in the increase of value, or in the price of its services. The income of a lawyer, a doctor, a clergyman, a merchant, or a tradesman, is in this sense as much produce as the proceeds of a farm. . . . But anything which yields produce that will sell for money is property, although it may be itself inalienable; consequently, all the free labourers, artizans, professional men, of the United Kingdom, having within them this power of production, are as essentially property as the things usually designated by that name. . . . Exclusive of all his external property, every man is worth something.[153]

It was a man's earning capacity that Farr argued should be taxed. This capacity was not understood simply in terms of a man's present earning. Farr recognized that this capacity depended on a man's age and social position and also on the amount of capital that had been invested in him. What he proposed to do then was to balance the probable future earnings of the individual against the capital expense in producing them. "The labour of the parents, and the expense of attendance, nurture, clothing, lodging, education, apprenticeship, practice, are investments of capital, at risk extending over many years; and the return appears in the form of wages, salaries, incomes, of the survivors. . . . The present value of the person's probable future earnings, *minus* the necessary outgo in realizing those earnings, is the present value of that person's services."[154] The differences in the salaries between social classes was justified, he believed, because salaries in general were proportional to the amount of capital invested.

To calculate the economic value of an individual at a given age one had to calculate the probable future earnings of the individual of that age and occupation, and deduct the probable future cost of maintenance or living expenses. The average cost of maintenance and the average wages could be obtained by observation, while the calculation could be made using a life table and appropriate actuary tools, the use of which for these purposes he had described earlier in his career.[155] In his article on taxation he showed how the calculation could be reduced to the application of wage and cost of living figures to life table entries.[156] By using a life table for a given occupational group he could take account of the mean afterlifetime at each age of a generation born simultaneously into a given occupation. If the average annual wages or salaries of persons of the occupation at age x were represented by w_x and the average annual living expenses in the same occupation at the same age by y_x, then $w_x P_x$ and $y_x P_x$ would represent, respectively, the total earnings and cost of living of the P_x persons of age x employed in the occupation. P_x was the average number of persons living through the year between the x and $x+1$ birthdays. If $W_x = P_x w_x + P_{x+1} w_{x+1} + \ldots + P_z w_z$ were the total future earnings of the occupational group of age x to the last age z in the life table, and Y_x were to represent the total future cost of maintaining the P_x persons, then $W_x - Y_x$ would be the annual excess of earning over cost of living to be expected for all persons who obtained the age of x out of the original number in the life table. $W_0 - Y_0$ was hence the total lifetime profit of the generation of workers in that occupation. If Q_x were the number of persons at age x or above in the lifetable, then $(W_0 - Y_0)/Q_0$ would be the annual profit per head for the entire generation. $(W_x - Y_x)/Q_x$ hence became the excess of probable future earnings over expenses for a person of age x in a given occupation or a measure of his economic value. Farr accepted this figure as the economic measure of the human unit.

One consequence of Farr's views was that economic value of men varied with age as well as social class. Although the cost of subsistence was relatively constant for various period of life, earning capacity was at first nil; later it increased rapidly with age, and finally declined slowly. For his article on the income tax, Farr traced the changing economic value of a Norfolk farm laborer. At birth the economic value of such a male child was £5.37; it rose to a maximus of £246.35 at the age of 25, and by the age of 80 was £ – 41.01.[157] The maximum economic value of a professional man was reached at a later age, owing to the longer period of training and hence the greater initial capital investment prerequisite for such an occupation.[158]

The concept of human capital had been used by several of Farr's predecessors in discussing matters of state and finance. In the seventeenth century William Petty was led to consider human capital in dealing with tax reform, but came rather quickly to use the concept in demonstrating the power of England, the economic effects of migration, and the economic losses from war and death.[159] Farr's contemporary Adolphe Quetelet calculated the cost of raising an abandoned child and used this value as a measure of the financial debt every child owed society.[160] Farr followed this tradition in recommending several applications of the concept of human capital. He suggested that the economic value of the individual should be the basis for settling claims in railway accidents.[161] Compensation for injury to any part of the body should be in proportion to the value of the whole life. He also suggested an application that was later to be fruitfully pursued, the study of emigration as "a transfer of living capital from one land to another."[162]

It was in describing the financial losses from disease that Farr most often applied his idea of the economic value of man. Here once again he had recent predecessors. During Farr's early career Edwin Chadwick and John Ramsay McCulloch had tried to estimate the financial cost of disease.[163] Farr recognized the power of such arguments. Excess mortality, he reasoned, should be counted a direct monetary loss. "It may be said that the nation loses the money value of the excess of mortality existing in its general population over that of the population in healthy districts."[164] The premature death of men such as soldiers in whom the nation had invested much was an especially great loss. But nonfatal illness, Farr recognized, caused financial waste as well. In both his article on vital statistics in McCulloch's volumes and in a later paper for the London statistical society Farr collected information from a variety of sources in order to calculate the number constantly sick or the average number of days of sickness per man per year in various trades.[165] From these figures the loss of productivity could be estimated.

But the cost of disease to the community did not stop there. Farr recognized the total price included the labor and cost involved in caring for the sick. In this regard diseases differed drastically in their effect on the community. Farr calculated that the first cholera epidemic in Paris caused 158,118 days of sick time or 5 hours sickness per person, whereas if the same number of people had been attacked by consumption, 73,600 years of sickness would have resulted.[166] Potentially, then, consumption was socially more important than cholera in spite of the drama of cholera attacks.

In the *Twenty-fifth Annual Report* he turned to fever. From the records of the London Fever Hospital he obtained age-group case fatality rates for continued fevers and a figure for the average duration of fever cases. Applying these rates to the registered typhus deaths in 1848–1862, he concluded that caring for fever patients cost the nation 4,643,000 days' subsistence and required the equivalent of 127 hospitals of 100 beds each.[167] In the thirties Farr had also attempted to study the cost of care and confinement of the insane. This study was more limited in scope and was occasioned by a debate over the cost of a proposed enlargement of the County Lunatic Asylum at Hanwell, Middlesex. He collected information on the cost of operating the county asylums, on the number and duration of the stay of the inmates, and calculated the weekly cost of care and treatment in the various institutions, and the cost per patient of the building under consideration.[168]

The fact that maximum human economic value occurred in the middle years of life meant that the most costly modes of death were those that were most prevalent among people in those years of life: warfare, violence, accident, childbirth, typhus, consumption, cholera, plague, and smallpox.[169] These were the causes of death which, for economic reasons, society ought to seek to eliminate. By comparison a diminution in the mortality of children did not have the same immediate effect on national power.[170]

This calculation, Farr recognized, ignored the long term need of having a new generation in training; it also overlooked completely the imponderable emotional value of human life.[171] Farr did not abandon his highly-colored, even sentimental appeals for public health reform when he began these cold calculations; in fact, he often combined tactics in his appeals, recognizing apparently that some men had more sensitive pocket books than hearts. One example should suffice. In an 1841 article on smallpox, he followed an impassioned call for public action, a call that described the human misery caused by the disease, with the estimated cost of providing the coffins that would be necessary to bury the victims of the ongoing epidemic.[172]

FIVE

THE ZYMOTIC THEORY AND FARR'S STUDIES OF EPIDEMIC DISEASES

Farr's Zymotic Theory

It is well known that when Farr began his career, the doctrine of contagion was highly controversial and had been, for over a decade, sharply criticized by opponents of quarantine and certain advocates of sanitary reform. The development of anticontagionism has received some fine historical study. Erwin Akerknecht's Garrison Lecture of 1948 first drew attention to the pervasiveness and importance of the anticontagionist position in the early nineteenth century.[1] Ackerknecht's analysis has the virtue of stressing the internationalism of anticontagionism, its scientific respectability or at least plausibility, and its relationship to liberal or radical political ideas. Recently, Margaret Pelling has provided a detailed analysis of disease theory in mid-century England and has insisted, quite properly, that the appearance of a complete victory for anticontagionism even around 1840 is illusionary.[2]

We have no intention of trying to provide an extensive account of disease theory in early Victorian England. There are, however, several points which ought to be recalled before one considers Farr's ideas. First, one should not expect to find among Farr's contemporaries many who completely denied the existence of contagion. The transmission of smallpox, rabies, and syphilis by inoculation was simply too strong a counterexample. What was more common, however, was the application of the term "contagion" only to the very restricted case of transmission by direct contact, as in inoculation, and the separation, categorically, of the contagious from the epidemic diseases.[3] According to such schemes the contagious diseases were transmitted from person to person by a material substance, and this animal poison was their only known cause. Epidemic diseases arose primarily from local causes. Contagious diseases were held to be absolutely uniform in their symptoms from case to case. It was also known that the acute contagious diseases attacked an individual only once. On the other hand, it was thought that epidemic diseases might attack the same individual repeatedly and could exhibit a variety of symptoms. Unlike the contagious diseases, they predominated in certain localities and in certain seasons. Epidemic diseases attacked a large number of individuals simultaneously, but it did not follow that all diseases bearing this property were epidemic ones. Smallpox, Southwood Smith explained, was not an epidemic disease simply because at any one time a large number of people might suffer its attack.[4]

It was the nature of the epidemic diseases, especially fever, plague, yellow fever, and later cholera, that was at the heart of the debate over contagion. By defining contagion in the narrowest sense and by relying on common knowledge of the experience of communities with such diseases, the anticontagionists built a formidable list of facts contagion could not explain.[5] It could not explain why these diseases occurred regularly in certain seasons nor why they visited certain localities and not adjacent areas. It could also not explain why those attending the sick in well-managed hospitals did not contract epidemic diseases or why fever did not seem to spread from the sick in hospitals or even from the wandering plague victims of the Near East to other people. Contagion could also not explain why epidemics seemed to end abruptly after reaching their peak at a time when the possibilities for spreading the disease by contagion was the greatest. Taken to its logical extreme, the critics claimed, the theory of contagion implied that once a serious epidemic had begun in a community, it would not end until all men had died.

Such exceptions caused strong doubts, even in minds unwilling to abandon completely the doctrine of contagion. But far from ever winning the day, the anticontagionists simply helped discredit older, simple ideas of contagion. The majority of medical men adopted some form of compromise, a variant of contingent contagionism. As William Henry put it in a summary for the British Association, "NO ONE MALADY IS INVARIABLY AND UNDER ALL CIRCUMSTANCES CONTAGIOUS; in other words, . . . a CONTAGIOUS POISON IS SUCH ONLY IN A LIMITED AND QUALIFIED SENSE."[6] While Henry gave wide scope to contagion, considering not only smallpox but also plague and typhus to be contagious, he also preserved a large role for environmental influences, and in practical matters such as prevention he joined hands with the anticontagionists in opposing quarantine and advocating public sanitation.

Almost all authors attributed to the environment, particularly to the atmosphere, an important role in the appearance of epidemic disease. The idea is, of course, very old. The anticontagionists emphasized an aspect of that ancient tradition to explain the influence of locality on health and to justify a campaign against filth. We may use here as spokesman Thomas Southwood Smith, one of the most aggressive British anticontagionists. "The immediate, or exciting cause of fever, is a poison formed by the corruption or the decomposition of organic matter. Vegetable and animal matter, during the process of putrefaction, give off a principle, or give origin to a new compound, which, when applied to the human body, produces the phenomena constituting fever."[7]

He went on to explain that the nature of that poison, or animal malaria, was not known, but he was able to demonstrate, using the observations of several medical authorities including Sir John Pringle and Richard Mead, that persons exposed to airborne organic poisons or miasmata soon developed fevers.[8] Both living bodies as well as dead organic material might be a source of miasmata, and the confining of air exposed to such pollutants merely concentrated the poison and magnified its potency. After recounting Mead's description of the traditional home of plague in the Nile valley, Southwood Smith went further to claim that similar conditions could be created artificially at home.

But by far the most potent febrile poison, derived from an animal origin, is that which is formed by exhalations given off from the living bodies of those who are affected with fever, especially when such exhalations are pent up in a close and confined apartment. The room of a fever-patient, in a small and heated apartment in London, with no perflation of fresh air, is perfectly analogous to a stagnant pool in Ethiopia, full of the bodies of dead locusts. The poison generated in both cases is the same; the difference is merely in the degree of its potency. Nature, with her burning sun, her stilled and pent-up wind, her stagnant and teeming marsh, manufactures plague on a large and fearful scale: poverty in her hut, covered with her rags, surrounded with her filth, striving with all her might to keep out the pure air, and to increase the heat, imitates nature but too successfully; the process and the product are the same, the only difference is in the magnitude of the result. Penury and ignorance can thus at any time, and in any place, create a mortal plague. And of this no one has ever doubted. Of the power of the living body, even when in sound health, much more when in disease, and above all, when that disease is fever, to produce a poison capable of generating fever, no one disputes, and the fact has never been called in question. Thus far the agreement among all medical men, of all sects, and of all ages, is perfect.[9]

That section is marvelously representative. It illustrates how close the contagionists and their opponents could be at times. Southwood Smith denied that fever was contagious, but he recognized that those who visited a slum flat where fever was raging might contract the disease. However, he denied that this was an instance of contagion. He introduced at this point in the debates a distinction which seems to blur completely the differences between two camps. He explained there were contagious fevers, epidemic fevers, and contaminative fevers. Typhus fever was of the last sort.[10] The typhus patient contaminated the air of the room. A visitor exposed to that air might contract a similar fever. Southwood Smith insisted that the visitor's case would not be identical to the first patient's. This difference helped establish that the second case did not arise from contagion. He also insisted that visitors to a well-managed fever hospital which has an abundant supply of fresh air would not contract fever. The difference between the two situations seemed to establish that modification of the atmosphere and not contagion was responsible for such apparent transmission of fever.

This quotation from Southwood Smith also helps to illustrate the practical bent of the English anticontagionists. They were poor theorists, or were perhaps indifferent to the fine points of medical theory.[11] They were not ashamed to appeal to common prejudicies or passions to score a point, as when Charles Maclean suggested the doctrine of contagion had originally been formed as part of a papal plot, and that it had been maintained ever since as an instrument of arbitrary power and propagated as a "medical religion" in the universities and schools of physic.[12] Dogmatic anticontagionism was nurtured to meet the needs of campaigns to change official policy: first to abolish quarantine and then to initiate programs of public hygiene. Many of its documents were intended for public consumption and had as their main aim the guidance of public action. Consequently, it was those proximate causes of disease which were "palpable, definite, and capable of complete removal and prevention"[13] that received the most attention. The precise mechanism of disease causation was of little interest to the sanitarians.

Finally we must notice, nevertheless, that there were in the English medical profession many who were interested in just such disease mechanisms or processes. This theoretical interest and scientific preoccupation sets apart the approach of such individuals from that of the dogmatic sanitary reformers. Although they might agree with the practical measures the sanitarians proposed, they were unlikely to be satisfied with the sanitarians' explanations: with perfunctory appeals to science, such as Southwood Smith's references to Priestley's experiments with animals in closed jars, or Chadwick's breathtaking pronouncement, "All smell is disease."[14] To the more theoretically engaged, to the seriously science-minded, chemistry, especially the work of Justus Liebig, had great appeal. It offered to make the old medical analogy between fermentation and fever scientifically precise, and as Pelling has put it, to reduce the "dichotomy between sanitary generalization and medical science."[15] In the forties and fifties Liebig's ideas had great currency in British discussions of disease. Many, including William Farr, found in Liebig important suggestions.

Within the spectrum of medical opinion, Farr was a moderate who believed the doctrinarians of both schools were fanatical.[16] Although disease theory was not his major preoccupation, Farr kept well-informed of medical discoveries and because of his eclectic and systematic intellectual habits, he produced a very reasonable synthesis. It was probably representative of the position taken by many members of the medical profession at mid-century. It was scientifically plausible and useful as a guide for research and preventive programs.

Farr accepted the contagious nature not only of diseases like smallpox that could be transmitted by inoculation, but also for the more controversial cases of typhus or cholera, in which, he alleged, the contagion could be passed insensibly through the atmosphere.[17] In this regard he adopted the position taken nearly a decade earlier by William Henry. But Farr denied that the traditional understanding of contagion could adequately explain all known phenomena, even of diseases like smallpox, which no one denied was contagious.

Small-pox is admitted on all hands to be contagious. It is communicated by inoculation, or by the inhalation of the vapour given off by a small-pox patient. . . . Will the simple principle of contagion then explain the rapid propagation of the epidemic?—Not exclusively; for the disease is always contagious, and a certain number of deaths are caused by it in all seasons, and in every county of England. The facilities of intercourse, and the frequency of contact with the sick, are not greater when the disease is increasing, or is at its height, than when it is stationary or declining. The fact that 2,513 died in the first period, 3,289 in the second period, and 4,242 in the third period, must therefore be accounted for either by assuming that the disease had its origin in some spreading physical cause; that the contagious principle grew more virulent, and was conducted with greater facility by the atmosphere; that the susceptibility of the population increased; or, finally, that the tendency of the organization to fall into this peculiar pathological state augmented spontaneously.[18]

Like his contemporaries, Farr believed such explanations would be found in physical or environmental influences, especially in changes of the atmosphere. In the *Third Annual Report* he compared temperature readings with deaths registered for various diseases in the metropolitan districts during the years 1838 to 1841.[19] In this study he illustrated the seasonal variation in the causes of death and showed that the deaths for pulmonary diseases bore some relationship to daily mean temperatures. But he was aware that by itself temperature explained very little. He had pointed out in the previous year that a smallpox epidemic seemed to move like a series of small local epidemics whose appearances were not dependent on temperature. An epidemic might be at its peak in one area, while in nearby localities experiencing the same temperature, the epidemic may have already subsided or may not yet even have begun.[20] Temperature acted indirectly by influencing either seasonal employment and hence the availability of the means of subsistence, or the rate at which organic material decomposed. "As the temperature advances, and autumn comes on, dead vegetable and animal matter undergoes rapid decomposition; the living are infected; and, where the miasmata are concentrated in cities, or in undrained lands, remittent fevers, dysenteries, plagues, and malignant maladies, are generated."[21]

Farr's earliest systematic accounts of his disease theory are found in the *Fourth* and *Fifth Annual Reports.*[22] Both statements occur in the discussion of some more practical problem, the classification of diseases or the explanation for the high mortality of towns. In discussing why the mortality of urban districts was usually higher than that of rural or suburban districts, Farr began by considering the possible effect of population density and income.[23] He then dealt with the effects of the atmospheric impurities a city produces.[24] First came various gases, especially carbonic acid (carbon dioxide). Farr estimated the quantity of carbonic acid produced daily in London by animal respiration and by the combustion of coal. Using the work of recent chemists, especially Thomas Graham's research on the diffusion of gases, Farr argued that carbonic acid and other gases such as carbureted hydrogen (methane) and sulphureted hydrogen (hydrogen sulphide) were diffused too quickly to present any risk to human health under normal circumstances.[25] Such was not the case, however, with the heavier, inelastic particles suspended in the air. These were not easily diffused and might therefore accumulate in city air in hazardous concentrations. He mentioned briefly inorganic particles, such as coal dust and soot, but he was especially concerned with airborne animal matter.[26]

Every population throws off insensibly an atmosphere of organic matter, excessively rare in country and town, but less rare in dense than in open districts; and this atmosphere hangs over cities like a light cloud, slowly spreading—driven about—falling—dispersed by the winds—washed down by showers. It is not *vitalis halitus*, except by origin, but matter which *has lived*, is dead, has left the body, and is undergoing by oxidation decomposition into simpler than organic elements. The exhalations from sewers, churchyards, vaults, slaughter-houses, cesspools, commingle in this atmosphere, as polluted waters enter the Thames; and notwithstanding the wonderful provisions of nature for the speedy oxidation of organic matter in water and air, accumulate, and the density of the poison (for in the transition of decay it is a poison) is sufficient to impress its destructive action on the living.[27]

This animal matter was given off by the lungs in respiration and through the skin as well as during the process of putrefaction or decay.

The discussion in the *Fifth Annual Report* presented one aspect of Farr's disease theory, the one most relevant to the sanitary movement. His comments in the *Fourth Annual Report* are theoretically more complete.[28] Here he first introduced his zymotic theory. This theory suggested that instead of being entirely distinct in their causation, as many authors in the recent past had suggested, the epidemic, endemic, and contagious diseases in fact resembled each other in their etiology. They were all caused by the introduction into a susceptible person's blood stream of an animal poison that was specific for each disease. It was apparent from the manner in which he introduced his discussion that he had in mind the cases of inoculation or of chemical poisoning where the introduction into the body of a sufficient amount of some material was followed by a specific sequence of pathological changes.[29] But the animal poison that produced these diseases was unlike ordinary poisons or even animal venom in that during the course of the disease it was reproduced in the blood. This fact seemed crucial to many of the early nineteenth-century writers.

Like other English medical men of the forties, Farr was also much impressed with Liebig's researches and with the German chemist's suggestion that disease processes might be considered forms of fermentation or putrefaction. The analogy promised to explain a great deal, including the reproduction of the contagion. Farr cited Liebig repeatedly in this first account and also found some precedent for his theory in the works of the seventeenth-century English authorities Thomas Sydenham, Thomas Willis, and Richard Morton. Farr suggested that the "pathological transformations" that occurred during the attack of an epidemic, endemic, or contagious disease were of a "chemical nature, and analogous to fermentation."[30] He chose the word "zymotic" to indicate this analogy, and did much to make the word commonplace in Victorian medical literature.[31]

Only a limited amount was known, Farr believed, about the zymotic principles. They might be either fixed or volatile, depending on external circumstances. Their chemical composition was unknown, although Farr entertained the hope that the investigations of Liebig and Dumas might throw light on the subject.[32] What could not be known from the "rough analysis of artificial chemistry," might be inferred from the effects of the zymotic principles on the human body. In the meantime Farr proposed to name these agents according to the pathological changes they were known to cause: varioline for smallpox, vaccine for cowpox, syphiline for syphilis, lyssine for hydrophobia, rubeoline for measles, cholerine for cholera, typhine for typhus, pestine for plague, and similarly for the causal agents of erysipelas, puerperal fever, scarlet fever, whooping cough, influenza, and several others.[33] He suggested similar zymotic principles could be inferred for other diseases such as gangrene, diphtheria, and tetanus.

Farr's creation united some of the most promising explanatory features of both traditional contagionism and the miasmatic and environmental notions of the anticontagionists and the sanitary reformers. It could account for both the known or suspected cases of contagion and for the geographical movement of epidemic disease. But it also reserved a large role for environmental conditions, working primarily through the agency of the atmosphere, in determining the prevalence and severity of the zymotic diseases. He suggested, for example, that atmospheric changes were probably responsible for the fact that at certain times zymotic principles seemed very active and humans particularly susceptible, while at other times few suffered from zymotic diseases.[34] In his early career he could agree with the most dogmatic sanitarians that filth and the resulting accumulation of miasmata were absolutely pernicious. Such airborne materials, he explained, could serve as a vehicle for the zymotic principles, "to connect by a subtle, sickly, deadly medium, the people agglomerated in narrow streets and courts, down which no wind blows, and upon which the sun seldom shines."[35] For some of his contemporaries Farr's disease theory had the added appeal of being consistent with current trends in scientific speculation about the cause of disease, especially in its use of Liebig's ideas.

In retrospect it seems that Farr's success in joining the two irreconcilable doctrines, contagionism and anticontagionism, depended on his blurring the distinction between the miasmatic and the zymotic materials. This was quite easy to do. In the first place he suggested that although the zymotic materials were specific for individual diseases, they were not entirely distinct from one another. It seemed apparent to him that the zymotic materials of smallpox and cowpox must be closely related, and he entertained the possibility that one zymotic material could be converted into another.[36] With the acknowledgment of such transformations within the zymotic group, it was only a short step to assuming a direct role for miasmata in the causation of zymotic disease. The two types of materials were much alike. Both were organic, nonliving substances, the products of fermentation, putrefaction, or analogous disease processes. Each could serve to initiate chemical change in appropriate material. Farr believed that the similarity ran even deeper. Not only did miasmata weaken the human body and make it more susceptible to the action of zymotic materials, but also, Farr asserted, in the most squalid conditions where miasmata were produced in abundance, zymotic material might be produced even without the previous occurrence of a case of the disease.[37] As late as 1866 he wrote, "Erysipelas, pyaemia, and gangrene are generated, when wounded soldiers are crowded in military hospitals; and the specific matter of each of these diseases produces the same specific diseases in other soldiers."[38] It was a short step from Farr's claim that the conditions which produced the most abundant and powerful miasmata might also produce zymotic materials *de novo* to Chadwick's assertion that smell, if it is intense enough, is disease. Farr's views not only served to effect a compromise on the question of contagion, but also to offer support for some of the observations Victorian reformers considered most important. Any complete disease theory had to explain the observed connection between poverty, filth, and crowding and prevalence of epidemic, endemic, and contagious diseases. Many men believed that in extreme conditions disease could be spontaneously created.

Farr's views were not only very reasonable when seen in their context, but because of Farr's sensitivity to scientific research, they also proved to be extremely flexible, and capable of accommodating major changes in attitudes. Disease theory was revolutionized during his career. Chemical and microscopic researches played important roles in bringing about this change, as did the experience of the three major epidemics of Asiatic cholera that occurred between 1848 and 1866. As originally set forth, Farr's theory emphasized the atmosphere's role in the causation of zymotic disease. In the absence of very firm evidence to the contrary he assumed the atmosphere was the medium for the propagation of the zymotic material. The first substantial change in his theory occurred on this point.

By the middle fifties Farr had become convinced that cholera could be propagated through either air or water.[39] We will soon discuss the reasons why he adopted this view. By this time he had de-emphasized the role of the atmosphere in his nosologies. In the classification he proposed for international use, he divided the zymotic diseases into three groups, only one of which was miasmatic.[40] But his de-emphasizing of the atmosphere's role went even further. He now defined the miasmatic diseases as those which were diffusible through air and water.

J. K. Crellin has shown recently that in the 1860s explanations of contagious or epidemic disease followed the scientific vogue of looking to particles as the fundamental units of biology.[41] A number of explanations of disease were advanced in Britain that relied on various sorts of infectious particles. Farr's zymotic theory was quite representative. In his earlier statements Farr spoke of zymotic principles or of zymotic matter without suggesting anything of their composition. But following the great epidemics of the middle sixties, cholera and cattle plague, Farr's attention was drawn to contemporary microscopic research and to the organic particles biologists were discussing. In a section of his monograph on the 1866 cholera epidemic, Farr discussed the scientific evidence for the zymotic theory. The older authorities, the chemists Liebig, Dumas, and Thomas Graham, had given way to the microscopists and pathologists: Filippo Pacini, Lionel S. Beale, John Burdon-Sanderson, August Chauveau, and Louis Pasteur.[42] Farr interpreted their work, especially their attention to microscopic particles, in zymotic terms. He had come to consider the agent of zymotic disease a specific particle.

To sum up the zymotic theory. It is now held by naturalists that each organ of the body has its proper life; and that it consists of minute centres of action, which have been called cells, globules, organic units, germs, granules, and other names. The cells like the supposed vesicles of the clouds are now shown to be solids, and Beale proposes to call them "germinal matter," which is perhaps a description rather than a name. "Monad" would serve to designate these living particles, but as it, as well as the other names proposed, have been already appropriated, these units of force and life may be designated *biads*.

. . . .

It is only with particular kinds of these *biads*, then that we have to do in *zymosis*; and, to give definite form to the theory, while *vaccine* lymph may be briefly called *vaccinine*, the granules of Chaveau may be named *vaccinads*; while those of *varioline* (smallpox lymph) are named *variolads*; those of *syphiline, syphilads,* and those of *cholrine, cholrads*,—the "choleragenic molecules" of Pacini.[43]

A few years later he named these disease-producing "biads" or zymotic molecules "zymads."[44]

The zymotic theory had undergone a significant change from the 1840s. The consideration of zymads reflects the increasing reliance on biology rather than on chemistry as the model for explanations of disease. Farr was well aware of the potential value of biology to students of disease. Immediately after the publication of Charles Darwin's *Origin of Species* Farr suggested that the evolutionary theory was applicable to the study of disease, since disease, a state of the human body, should participate in any evolutionary changes the body undergoes.[45] In this way the appearance of new diseases could be accounted for, and these could be expected to be recognized at first as varieties of older types and then as distinct species. In the 1860s the particulate nature of Darwin's theory of inheritance, pangenesis, caught Farr's attention. He did not miss the opportunity to point out the similarity between his zymads and Darwin's gemmules.[46] Both were elementary biological units having a corpuscular life but not an independent existence.

One of the most interesting features of the development of Farr's zymotic theory is the way during the next few years he endowed the zymads with more and more properties of life, until they became indistinguishable from minute organisms. In this manner the zymotic theory became for some a convenient bridge to the germ theory. As early as 1840 Farr was aware of animalcular theories, and in his second annual letter to the registrar general he mentioned the minority opinions of Jacob Henle and Henry Holland.[47] But it was only in the 1860s that Farr began to seriously consider the animalcular hypothesis. In his report on the cholera epidemic of 1866 and in the next annual report he called attention to the importance of Pasteur's work on fermentation and on the diseases of silkworms.[48] Pasteur's work seemed to strengthen his conviction that disease processes resembled fermentations and served to demonstrate that the biads were reproduced in the process.

Each fermentation has at least one specific chemical product, be it alcohol, acetic acid, lactic acid, or butyric acid; and also one ferment. It is the great merit of Pasteur to have established by ingenious and experimental research, that all these ferments consist of organic molecules, propagated from previous molecules of the same kind. He has shown not that spontaneous generation is impossible, on the confines of the three kingdoms, under every possible condition, but that the fermentations in all the cases he examined were set in motion by specific pre-existing germs; multiplying indefinitely by reproduction under given conditions.[49]

At this time he did not believe the zymads, those pre-existing germs of disease, had an independent life, although they had some properties of living things such the ability to reproduce. Unlike known disease-causing parasites, they did not have a "well defined, independent existence, and a distinct place in the animal and vegetable kingdom"; they seemed to occupy instead "a sort of border land on the confines of the three kingdoms [of nature]."[50]

Farr's conversion to the germ theory took place in the 1870s when he was in his sixties. The change required merely the admission that the disease-producing zymads were in fact independent organisms. In his letter published in 1870 Farr was prepared to admit that the zymads behaved "as if they possessed an independent life,"[51] and three years later was willing to grant them this autonomy.[52] By 1875 he equated the zymads with disease germs.[53] In his letter of 1878 Farr makes the rather ambiguous suggestion that zymotic diseases were referable to "extraneous organisms."[54] Since he was writing before the string of discoveries of pathogenic microbes by Koch and his students, it is not surprising that Farr's understanding of the germ theory was not entirely modern. It does seem clear that by the end of the 1870s Farr had accepted the major features of the germ theory simply by changing his understanding of the nature of the zymad.

The decade was full of soul-searching and conversions among English students of disease. Several decades ago Winslow summarized the way John Simon came to accept the basic features of the germ theory during his career as Medical Officer of the Privy Council.[55] Around 1850 Farr and Simon held similar views on disease causation. Over the next two decades their understanding changed in comparable ways. During the sixties the experience with the epidemics of cholera and cattle plague and the results of microscopic pathological research, mainly on the continent, encouraged Simon to re-examine his theory. By the late 1870s he had come to accept the view that most of the zymotic diseases were caused by minute organisms, which had not yet been discovered, and which reproduced themselves in the body of the sick man. Such changes in disease theory did not immediately revolutionize all aspects of the program to prevent disease. As we shall see in the next chapter, Farr continued throughout his life to advocate essentially the same means of preventing zymotic disease and of lowering mortality. Many of his preventive measures had lost their original justification by the seventies, but they had either acquired a new rationale or were retained because they had been for so long an essential part of the sanitary campaign. Also unchanged was Farr's fundamental belief in the regularity of biological processes, including those of disease. We have already suggested that Farr used this regularity to justify his statistical approach. In the remainder of this chapter, we will consider several examples of his statistical studies of major epidemic and epizootic diseases: smallpox, cattle plague, and cholera. In these studies, especially the ones he undertook of the cholera epidemics, one can easily see the operation of two theoretical forces: Farr's zymotic theory, and his notion that statistics could be used to elucidate the obscure regularity in the course of major diseases.

Sickness Tables and the Law of Disease

There is little question but that the statistical study of zymotic disease was one of Farr's major preoccupations. His work on this subject began well before he joined the General Register Office. His ultimate purpose was the discovery of the laws that regulated the course of disease. As we have seen, he had no doubt that the diseases were law-abiding and that this fact was the key that would unlock the secrets of their nature. During his career he wrote statistical laws of disease that were of various sorts: laws giving an individual's chances of recovery or death during an illness, laws describing the course of an epidemic over time, and laws illustrating the effect of some environmental circumstance on the course of disease.

We can not be absolutely certain of the origin of Farr's idea of a law of disease. It may have come from his medical study in Paris. Some students of Pierre Louis acquired such a notion from their teacher's studies.[56] George Rosen has suggested that around 1840 Jacob Henle's work helped turn Farr's mind to the idea;[57] however, the particular form of Farr's laws suggests another strong possibility. His first laws of disease were derived from sickness tables, which were formed according to the procedures for constructing life tables. The law of disease seems to have been a direct borrowing of the law of mortality which the actuary Thomas Rowe Edmonds used to construct theoretical life tables.

In the middle thirties Edmonds had begun to apply his ideas to the study of sickness. In *Lancet* articles for 1835–1836, Edmonds showed how laws of sickness could be deduced from hospital and friendly society records by his techniques.[58] Furthermore he believed he could demonstrate a relationship between morbidity and disease mortality, and that he could describe numerically the course of illness among a group of patients. The statistics of the London Fever Hospital suggested to him that "a given number living at every year of age suffer the same number of attacks of sickness; and that the duration of each case of sickness, at any age, is proportional to the mortality at that age."[59] The most striking feature of this study was Edmonds's demonstration that the changes in mortality from fever with age could be described by the numerical formula.[60] Farr was impressed by these results. In several publications from the thirties to the fifties he called his readers' attention to Edmonds's articles.[61]

By the time Edmonds published these articles on disease, Farr had already realized that Edmonds's technique of deducing a law of mortality from a series of mortality rates and using it to construct a theoretical life table could be used to study disease. He set to work collecting data from hospital records.[62] In 1837 and 1838 he published three articles that announced the discovery of laws for recovery and death in smallpox.[63] These articles show very clearly the impact of the actuary techniques he learned from Edmonds.

For this study Farr collected the records of nearly eight thousand cases of smallpox at the Smallpox Hospital in two periods, 1780-1799, before vaccination was widespread, and 1825-1835, after the practice was more common. He then used the records of 4,915 of these cases to construct what he called a sickness table, a survivorship table in contemporary usage, for a group of 100,000 patients between the ages of 10 and 35.[64] The table showed the number sick, the number dying and recovering, and the number who would recover or who would die in each consecutive 5-day period from 5 to 105 days. It was, in fact, exactly analogous to a theoretical life table, except that instead of two basic columns, living and dying, it had three: the sick, the recovering, and the dying. From the table one could easily see how the fatality from the disease increased rapidly in the early stages, reached a peak between the tenth and fifteenth days, and then declined thereafter.

The table demonstrated in fact two laws: a law of mortality and a complementary law of recovery. Farr found that the rates of recovery or of death in consecutive periods of disease formed geometrical series which he could approximate by several formulae for separate intervals of the illness.[65] Like Edmonds before him, he compared his theoretical series generated by those formulae to the set obtained by observation.[66] In the first two articles Farr did not consider the effect of age or of sex on the outcome of smallpox cases. But in his third paper he showed how the mortality of smallpox varied with age. From a peak in infancy smallpox mortality dropped to a minimum at puberty and then increased by about one-third every ten years of age thereafter. The form of the law of mortality for smallpox by human age was thus the same as the law of mortality in a life table.

Farr believed this approach which he named "nosometry" would be a valuable tool of medical research.[67] The following year he extended the method to Asiatic cholera using records of 9,372 cases from Rome in 1837 which Sir James Clark had brought to his attention.[68] Nosometry, Farr believed, might become a means of reforming clinical medicine. If sickness tables were constructed for the major diseases and were based on a large number of cases, they would serve as standards and references for medical judgment. He showed how, from such a table, one could easily determine the chances of recovery or of death and the probable future duration of the illness at each period of the disease.[69] Such information would do much to place prognosis on a sure footing.

The construction of sickness tables would also help evaluate the effectiveness of therapy. One could only make such judgments, Farr claimed, by determining whether a particular treatment either increased the probability of recovery or shortened the course of sickness.[70] Sickness tables would provide such information and therefore would serve as balances "neither vague, influenced by prejudice, nor falsified by an imperfect perception of general relations beyond the grasp of unassisted reason. Nothing is so well calculated to extinguish the abounding quackery of the day."[71]

Nearly a quarter-century later Farr repeated this recommendation in a paper to the British Medical Association.[72] He used the data from his smallpox study of 1837 to show how the inductive approach might bring greater certainty to medicine. It would silence cynics who claimed medicine could do nothing, and serve as a corrective to the claims of empirics and sectarians who pointed to the recovery of any of their patients as a vindication of their system. In the present state of pathological knowledge other diseases besides smallpox might be studied by this method. He mentioned measles, scarlatina, diphtheria, croup, whooping cough, typhus, erysipelas, metria, and carbuncle. He did not suggest the formation of control groups. The object of medicine was to heal. It would be "impossible and wrong" to form such sickness tables for cases that were left to run their natural course.

About the same time these first articles on recovery or deaths in smallpox and cholera appeared, Farr used this approach again. It occurred in his study of the institutional care of the insane. Originally the work appeared in his own journal, but he used it again as the basis for his first paper to the Statistical Society of London.[73] He exhibited in tables the rates of cure and relapse, and the mortality rate for inmates in various institutions. In the later paper, he constructed a "Nosometrical table" for the inmates of the Hanwell asylum that showed for each of the first 7 1/2 years of residency the number who would recover or die, and the number of cases terminating, distinguishing those recovering from those dying out of an original group of 1,000 inmates.[74] He illustrated the numerical laws of death and recovery revealed in the table by comparing the observed and the calculated series. Once again he showed how the table could be used to calculate the probabilities of recovery or of death and the probable future duration of insanity. The findings confirmed the suspicion that the longer a patient had been insane the less likely it was that he would recover. Farr also suggested such tables could be used to judge the efficacy of treatment.

As a clinical tool, Farr's technique was promising. Judged solely as a statistical method it was more sophisticated than the numerical studies of Pierre Louis. Its medical implications were more fully developed in Farr's than in Edmonds's hands. Farr had at least one medical imitator in England. Farr's friend and collaborator, R. Dundas Thomson, recommended that Farr's approach be used to study the case histories of cholera patients to discover laws of that disease.[75] But in general, Farr's medical contemporaries did not show much appreciation for his method. In the thirties it was not easy to find adequate clinical records. Furthermore, it is doubtful if many physicians or patients placed much value in the abstract, impersonal probabilities Farr's tables and laws revealed. Farr himself did not develop clinical statistics much further. When he joined the G.R.O. he suddenly had an abundance of mortality data, but by themselves they were of little help in continuing this line of research.

He certainly did not abandon interest in morbidity statistics. Occasionally he could turn the national mortality statistics to advantage. This is most obvious in his famous studies of the cholera epidemics. In his first special cholera report, the one for the epidemic of 1848–1849, he constructed a sickness table for cholera.[76] Since his information was drawn from the register of deaths, from the entries for the cause of death and the duration of last illness, the table listed only fatal cases, and in three columns it showed for each day of the illness and for six-hour intervals during the first day the number of persons, the males, and the females, surviving and dying. He also found the average duration of fatal cases of cholera and diarrhea, separately by age groups. In his third cholera study, the one for the 1866 epidemic, Farr combined his data for the last three epidemics to show how cholera mortality increased by decennial age groups according to an exponential law.[77] Farr also considered other major diseases. In 1864, for example, as a sequel to Edmonds's study, he used the recorded fever deaths from 1848 to 1862 and the records of the London Fever Hospital to find a law that determined how the case fatality from fever increased with age.[78]

The Law of an Epidemic

Farr's best-known studies of disease were his studies of epidemics. In his memorial volume, Humphreys emphasized this aspect of Farr's work, especially his cholera studies, to the total omission of the early papers on recovery and death in smallpox and insanity.[79] There seems little reason to modify the assessment John Brownlee offered in 1915, that Farr was the first person to adequately describe an epidemic numerically.[80] He did this by extending the actuary's technique of discovering the law of mortality in a life table.

The first epidemic he studied was smallpox. An epidemic was already in progress when civil registration was established, and by the end of 1839 the deaths of nearly 31,000 people had been attributed to that disease in the first 10 quarters of registration. In the *Second Annual Report* Farr described the course of the epidemic and showed how the rate of mortality from smallpox for the entire population and the number of smallpox deaths for the nation and for certain regions declined in a predictable manner.[81] He found, for example, that if he took the mean number of smallpox deaths in consecutive quarters, a series of figures was produced which he could describe by a statistical law. Using the smallpox deaths registered in all England and Wales, he showed that by taking the mean deaths in the third and fourth quarters as the figure for a first period, the mean deaths for the fourth and fifth quarters as the figure for the second period, and similarly through the tenth quarter of registration, a series of seven figures was produced which described the decline of the epidemic: 4,365, 4,087, 3,767, 3,416, 2,743, 2,019, and 1,631.[82]

The rate of decrease, he explained, itself increased with each successive period. The rate of decrease for the first period was 1.052, and it increased in each successive period by a factor of 1.046. Farr called 1.052 the rate of decrease and 1.046 the constant. By successive multiplications beginning, apparently, with the third period, he produced the series: 4,364, 4,147, 3,767, 3,272, 2,716, 2,156, 1,635. The agreement with the observed series was close enough to satisfy him. Using the same means, Farr went on to find figures for the rates and constants to describe the decline in the epidemic in the metropolis and in Wales and the western countries of England.

In this report Farr made brief mention of the quarterly increase in the smallpox deaths in the first stages of the epidemic. He pointed out that in England and Wales the deaths in the first three quarters of registration were 2,513, 3,289, and 4,242. The rate of increase seemed to be about 30 percent. In the next period the increase dropped to 6 percent before an absolute decline in smallpox deaths occurred. After explaining that several epidemics would have to be studied before definite conclusions could be reached, he offered some tentative observations on the rise and fall of a smallpox epidemic: "It appears probable, however, that the small-pox increases at an accelerated and then a retarded rate; that it declines first at a slightly accelerated, then at a rapidly accelerated, and lastly at a retarded rate, until the disease attains the minimum intensity, and remains stationary."[83] He had the figures to be much more precise. With the benefit of hindsight we can see that the quarterly smallpox deaths for the metropolis conform quite closely to a normal curve: 257, 506, 753, 1,145, 1,061,

858, 364, 117, 65, 60.[84] Farr, however, did not seem to notice this fact. He dropped one tantalizing suggestion. After describing how the rate of increase of deaths declined, he said it reached a level of 6 percent, "where it remains stationary, like a projectile at the summit of the curve which it is destined to describe."[85] The figure of speech suggests more to us than it did to Farr. Neither here nor in other cases did he point out that his data conformed to Quetelet's law of error. His perspective and computational method made it very unlikely that he would consider his data in the way implied in Quetelet's work or made explicit by late nineteenth-century statisticians, as a problem of distribution.

The discovery of these laws raised the possibility of predicting the course of an epidemic. Farr attempted to do this several times. The first time he was very cautious—making the prediction only after the fact. In the late fall of 1840, smallpox deaths were found to be increasing, and it looked as if another epidemic were on the way. In an article in the *Lancet* Farr determined the rate at which metropolitan smallpox deaths had increased in the first four quarters of the last epidemic, and he found that if he had used that rate to predict the rise of the present epidemic, he would have been very close to the mark.[86] The series of registered deaths was 60, 104, 170, 253, and the calculated series was 60, 99, 163, 267. Farr went on to recommend universal vaccination, and to criticize the Poor Law authorities for the failures in the vaccination program.

On one other occasion Farr tried to predict the future course of an epidemic. As the Cattle Plague grew more serious during the winter of 1865-1866, Robert Lowe stood in the House of Commons to forecast disaster for English agriculture. Farr responded with a letter to the *Daily News* in which he predicted the epidemic was about to subside.[87] It was a bold prediction because he had only four monthly figures: 9,597, 18,817, 33,835, and 47,191. While the number of cattle dying of rinderpest was still increasing, the rate of increase was dropping. This fall in the rate suggested to Farr that the epidemic was about to reach its peak and that deaths would soon diminish. In the basis of those four figures alone Farr derived a law for the epidemic and predicted the cattle deaths for the next five months: 43,182, 21,927, 5,226, 494, and 16. Although the epidemic did decline, his forecast was not entirely accurate. The actual cattle deaths were 57,004, 27,958, 15,856, 14,734, and about 5,000.[88] In making the predictions Farr took consecutive orders of differences of the logarithms of the first four figures. Since he had only one third order value, he simply assumed third order differences would be constant. He generated the series in his prediction on that bold assumption. It was a procedure which could only have been used by a man who was thoroughly convinced that the course of epidemics could be adequately described by geometrical series.

Farr's most comprehensive studies of epidemic disease were his famous reports on the cholera.[89] In these volumes one can not only see his idea of a law of disease elucidating causes of epidemics, but one can also trace significant changes in his theory of disease. His first cholera report was a separately published volume for the epidemic of 1848 and 1849.[90] It was a major work, comprising Farr's hundred-page introduction followed by three hundred pages of plates and tables. It established a pattern that his later studies followed. Farr discussed the history of cholera, traced the course of the present epidemic, and noted the characteristics of local outbreaks. Besides his statistics of the epidemic, Farr also offered a discussion of the theories and analogies that had been proposed to explain epidemics of the disease, and he offered suggestions for prevention.

The statistical portion of the report contained some analyses that Farr had offered for other diseases: mortality rates for the disease by age group and sex, and the construction of a sickness table.[91] He also plotted on circular graphs meteorological data from the Greenwich observatory and daily cholera deaths, finding no significant relationships.[92] He did discover that most cholera deaths occurred Sunday through Wednesday, a finding he regarded as coincidental or dependent on human habits, such as the drinking practices of the working class.[93]

The mortality statistics did suggest that the epidemic was particularly severe in certain geographical areas. Farr identified nine areas of intense cholera mortality, "cholera fields" he called them, each one having a large port city as its center. Both his figures and his ideas about the causes of epidemics led him to believe that some features of certain localities accounted for these high cholera mortality rates. He began a topographical analysis of his data. He found that nearly 80 percent of the 53,000 registered cholera deaths in 1849 occurred among four-tenths of the population living on one-seventh of the land area. On an average, coastal districts had three times the cholera mortality of inland districts.[94]

To discover what factors were responsible for the high local cholera mortality, he turned to the registration districts of London.[95] He found that the order of districts by cholera mortality was very similar to their order according to deaths from all causes in other years. There also seemed to be an inverse relationship between income, determined by taxable property, and cholera mortality. But he failed to find an expected relationship with population density. It was only when he considered the elevation of the soil that Farr reached statistically satisfying results.

He arranged the districts of London into terraces according to their mean elevation above the Thames high water mark. Each terrace had a range of twenty feet, 0–20, 20–40, etc. The cholera mortality per 10,000 for consecutive terraces declined in a series 102, 65, 34, 27, 22, 11—roughly the same series as one would obtain by dividing 102 successively

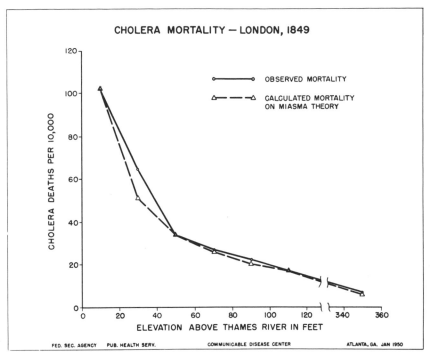

Figure 4. Alexander Langmuir's graph illustrating Farr's elevation law for the 1849 cholera epidemic. Alexander D. Langmuir, "Epidemiology of Airborne Infection," *Bact. Rev.* 25 (1961): 174.

by 2, 3, 4, 5, and 6. When he considered the cholera mortality for districts of specific mean elevation, Farr found he obtained a decreasing series which was adequately represented by the formula $C = C' \cdot (e' + a)/(e + a)$ where C and C' are cholera mortality rates per 10,000 in two districts having mean elevations e and e', and a is a constant, approximately 13.[96] Using the formula, he calculated for the elevations 0, 10, 30, 50, 70, 90, 100 and 350 feet, a theoretical series (174, 99, 53, 34, 27, 22, 20, and 6) that closely agreed with the series of recorded figures (177, 102, 65, 34, 27, 22, 17, and 7). Alexander Langmuir has plotted the observed values and Farr's calculated ones to show the close agreement.[97] (See fig. 4.) Farr offered a diagram of his own to illustrate the relationship between elevation and cholera mortality.[98] (See fig. 5.)

This discovery must have delighted Farr. Not only did it conform to his notion of a statistical law, but the implications of the law were consistent with his disease theory. The soil at low elevations, especially along the margins of the Thames, held abundant organic material for the production of miasmata. The concentration of these deadly atmospheric

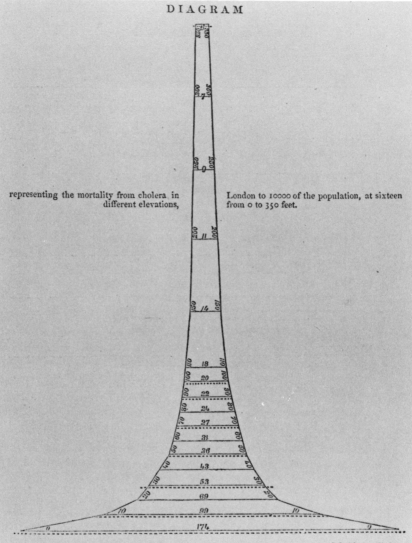

representing the mortality from cholera in different elevations,

London to 10000 of the population, at sixteen from 0 to 350 feet.

The figures in the centre express the number of deaths from cholera to 10000 inhabitants living at the elevations expressed in feet on the sides of the diagram.

The length of the *black horizontal lines* shows the *calculated* relative fatality of cholera in districts at relative elevations indicated by the height from the base of the diagram. The *dotted lines* indicate the mean mortality *observed* in the elevations given. Thus:—in districts at 90 feet above the Thames, the average mortality from cholera was 22 in 10000 inhabitants.

Figure 5. Farr's diagram for the elevation law for the 1849 cholera epidemic. William Farr, *Report on the Mortality of Cholera in England, 1848–49* (London, 1852), p. lxv.

pollutants could be expected to be much greater at lower than at higher elevations. The law for the relationship of cholera mortality and elevation therefore appealed to Farr for at least two very basic reasons. It is extremely interesting to notice the fate of the elevation law as Farr's understanding of the cause of cholera changed.

When the epidemic began in 1848, Farr considered only the atmosphere as a medium for transferring cholerine, the zymotic material of cholera. But before his own study of the epidemic appeared, John Snow had suggested an alternative explanation.[99] Snow, as is well-known, suggested that cholera was transmitted when material from the intestines of a cholera patient found its way to the digestive tract of another person, either through contact or via drinking water or food. We can be certain that Farr knew of Snow's work by the time he wrote his own report, because he offered a summary of Snow's conclusions and a discussion of some of their implications.[100] He compared the cholera mortality of the districts served by the London water companies, and he recognized that the districts where cholera was most often fatal were not only those of lowest elevation but also ones served by the Southwark and Lambert water companies that drew their water supply downstream in the polluted tidal waters of the Thames. He also recognized that of two cities on the same river the one further downstream almost invariably had a higher cholera mortality and that it inherited the sewage from its neighbor upstream. These discoveries, however, suggested to Farr that sewage-contaminated water, like other factors such as income, was merely a modifying influence. Water's role did not seem so certain or decisive as elevation. It is fairly clear that Farr regarded the polluted river water as but another source of miasmata. He attached considerable importance to Glaisher's estimate of the amount of water evaporated from the Thames in London.[101] Along with the water vapor, organic material entered the air from the polluted river water.

Although Snow's theory was by no means generally accepted, it had made water purity an issue in discussions of cholera. When the disease returned in 1853, informed members of the medical profession looked for a way of testing Snow's theories. A nearly perfect opportunity presented itself.[102] John Simon, John Snow, and William Farr all recognized its value. The Metropolis Water Act of 1852[103] required that by August 1855 all river water supplied commercially for domestic use must be drawn from the Thames above Teddington Lock or from one of the river's tributaries above tidal influence. By the time of the 1853–1854 epidemic only the Lambert Waterworks Company had complied with the new regulations. With this change came a dramatic improvement in the quality of the company's water. The Lambert Company had formerly supplied some of the most polluted water. Now it pumped some of the least contaminated. But most important was the fact that in a number of South London districts the Lambert company competed directly, street by street, house by house, with the Southwark and Vauxhall company, which continued to supply water highly contaminated by sewage. The quality of their drinking water was the only apparent way in which the social and sanitary conditions of the two companies' patrons differed. A simple comparison of the mortality from cholera between the two groups gave striking results. In 1848-1849 the rates for both groups were very high, 11.8 per 1,000 for the Southwark and Vauxhall company and 12.5 for the Lambert company. In the next epidemic the rate for the Southwark and Vauxhall company had increased to 13.0 while that for the Lambert company had fallen dramatically to 3.7. Faced with this striking result, medical opinion on the cause of the disease began to change.

Farr was a member of the General Board of Health's Scientific Committee that investigated the cause of the 1853-1854 epidemic. Farr's influence, especially in the statistical section, is evident in the committee's report.[104] Farr did not publish a major study for this epidemic. His volume for the previous epidemic had appeared only the year before. He had published observations on the epidemic in the registrar general's weekly reports, and he summarized these in his letter in the *Seventeenth Annual Report*.[105] The analysis is much like the one in the previous publication. The tremendous variation in cholera mortality rates, ranging among the London districts from 2 to 211 deaths per 1,000 suggested, Farr claimed, that the "cause of the intense form of cholera is local, and circumscribed in its action."[106]

What distinguishes this discussion from its predecessor is the increased attention to the relative cholera mortality in London's water fields, the areas served by each of the private water companies. Farr began his investigation of the effects of the water supply early in this epidemic. On October 13, 1853, the General Register Office addressed a letter to each water company requesting information on the source of its water, the area of the metropolis it served, and any changes it had made in the water quality or service since 1849.[107] Farr was eager to investigate Snow's hypothesis. John Simon later recalled that it was Farr who urged the General Board of Health's Scientific Committee to study the water supply and cholera mortality in South London.[108]

The results of the water field studies convinced Farr that polluted water played a large role in determining the character of London's cholera epidemics, and that his zymotic theory required modification. He ended his discussion by saying "the cholera matter or *cholerine*, where it is most fatal, is largely diffused through *water*, as well as through other channels."[109] But this did not mean that Farr had embraced Snow's theory wholeheartedly or abandoned the airborne explanation. He seems to have continued to regard the airlung route as the major mode of causation. It seemed to him that cholerine, diffused in water, was most likely to be deadly when it entered the air by evaporation from cisterns, taps, drains, and local reservoirs. The water "comes into contact with the body in many ways and it gives off incessantly at its temperature . . . . vapors and effluvia into the atmosphere that is breathed in every room."[110]

Such partial accommodation to Snow's theory was quite common. The General Board of Health's cholera committee concluded that the unknown cause of cholera acts as a ferment and "that it therefore takes effect only amid congenial circumstances, and that the stuff out of which it brews poison must be air or water abounding with organic impurity."[111] John Simon equally blamed fecalized air and fecalized water.[112]

The epidemic of 1866 proved decisive in establishing the water-borne theory for cholera. By that time the climate of medical opinion had changed in important ways. We noted earlier that in his report on this epidemic Farr gave serious attention to recent microscopic and pathological studies, especially those of the intestines and stools of cholera patients.[113] This report, like Farr's first cholera report, was book-length, and in some ways it was the most sophisticated of Farr's three cholera investigations. Like its predecessors it analyzed the epidemic as a complex social and medical phenomenon. Once again he considered the effects of income, occupation, population density, age, sex, and weather. This time, however, such factors were passed over rather quickly.[114]

The bulk of the report on the 1866 epidemic was given over to demonstrating the role of sewage-contaminated water. By the time he wrote the report Farr became convinced that although water was not the only means of transmission for cholera it was certainly the most important. The *Lancet* concluded that his investigation made the water-borne theory "irresistible."[115] The heart of the study was a water field analysis of London, which placed most of the blame for the epidemic on the operation of the East London Waterworks Company.[116] Early in the epidemic it became clear that mortality in that company's water field was excessive. A series of official investigations followed, and these showed that the East London Waterworks Company had been illegally supplying water from its reservoir at Old Ford which had been contaminated by the discharge from the recently completed sewage system of West Ham.[117]

For his water field study Farr divided the 135 subdistricts of the metropolis into 15 groups, 8 receiving their water exclusively from one of London's water companies, and 7 having mixed supplies. The cholera mortality rates for the former 8 fields pointed unambiguously to East London. The death rates per 10,000 over the entire epidemic for each of the other 7 groups having a single source of water were 3, 4, 4, 6, 7, 8, and 15, while the rate for the East London company field was 72. In the subdistricts supplied wholly or in part from the Old Ford reservoir the rate was even higher. Furthermore while the cholera mortality rates for other parts of London had steadily fallen as the water quality had improved, falling in South London, for example, from 122 to 94 to 8 over the past three epidemics, the mortality in East London had gone from 59 to 34 to 72. The turnabout between 1854 and 1866 seemed to have been due to the pollution of the River Lea.

Farr also used his idea of a law of the epidemic, a numerical description of the manner in which mortality from the disease increased and fell over time, to add support to his conclusions about the role of water.[118] He showed that although the absolute number of deaths in the metropolis in 1866, except for East London, was greatly reduced from previous cholera epidemics, the general course of the epidemic was very much like that of its predecessor. In East London, on the other hand, the decline in the epidemic was much more abrupt than in the previous epidemics or than what the law of the epidemic for East London, deduced from earlier 1866 weekly mortality figures, would have suggested. Farr believed this sudden change in the law of the epidemic was due to the changes the company made in its supply, when attention was drawn to the cholera fatality among its patrons.

Farr concluded that cholera was propagated by cholera flux, the intestinal discharges of cholera patients. He now recognized four means of disseminating cholerine from cholera flux: (1) personal contact, (2) air, (3) sewer vapor, and (4) water. While the first three sources exerted some influence, estimated for London at a rate of 5 deaths per 10,000 population, he maintained that in an industrial society like England these other sources were insignificant in comparison to contaminated water.[119] As we have suggested, the 1866 epidemic was a turning point in the development of Farr's disease theory. It marked the decline of the role he assigned to the atmosphere in epidemics and it strengthened the case for contagion.

Although his disease theory was changing, his belief in statistical laws for disease was not. Farr's third cholera report, like the first, was devoted in part to the discovery of statistical laws of the disease which would explain such relationships as that between the relative mortality of an epidemic and the average duration of its fatal cases.[120] Once again the law sought was a numerical relation that permitted one to construct a series of numbers approximating the observed figures. That Farr strongly believed in such laws is evidenced by his retention of the elevation law in the second and third cholera reports, despite the abandonment of the miasmatic theory—the theory which had probably encouraged Farr to consider such a relationship in the first place, and which could explain such a relationship. Farr apparently believed that a relationship that could be demonstrated so clearly in a numerical law revealed some fundamental feature of the disease that must not be overlooked, even though medical explanations for it might change. Farr never accepted John Snow's conclusion that the elevation law was founded on coincidental circumstances of 1849.[121]

In the 1853–1854 epidemic Farr discovered that the elevation law did not seem to hold in its original form. He found, however, that if figures for both epidemics were combined, a law of similar form could be deduced.[122] His task in the report for the 1866 epidemic was much more difficult. Once again the amassed mortality data did not conform to his law; but furthermore, the rationale for looking for such a law all but vanished with the acceptance of Snow's theory. London had only one atmosphere, but it had several water supplies. Farr made a discovery that saved the elevation law. Although the law no longer held for the metropolis as a whole, it seemed to hold within individual water fields and to hold better as the water supplied was more heavily contaminated.[123]

Farr thought he could explain both this new application of the elevation law and its current failure to describe the distribution of cholera deaths in the entire metropolis. This explanation, like its predecessor, depended on the distribution of cholerine in its medium, but now the medium was water, not air. Early in his report for the 1866 epidemic Farr carefully explained Professor Frankland's observation on the distribution of cholera flux in glass tubes of distilled water. By analogy, London's water pipes could be thought of as Frankland's tubes, in which the flux settled to the lower end of the vessel.[124] Farr suggested that households drawing their water from mains at lower elevations would therefore receive more suspended cholera material than those whose taps were at higher elevations. We should recall that at this time water was pumped to homes intermittently, rather than under constant pressure, and that under such conditions Farr's explanation was a bit more plausible.[125] He reasoned that since the companies supplied water of different degrees of purity, the cholera law could be observed only within a cholera field. The influence of elevation was more obvious with more highly contaminated water, because in that case the differences in the relative density of cholerine in suspension at different elevations would be more pronounced.

But why had the elevation law applied to the entire metropolis in the past? In 1848–1849, Farr explained, all London's water was highly and universally contaminated, so that the entire area could be considered a single water field. By 1854 the quality of some companies' water had improved, and this change produced the disturbance in the elevation law for the entire region. By 1866 the amount of cholera material in the water of most companies had been so drastically reduced that the effect of elevation was hard to detect and could be demonstrated only within a water field. Farr was certain, however, that when deaths within a water field were considered and when elevation was measured from the level from which water had been pumped, cholera mortality declined with elevation in a way predicted by the elevation law.

Farr saved both the elevation law and his modified zymotic theory. The incident is extremely revealing. It shows Farr's firm belief in the value of statistical laws, and in the potential value of the studies he undertook to discover them. His cholera studies, especially the third, helped establish Snow's theory. His cholera work also demonstrates that Farr kept well-informed of contemporary research in medicine, and that he remained receptive to new evidence and theories. Although he might have held firmly to a position he believed was well-established, he cannot be accused of being closed-minded or doctrinaire. Certainly his cholera studies demonstrate some of the dangers in statistical work that tries to deduce causes from amassed data. The longevity of the elevation law is both a tribute to human creativity and a monument to the dangers lurking in statistical inference. Finally, in Farr's studies of the cholera we get a glimpse of techniques Farr was to use in other studies: comparisons of death rates for groups of individuals differing, for example, in place of residence, manner of life, age, sex, and income. From such information Farr undertook to study some of the most pressing social problems of the industrial age. His studies of the health of urban man are the subject of the next chapter.

THE WELL-BEING OF URBAN MAN

SLUMS, ILLNESS, AND PHYSICAL DEGENERATION

Establishing the Case for Sanitary Reform

How the people of England live is one of the most important questions that can be considered; and how—of what causes, and at what ages—they die is scarcely of less account; for it is the complement of the primary question teaching men how to live a longer, healthier, and happier life. Armed with this golden bough, we may enter the gloomy kingdom of the dead, whither have gone in twenty years nine thousand thousand English children, fathers, mothers, sisters, brothers, daughters, sons. . . each having left memories not easily forgotten; and many having biographies full of complicated incidents. Here, fortunately for this inquiry, they appear divested of all colour, form, character, passion, and the infinite individualities of life: by abstraction they are reduced to mere units undergoing changes as purely physical as the setting stars of astronomy or the decomposing atoms of chemistry; and as in those sciences so in this, the analysis of the elementary facts observed in their various relations to time and place will shed new light on the more complicated phenomena of national life.[1]

With these words Farr opened the *Supplement to the Thirty-fifth Annual Report.* He was then sixty-eight years old, and the work he was presenting was perhaps his most comprehensive single production. In this supplement he returned for a last, sustained look at an issue that had occupied his attention at intervals throughout his long career: the statistical analysis of the health of the urban poor. Throughout his career Farr undertook statistical investigations of several important public health problems. His studies of occupational mortality and of the effectiveness of smallpox vaccination could be mentioned specifically.[2] But it was the high death rates of cities that commanded his greatest attention. It seems wise, therefore, to discuss his studies of this problem in some detail to illustrate the interplay of his disease theory, his statistical methods, and his reform ideas.

In his first letter to the registrar general, Farr made it very clear that he intended to make the national register of deaths serve the interests of public health. After explaining how an analysis of the causes of death could help improve medical practice, he turned to public health and the high mortality among urban populations.

Any improvement in the treatment of disease, and any addition to medical science, will tend ultimately to the dimunition of human suffering; but the registration of the causes of death is calculated to exercise a still more direct influence upon public health. Diseases are more easily prevented than cured, and the first step to their prevention is the discovery of their exciting causes. The registry will show the agency of these causes by numerical facts, and measure the intensity of their influence. The annual rate of mortality in some districts will be found to be 4 percent, in others 2 percent; in other words, the people in one set of circumstances live 50 years, while in another set of circumstances, which the registration will indicate, they do not live more than 25 years. In these wretched districts, nearly 8 percent are constantly sick, and the energy of the whole population is withered to the roots. Their arms are weak, their bodies wasted, and their sensations embittered by privation and suffering. Half the life is passed in infancy, sickness, and dependent helplessness. In exhibiting the high mortality, the diseases by which it is occasioned, and the exciting causes of disease, the abstract of the registers will prove, that while a part of the sickness is inevitable, and a part can only be expected to disappear before progressive social amelioration, a considerable proportion of the sickness and deaths may be suppressed by the general adoption of hygienic measures which are in actual but partial operation. It may be affirmed, without great risk of exaggeration, that it is possible to reduce the annual deaths in England and Wales by 30,000, and to increase the vigour (may I not add the industry and wealth?) of the population in an equal proportion; for diseases are the iron index of misery, which recedes before strength, health, and happiness, as the mortality declines.[3]

This paragraph deserves careful reading because it reveals a good deal about Farr. We see here his optimism about the possibility of a genuine and lasting improvement in human health and well-being. The statement also illustrates his belief in the existence of a direct relationship among mortality, sickness, and quality of life. Finally, his examples indicate the methods he intended to use in these studies. We will discuss each of these features momentarily.

The studies of high urban mortality rates Farr published in the first five *Annual Reports* have been described by M. J. Cullen. Cullen points out that Farr's statistics were compiled to verify pre-formed conclusions. "What is striking about all this [Farr's early study of the health of towns] is not so much its humanity as how little the tediously collected and collated statistics were required. The real function of the General Register Office was to be another government-sponsored pulpit for reforming ideas."[4] It is certainly true that Farr used his statistics to serve his reform interests. We should be surprised at this only if we believe the Baconian slogans that the statistical societies issued in the thirties. But Farr deserves comparison with other Victorians who used numerical arguments in policy discussions. He was never as self-serving as the industrialists in the Manchester Statistical Society; nor was he as inflexible as Edwin Chadwick or Florence Nightingale, with both of whom he shared many concerns. The minds of Chadwick and Nightingale, once fixed upon a reform strategy, never budged or even considered contrary evidence. By contrast, the fate of his disease theory illustrates that Farr could modify even firmly established views when faced with convincing evidence. Farr was broadminded; he had a sense of perspective, and he remained informed. Such qualities kept him from many of the worst sins of a bigoted crusader.

Farr believed cities of his day were unhealthy places. The idea was, of course, a commonplace and very old one.[5] Much evidence gave credence to the view. Rapid urban growth was one of the most important of social realities during the whole of Farr's lifetime.[6] Between 1821 and 1831 Manchester and Salford increased by 47 percent, West Bromwick by 60 percent, and Bradford by 78 percent, while the population of Dukinfield tripled. In the two decades between 1851 and 1871 the number of towns in England increased from 580 to 938, while the town population grew from nine to fourteen million. The results are familiar to most readers of historical subjects.

Housing and sanitary facilities could not keep pace with such growth. Customs, technologies, and administrative practices that might have been adequate in older cities or in small villages proved grossly insufficient in the industrial cities.[7] The results were enormous problems in disposing of human and animal waste and in providing housing. These were problems contemporaries recognized. Less well appreciated at the time were occupational hazards and the effects of improper diet. The consequences could be detected even in the imperfect vital statistics of the early nineteenth century. The national death rate which had been falling in the second half of the eighteenth century seems to have risen gradually in the early nineteenth as the town population grew.[8]

Farr sought to demonstrate the extent to which the urban environment undermined the public health. In doing this he compared district mortality rates, a method he used in a variety of studies. In this case he typically compared urban with rural or with suburban districts and also poor with wealthy urban districts. He usually explained the higher mortality rates of the urban poor in hygienic, not economic, terms. His disease theory, in fact, supported his social and political biases.

The existence in the atmosphere of organic matter is therefore incontestable; and as it must be most dense in the densest districts, where it is produced in greatest quantities, and the facilities for decomposing it in the sunshine and sweeping it away by currents of wind are the least, its effects—disease and death—will be most evident in towns, and in the most crowded districts of towns.

It is to this cause, it appears to me, that the high mortality of towns is to be ascribed; the people live in an atmosphere charged with decomposing matter, of vegetable and animal origin; in the open country it is diluted, scattered by the winds, oxidized in the sun; vegetation incorporates its elements, so that, though it were formed, proportionally to the population, in greater quantities than in towns, it would have comparatively less effect.[9]

This is not to suggest that Farr ignored the role of want and privation. We have already seen that in the *First Annual Report* he attributed sixty-three deaths in the metropolis to starvation and privation, an incautious claim that he could not defend against the criticism of the Poor Law Commissioners and Chadwick.[10] In the middle forties he looked for a relationship between the price of wheat and the national mortality rate.[11] He used the London Bills of Mortality, Rickman's returns for 1780 to 1830, as well as Tooke's study of wheat prices in the eighteenth and nineteenth centuries, and seventeenth- and eighteenth-century market records. He found evidence, he believed, that in the seventeenth and eighteenth centuries relatively high prices of wheat were accompanied by an increase in mortality in London. The first five years of civil registration seemed to verify this same tendency.

Although he recognized that privation had a hand in producing high mortality, he believed its role was less important than insanitation and the results of human ignorance or indifference. In the *Fifth Annual Report* he wrote a hypothetical equation to explain what he believed was the relative importance of income and hygiene in producing high mortality. He suggested that $m' = m \cdot d \cdot o \cdot s$ where m' is the observed rate of mortality; m, the ideal rate (i.e., the rate under perfect conditions); d, the population density; o, a measure of the number of organic particles entering the air in a given time; and s, what he called the reciprocal of the coefficient of subsistence.[12] The factor s was a measure of the population's ability to procure the necessities of life: $s = C/N$, where C is the market price of all necessities of life in that area and N the mean income in that district or among that class. According to this scheme, only when C was greater than N did low income exert an important influence on mortality. Under other circumstances hygiene was more important.

This was a hypothetical scheme. Farr did not have the statistics to demonstrate it, nor did he pursue this line of argument further. He had in fact reached the same conclusion several years earlier without the equation.[13] At various times in his career he did compare the longevity of members of various classes or professions in order to illustrate the effect of social position on mortality. In his report on his first national life table he compared the mean age and the mean duration of life of continental monarchs, the pope and cardinals, and the English bishops and peers with the mean age and duration of life of all Englishmen.[14] Wealth and social privilege seemed to grant no longer lives to those upper class men.

Poor hygiene, insanitation, and other environmental defects were the factors Farr blamed most consistently for the high mortality in cities.

He was an advocate of sanitary reform before Chadwick, and he continued to support the cause some thirty-five years after Chadwick had been forced out of public office. If, for example, we consider his letters to the registrar general which were published before 1842, years in which Chadwick was gathering his evidence, we find Farr recommending that public action be taken to eliminate the accumulation of organic wastes in the vicinity of the living by the construction of sewage systems, by paving and street cleaning, and by the reform of practices of burying the dead and slaughtering animals, as well as by making arrangements for better ventilation through widening streets, creating more parks, and prohibiting dense living arrangements.[15] In his *Second Annual Report*, Farr even suggested what was later to become Chadwick's hobbyhorse, the sale of manure from city sewage systems as agricultural fertilizer.[16]

But unlike the most dogmatic sanitarians Farr never reduced health reform to a single program. Unlike Chadwick, he recognized that civil engineering alone was not sufficient. Many other factors besides the removal of human excrement must be involved. At the end of his article "Vital Statistics" in McCulloch's statistical digest of 1837 Farr recommended a number of ways in which the public health could be improved.[17] The importance of sanitary reform was only implied in this list under the obligation of the government and municipal corporations to make towns serve the needs of the human organization. But he specifically recommended other measures: the keeping of statistics in order to discover the causes of disease, the teaching of the basic principles of individual hygiene, and the reformation of medical education and institutions to improve medical knowledge and to encourage physicians to assume responsibility for preventing illness. In other places Farr pointed out that sedentary habits and psychological states exercised an important influence on health and might be partly to blame for the high mortality in prisons.[18] He consistently recommended vaccination.[19] After he had learned the lessons John Snow taught about cholera, he also stressed the importance of procuring uncontaminated water.

In short, as much as Farr might preach the sanitary doctrine, he was no single-minded reformer. He had the perspective of a broad-minded medical man on public health. His opinions on this matter resemble those of John Simon more closely than those of Edwin Chadwick. Farr's career at the G.R.O. spanned the health administration of both Chadwick and Simon. Farr's own ideas about public health developed in much the same way as did the health policies of the nation. He was in a certain sense a microcosm of the larger public health movement. In the forties he stressed the need for sanitary reform and used fairly crude statistical means to demonstrate the differences in the health of various places. By the sixties, his statistics were more refined, his understanding of the causes of disease and premature death more inclusive, and his recommendations for prevention more diverse. Farr, of course, benefited by improvements in the medical understanding of disease. But we should recall that he contributed significantly to the development of that knowledge. He helped supply much of the factual material on which the English public health program developed. He also helped interpret that material for the public and for the medical profession.

Farr equated length of life with quality of life. This assumption lay behind many of his studies of the health of cities. It was furthermore an assumption he freely acknowledged. Mortality rates indicated the rate and the manner of dying, but they also, he believed, served as broader indices of well-being and happiness. In 1837, while still a medical journalist, he wrote: "For death is the exponent of misery; a merciful God has established a direct relation between pain and the cessation of sensibility—between happiness and long life: he has never chained together eternal life and suffering in the organic world vouchsafed to our observation."[20] As we have seen, he parodied David Ricardo in calling diseases the "iron index of misery."[21] Three and a half decades later Farr made the same claim. "There is a relation betwixt death and sickness. . . . There is a relation betwixt death, health, and energy of body and mind. There is a relation betwixt death, birth, and marriage. There is a relation between death and national primacy. . . . There is a relation betwixt the forms of death and moral excellence or infamy."[22]

There was certainly some criticism of this assumed connection between length of life and quality of life. Perhaps the most articulate spokesman was Charles Dickens. In commenting on proposals to register cases of sickness, he suggested: "So far as care of the body goes, it concerns a man more to know his risks of the fifty illnesses that may throw him on his back, than the possible date of the one death that must come, and of which the time is to him personally—in spite of libraries full of statistics—utterly unknown and uncertain."[23] Such reservations were, as we shall see, shared by some physicians as well. But many of Farr's contemporaries, in particular those most keenly interested in public health, accepted length of life or the more easily obtained mortality rate as an index of well-being. Benjamin Ward Richardson may be taken as a late Victorian proponent. In commenting on Farr's work he concluded:

So completely applicable to sanitary and economic purposes have these mortality tables become, that, now, towns are calculated up as salubrious or insalubrious by the death-rate returns which they present. Give one of us who has mastered these tables the death-rate of a place and the prevailing causes of death for a sufficient period to prove that the regular death-rate is before us, and we can determine, with fair exactitude, what is the state of the drainage, the water-supply, the general condition of the inhabitants, and the number of public-houses, although we may never have set foot in the place or its neighborhood, nor have read nor heard of it beyond the tale of the register. The proverb that "pestilence walketh in the dark" is no longer true; pestilence measured and registered, walketh, at last, in the open day.[24]

Farr played a major role in establishing mortality rates as criteria of human welfare. He used most of the statistical techniques we discussed in Chapter Four. He computed crude mortality rates for whole cities or counties and for individual registration districts. He also calculated more select death rates for either sex, for age groups, and for various diseases or causes of death. He constructed life tables for certain geographical areas and compared values for such phenomena as life expectancy and mean age from those local tables with figures from the current national table or from other local tables.

During his first several years in the civil service Farr produced a series of papers on urban mortality. In these studies he presented his theory of disease, his mortality statistics, and his recommendations for reform. The theory, the data, and the recommendations were mutually supportive. His statistical demonstration relied on a comparison of mortality rates for groups of urban and rural districts. His section "Diseases of Towns and the Open Country," in the *First Annual Report* established the pattern he followed for several years.[25] This study was based upon the deaths recorded in the *First Annual Report,* the six months July 1 to December 31, 1837, and the following six months, and upon an estimation of the population derived from the rate of growth over past census periods. Farr first compared figures for the metropolitan districts with those for rural Devonshire, Dorsetshire, Wiltshire, Cornwall, and Somersetshire, the counties soon to be designated the South Western Districts.[26] Both groups of districts had about the same population, but in the metropolis that population was concentrated in a much smaller area. In this first report Farr simply compared deaths and found that out of approximately equal populations, 53,597 died in the metropolis, while only 34,074 deaths occurred in the five rural counties. He suggested that rural areas might be even healthier than these figures suggested, because these particular counties contained a number of large towns such as Bath and Exeter where epidemics of smallpox were in progress.

He next compared twenty-four urban districts and seven rural counties: Essex, Gloucester, Hereford, Norfolk, Suffolk, Sussex, and Westmoreland.[27] For this comparison he excluded the population and deaths from Norwich, Bristol, and Clifton to make these counties more rural and to bring their population to the level of the cities (3.5 million). He compared not only total deaths (47,953 against 29,693) but also the number of deaths returned for a variety of causes, arranged according to his statistical nosology. The comparison showed that the fatality from all diseases was greater in the cities, but that certain diseases were much more often fatal in urban areas. Among the latter the zymotic diseases and diseases of the respiratory organs were responsible for about twice as many deaths in the cities as in the counties (12,766 against 6,045 for the zymotic and 12,619 against 7,847 for diseases of the respiratory organs).

He also found significant differences in the relative importance of other causes of death. Three causes of death that affected mainly people in the prime of life, 15 to 65 years of age, all increased in fatality in these urban districts, but they did so at different rates. Consumption increased by 39 percent, childbirth fatality by 71 percent, and the fatality of typhus by 221 percent. He also believed his figures suggested that the relative importance of the zymotic diseases and the respiratory diseases varied according to the absolute mortality of the area. In districts having low mortality, deaths from respiratory disease outnumbered those from zymotic disease, but when deaths from zymotic diseases equaled or exceeded those from respiratory disease, the total mortality was certain to be high.

Farr did not point out one anomaly in his tables: deaths from diseases of digestive organs were also nearly twice as numerous among the urban population. This high fatality from diseases of digestive organs in large cities would be noticed again later and would be regarded as highly significant in John Simon's administration. The reason Farr attached so little importance to it in 1839 was probably the fact that it made little sense in the way he then understood the cause of disease. The high fatality from zymotic disease was an expected result. Earlier in this report he had explained that the prevalence of the epidemic, endemic, and contagious diseases was the "index of salubrity" and that among the classes of his nosology it varied most with time and place.[28] A high return under diseases of the respiratory organs might not have been expected, but it was at least plausible within a theory of disease causation that emphasized the role of miasmata. The same could not be said of a high return under diseases of the digestive organs.

Farr's study pointed to another expected relationship. Mortality seemed to increase as the population density increased. This entire section of the First Annual Report seems to have been designed to demonstrate this point. Farr opened the section by explaining that besides age, sex, and hereditary organization there were three classes of reasons why mortality rates differed among different groups of people: occupation, the supply of warmth and food, and the "exposure to poisonous effluvia and to destructive agencies."[29] The tables that followed would, he claimed, exhibit the influence of the "contaminated atmosphere" of cities, and in the following pages he gave almost no attention to the role of the other influences. After making the two comparisons of town and country districts just mentioned, he offered one of his earliest statements of a miasmatic theory and made recommendations for sanitary reform.[30] Immediately following that short discussion he offered a third comparison that was designed to indicate the relationship between population density and mortality more exactly.[31] He ranked the thirty-two registration districts of the metropolis by annual female mortality. The rates ranged from 3.908 percent in Whitechapel to 1.785 percent in St. George, Hanover-square. He did not explain the reason for using female mortality rates here, but it became an often-used rate because it was believed to minimize the effect of occupation. In tables he then gave a measure of crowding, square yards of surface area per person in each district, and the mortality rates for seven groups of causes of death. The table showed that as a general rule mortality from all causes and mortality from the more important diseases increased as the area allotted to each person declined. The relationship held even more exactly when he compared average figures for three groups of Metropolitan districts, the first group comprising the ten districts with the lowest general mortality, the second group the next ten districts in order of general mortality, and the third group of the third set of ten districts.

These results were all of the sort he was looking for. In treating this topic over the next few years, he used the same comparisons and reached similar conclusions. His methods, however, became more complete, and he acknowledged a few of the limitations in his approach. In the *Second* and *Third Annual Reports* he not only compared deaths in his two groups of equally populous districts, but also gave the mortality rates and mean duration of life for both pairs of districts.[32] In addition he made some attempt to correct his data. In the *Second Annual Report* he explained how he now corrected the female mortality used in the comparison of the metropolitan districts by subtracting the deaths which occurred in hospitals and by increasing the remainder by 4 percent to compensate for under-registration.[33] In the *Third Annual Report* he explained his mistake in the previous report of failing to subtract deaths for Bristol, Clifton, and Norwich from the county returns.[34] He also acknowledged for the first time that the age distribution of the population in town and country districts was different.[35] He did not elaborate on this important point, but he apparently intended it to suggest that towns were even more unhealthy than his figures indicated, since he believed that towns had a disproportionately high number of people in their middle and healthiest years of life. Finally in this third report he also tried to explain his notion of the relationship between density and mortality more exactly. Strictly speaking, it was not the density of population but the density of the air-borne organic material that caused the increase in mortality in towns.[36]

The *Fifth Annual Report* offered Farr's most complete early study of the causes of high mortality in towns. Cullen has suggested that the G.R.O. put extraordinary efforts into this report because the staff was worried that registration might be curtailed or abolished. He called it a "ham performance of heroic dimensions wringing out every last drop of sympathy and support for the Office. Like most ham performances it concealed inadequacies."[37] The suggestion is plausible, although the judgment seems a bit severe. The *Fifth Annual Report* does contain Farr's most popular expositions of the value of national life tables and of the principles of sanitary reform. Occasionally its claims are extreme. But it is also obvious that the report was a long time in the making. The material and conclusions presented could not have been drummed up suddenly to serve immediate administrative needs, although the mode of presentation might have been altered somewhat for that purpose. Furthermore, long after the immediate crisis was past, Farr continued to rank this report among his finest. He forwarded a copy to Florence Nightingale in 1860, calling it "one of our best" and recommending particularly the section on the health of towns.[38]

The *Fifth Annual Report* offered a more comprehensive analysis of mortality than either its predecessors or its immediate successors. It gave an elaborate abstract of causes of death in groups of town and country districts for 1841 and for the four years 1838-1841.[39] Deaths were listed for each group of districts for all causes, for each of the twelve major divisions of his statistical nosology, and again for ninety-six separate subheadings. Farr gave, too, certain demographic information in this table: population, the rate of increase of females, and population per square mile.

In discussing these abstracts he explained that greater certainty could now be placed in comparisons of rural and urban mortality rates. Four full years of death registration were now available, and in addition a census had just been taken so that mortality rates could be more accurately calculated. Once again he used his data to illustrate what he believed was the extent of preventable mortality in towns. By totaling the figures for his select town and country districts and correcting for differences in the size of the populations, he calculated that 99,762 more deaths had occurred among the town population in those four years than among the equally numerous country population.[40] He estimated that if the metropolis had experienced the same mortality as the South Western Districts, some 10,000 to 12,000 lives would have been saved.

Thus far the approach was like that in the preceding reports. But Farr made two additions that set this report apart. After his second major discussion of his theory of disease,[41] Farr offered an extended treatment of the relationship between population density and mortality.[42] His disease theory explained why mortality should increase in more crowded urban areas. Now he tried to find a numerical expression for this relationship. By ranking the metropolitan districts by population density and female mortality rate he found that mortality seemed to increase as the sixth roots of the densities; in other words $m' = m \sqrt[6]{d'/d}$. The equation did not hold with the precision of some of his other formulae. He found that it held quite well for the ten healthiest and the ten least healthy districts, either collectively or among members of either group. It did not hold for the middle group of ten districts.

In discussing the utility of considering population density,[43] Farr pointed out that the use of density figures helped eliminate some of the ambiguities in analyses of the health of "town" and "country" districts. He repeated his warning that population density was only an indirect measure of the most important condition, the density of zymotic and other organic material in the air. Districts with similar population densities might have atmospheres of varying degrees of purity, depending on the provisions for drainage, ventilation, and other sanitary facilities. Until chemists learned to measure the density of the zymotic atmosphere, greater precision in these studies was unlikely, and the relative amount of organic material in the air would have to be inferred from the population density. Farr recognized that it would be more correct to measure the volume of air each person had at his disposal and not his relative share of the land's surface. But he suggested that in a city like London, where similar house construction was used over large areas and where the majority of human lives were passed indoors, his procedure was justified.

While Farr would have liked to have found a more exact statistical relationship, he concluded that his formula was adequate for sanitary inquiries, and he showed how it might be used to exclude the effects of population density when one was trying to determine the reasons for the differences in mortality in two districts.[44] As an example he compared the metropolis's most healthy district, St. George, Hanover-square, and its least healthy, Whitechapel. He stretched plausibility in trying to assign values, some to the fifth decimal place, to his equation $m' = mdos$.[45]

The second major innovation that appeared in the *Fifth Annual Report* was the use of local life tables to compare the relative health of places. We have already seen that Farr, F. G. P. Neison, and William A. Guy all criticized Chadwick's use of the mean age at death as a measure of health. They claimed that although the mean duration of life in a district was a good indicator of the health of the residents, the mean duration of life could only be obtained from an accurate life table. Without access to a life table, the investigator was advised to use mortality as the next best index of health. With the computation of English life table number one, which first appeared in the *Fifth Annual Report*, Farr was able to follow this prescription.[46] He presented in Graham's letter basic life tables and tables of the expectation of life for the English and Welsh people as a whole and for the residents of three areas chosen to represent the full spectrum of of salubrity: the metropolis, Surrey (excluding the metropolitan districts), and Liverpool.[47] He also gave a series of diagrams to illustrate

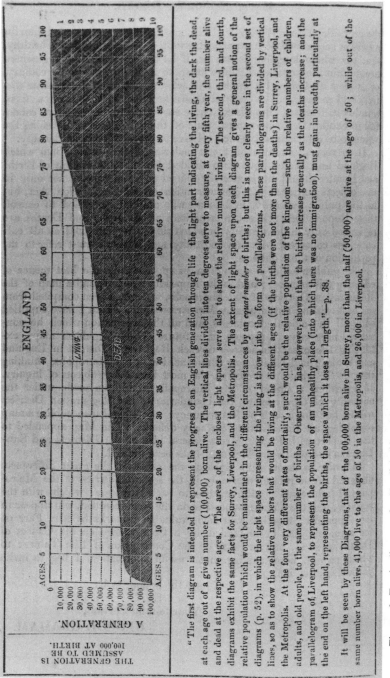

Figure 6. Farr's diagram for English life table no. 1; 5th A.R.R.G., pp. 50-51 [PP, 1843, XXI].

134

the numbers remaining alive or dying with each year of age and the age distribution of the population in these areas.[48] (See figs. 6-8.) The tables showed that very different laws of mortality were in operation in these three areas. The life expectancy at birth for both sexes in Surrey was 45.1 years. For the entire nation it was 41.16 years. In the metropolis the figure dropped to 36.7 years, while in Liverpool it was only 25.7 years. Even more striking was the exceedingly high fatality among infants in Liverpool, the least healthy industrial city. According to the tables only half the infants born in Liverpool were alive on their fifth birthday. In rural Surrey, on the other hand, it took nearly fifty years for half those born there to perish. The tables both demonstrated the waste of human life that occurred in cities, and gave some idea of the way in which the losses occurred.

The *Fifth Annual Report* represents the acme of Farr's early interest in the relative health of town and country districts. He not only produced satisfying results, but he also recognized some of the pitfalls in his approach. Districts might contain both rural and urban parishes. Town and country populations had different age distributions. Population density was only an indirect measure of the causes of high mortality in cities. Significantly, however, he never considered the extent to which differences in the accuracy and completeness of registering deaths might influence his results.

We should not leave the impression that this series of reports merely confirmed established opinions. It also illustrated new issues. Farr was certainly correct in claiming that until studies of this kind had been made, few people appreciated the extent to which mortality and longevity differed from place to place.[49] Men die at all ages in every place, and one can see men and women at advanced ages in all places. Vital statistics revealed demographic patterns that casual observation could miss. Farr also put his figures to use in determining the relative importance of various diseases in rural and urban areas. The discovery of a much higher fatality from consumption in urban districts probably came as a surprise. His observation, "sufficient attention has perhaps not been paid to the great excess in the mortality of consumption, caused by the insalubrity of towns," was both original and important.[50] The topic would not receive much attention for another fifteen years.

Following the publication of the *Fifth Annual Report*, Farr's attention went to other matters: life tables and their commercial uses, revisions of his statistical nosology, efforts at improving the registration procedure, studies of deaths in childbirth and the differences in mortality among various trades, and of course his first two studies of the cholera epidemics. Additional local life tables appeared over the next few years: one for Manchester in the *Seventh Annual Report* and another for Northampton the following year.[51] But the comparison of town and country mortality be-

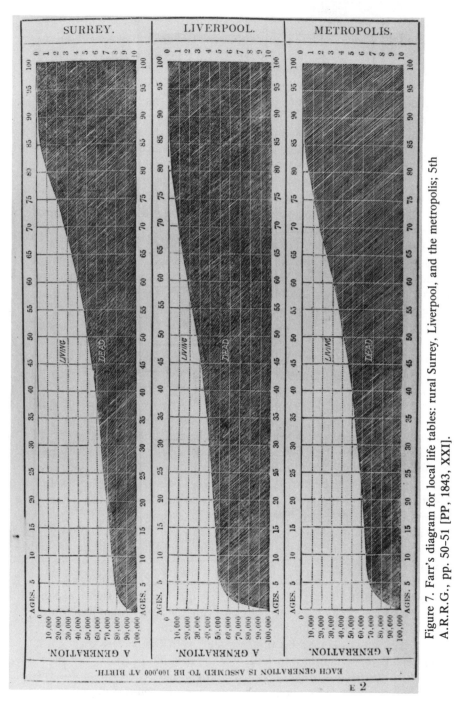

Figure 7. Farr's diagram for local life tables: rural Surrey, Liverpool, and the metropolis; 5th A.R.R.G., pp. 50-51 [PP, 1843, XXI].

136

came a more routine matter that was treated in the annual abstracts and in the *Quarterly Reports*.

The G.R.O. began to issue its *Quarterly Reports* in 1842. George Graham's letter in the *Fifth Annual Report* announced the beginning of this series for the 114 most populous districts. He declared that quarterly reports would be published promptly and would therefore "give immediate warning of any great increase in the mortality, and . . . have the further advantage of directing frequent attention to the particular districts . . . in which the mortality is above average."[52] It became in fact a routine procedure to use local mortality rates to monitor public health. Eventually the quarterly returns were reprinted in the *Annual Reports*, and someone on the G.R.O. staff, probably Farr, discussed the significance of the deaths registered in the quarter and went on to offer more general comments on the state of the public health and to make specific recommendations. Sanitarians seem to have taken these general mortality rates as an implicit reflection of the healthiness of places. This way of regarding local mortality rates was encouraged by the Public Health Act of 1848 which, by section eight, permitted the central health authorities to intervene and require sanitary improvements, should the average annual mortality rate of a place be above the then national average of 23 per 1,000.[53] The Act in effect established the rate of 23 per 1,000 as an arbitrary standard of health. For the next few years the comparison of general mortality rates was a fairly routine matter.

By the later 1850s Farr began once again to devote special attention to the mortality rates of towns. His attention may have been jolted back to this subject by changes that were occurring in the public health movement. John Simon had replaced Edwin Chadwick as the chief public health administrator. Simon and the men around him had medically more sophisticated views of public health reform than did Chadwick. The change in methods in Simon's group implied some criticism of the G.R.O.'s statistics. Edward Headlam Greenhow's famous report on the English death rates is representative of the change in attitudes and methods.[54] Simon may have encouraged the writing of this report; he certainly used it to his own advantage. Greenhow followed accepted statistical practice to a certain point. He used crude mortality rates to illustrate the general state of public health in local areas, and he seems to have accepted Farr's suggestion that mortality rates above 17 per 1,000 should be regarded as excessive.[55] But he believed that the diseases that caused the variation in the local mortality rates had not been sufficiently investigated, and that the excess mortality had been attributed to too few causes.[56] He was especially critical of the manner in which excess deaths were so easily attributed to zymotic disease.

Like several other medical authorities we have mentioned, Green-

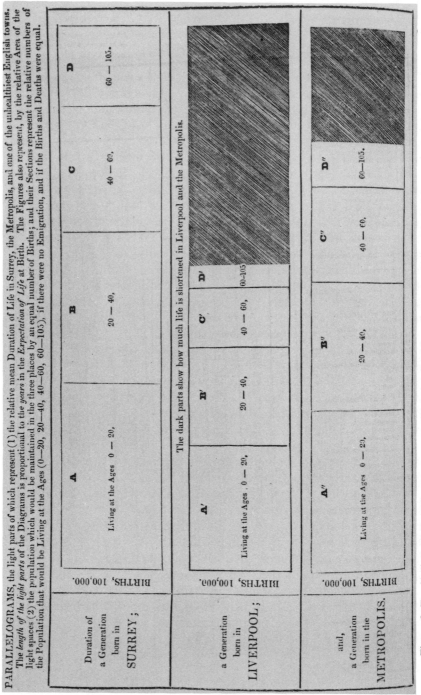

Figure 8. Farr's diagram for life expectancy and age composition of the population in rural Surrey, Liverpool, and the metropolis; 5th A.R.R.G., p. 52 [PP, 1843, XXI].

138

how was suspicious of Farr's zymotic class and of a mortality rate calculated for that whole class. It was not that his disease theory was fundamentally different from Farr's at this time, but he objected to the lumping together into one class diseases of such diverse character. In his own study of the mortality rates he used the G.R.O.'s unpublished records of deaths in 105 districts for the years 1848-1854, in which the census year 1851 was the midpoint. The districts were chosen to represent areas of low and high mortality and a wide range of prevalent occupations. In computing the mortality rates he dispensed with Farr's zymotic class and calculated rates for ten disease classes: pulmonary diseases (including consumption); contagious diseases (smallpox, measles and whooping cough, and scarlatina); alvine flux (diarrhea, dysentery, cholera, etc.), typhus and erysipelas; croup, influenza, and ague; strumous diseases (scrofula and tabes mesenterica); nervous diseases of children; apoplexy and paralysis; rheumatic fever and rheumatism; carbuncle and phlegmon. The most striking discovery was the importance of the pulmonary diseases as contributors to the high death rates. Farr had noticed this fact in his early studies but had left it as a passing observation. In the mortality research Greenhow later undertook for Simon, the former emphasized pulmonary disease.[57]

In this investigation Greenhow also showed that deaths from "the alvine flux" (dysentery, diarrhea and cholera) were major causes of high local mortality rates. This result was not unexpected, but it had not been effectively demonstated before nor used in public health administration. John Simon began the policy of monitoring local mortality rates from alvine flux and initiating special investigation of any sudden changes.[58] These studies are symptomatic of changes occurring in public health policy under Simon. Whereas Chadwick had relied on a few remedies and had used either mean age at death or general mortality rates to demonstrate their value, Simon instituted a comprehensive policy of preventive medicine that relied on special death rates. Simon believed the two major functions of his office were: first, to monitor changes in special death rates and to keep the facts of high rates from preventable diseases before the public, local authorities, and the legislature; and second, to undertake special investigations of high mortality rates and to interpret the results of those special statistical and field studies.[59] That procedure became the mainstay of Simon's administration. It placed new demands on the registration system and the G.R.O. and helped establish a more critical atmosphere for the development of vital statistics.

There may have been another reason for Farr's return to more extensive studies of urban death rates. The official mortality statistics and their interpretation were coming in for some rigorous criticism. The critics were often medical officers of health from industrial cities and from resort towns, two types of districts that consistently did poorly in any comparison of crude death rates. I have shown elsewhere that these spokesmen argued that the mortality of their towns was overstated by the G.R.O.'s figures.[60] In support of their claim they pointed to the known defects in the Registration Act, to the fact that municipal and registration district boundaries did not coincide, to the disturbing influence of hospitals and work houses, and especially to the differences in the ages of inhabitants of urban and rural districts. They found a more systematic critic in Henry Rumsey, who added to these complaints a stinging critique of the system for registering cause of death. The appearance of this criticism reflects both the success of the early sanitary reformers in making local death rates a sensitive issue and the evolution of the public health campaign. Some medical officers of health had now been on the job for nearly a decade and many had discovered the complexity of their tasks and the limitations of the early sanitary program. There is certainly some truth to Noel Humphreys's claim that these health officers were statistical neophytes who had just discovered problems with which experienced statisticians had been grappling for two decades.[61]

The urban critics' complaints actually could not be correctly leveled at Farr's best studies. Even in his first series of reports on the health of towns, studies which appeared nearly twenty years before these critics spoke, Farr had used life tables in comparing the health of places to take account of differences in age composition, and he tried to correct local rates for deaths in public institutions.[62] These corrections were rudimentary and not nearly as fully developed as those of Farr's later studies. They do certainly prove, however, that the health officers had not discovered the objections they raised in the years following 1860.

At the heart of these critics' complaints was the G.R.O.'s practice of ranking districts by crude mortality rate and the increasingly common assumption among the public that such figures accurately represented differences in health or in sanitary provision. They saw here both the narrowmindedness and the menace of dogmatic lay sanitarians. Chadwick was a favorite whipping boy. "Stating his belief, he asked for facts in support of it, and of course obtained them."[63] The evolution of public health administration both at the central agency and at the local level encouraged Farr to consider again the health of towns and to do so using more sensitive statistical methods. In his later studies Farr began more regularly to use specialized death rates: rates specific for disease or other cause as well as age-specific mortality rates. It was in these years he introduced the healthy district standard and used it rather than the mortality of "country" districts in assessing the health of towns.[64] He had already discovered, as we have seen, that by 1850 one-tenth of the registration districts, the ones he named health districts, had average annual mortality rates not exceeding

17 per 1,000. Farr suggested that this rate might therefore be taken as a safe estimate of the natural mortality of Englishmen, and that rates in excess might be attributed to unnatural or preventable causes. By subtraction he calculated the "degrees of insalubrity" for various districts, each degree representing 1 per 1,000 above the rate 17 per 1,000. He also calculated the number of preventable deaths in the district resulting from that degree of insalubrity.[65]

This was a brilliant publicity device, one that exhibited differences in mortality more dramatically than a comparison of crude death rates. It relied, however, on those crude rates and was therefore subject to the same objections. This use of the healthy district standard may well have fanned the flame of discontent among the medical officers of health. But Farr put the healthy districts to other, methodologically sounder, uses. He constructed a life table for these districts.[66] Using that table he was able to compute local death rates corrected for differences in the age distribution. Even before the healthy district life table was published, Farr illustrated this method. In the *Twentieth Annual Report* he printed a table that exhibited separately for the male and female residents of London the population, in each of twelve age groups according to the 1851 census, the deaths registered in the years 1849-1853, and the average annual mortality rate for each age group of either sex.[67] He also listed the average annual mortality for each age group in the healthy districts and computed the number of deaths which would have occurred in that age group in London, had London experienced the same law of mortality as the healthy districts.

This table was a preview of the techniques Farr would use more extensively in his two decennial supplements: the *Supplement to the Twenty-fifth Annual Report* for the decade 1851-1860 and the *Supplement to the Thirty-fifth Annual Report* for 1860-1871.[68] They are his most able studies of the differences in mortality among places and people, and they serve as an example of the statistical techniques Farr used in his later career. These supplements offer a number of extremely interesting studies. Besides assessments of the excessive mortality of towns, both supplements treat occupational mortality.[69] The *Supplement to the Twenty-fifth Annual Report* has a section on mortality of women of childbearing age.[70] The *Supplement to the Thirty-fifth Annual Report* offers magnificent statistical fare with a discussion of population growth, the Malthusian debate, and the relationship between the birth and death rates; a "hygienic topography," a survey of mortality in the registration divisions; suggestions for a method of calculating the effect on the general mortality rate of the elimination of a single disease as a cause of death; and comments on the economic importance of different diseases.[71]

Above all it is their recognition of the importance of age on mortality that sets these two reports apart. Life tables showed that mortality declined with each year of life until the ages 10 to 15, and then it slowly increased. In key sections of these decennial supplements Farr followed an English generation through life, down the columns of a national life table, and discussed its mortality in each of twelve age groups.[72] In his section on each age group he listed the annual mortality for each sex and the combined rate, and he commented on the manner in which the rate of mortality changed with each succeeding year. He also discussed the relative importance of various causes of death at each period of life and drew attention to anomalies in the local rates. Farr was aware both that mortality varied from one age of life to another, and that the relative chances of dying from a given disease also changed as age advanced. In the *Supplement to the Thirty-fifth Annual Report* he returned briefly to the subject of survival tables for illness.[73]

Assessments of the health of towns, Farr now insisted, must take account of peculiar age distribution of urban populations. For this purpose Farr took the nation as a whole and the healthy districts as standard populations whose age-specific mortality rate could be obtained from English life table number three and from the health district life table. Applying these age-specific mortality rates to the urban population at similar ages, he obtained what he believed was a fair measure of the excessive mortality in England's thirty large towns.[74] He computed that if the thirty large towns of England had experienced the same law of mortality as the Healthy Districts their mortality rate would have been 15.13 per 1,000 instead of the observed 28.01 per 1,000. Farr believed the actual mortality for the thirty large towns might have been even higher. But even assuming that 28.01 were correct, the higher rate meant that 327,354 unnecessary deaths had occurred in those town districts in the years 1851–1860.[75]

These comparisons of district mortality rates pointed once again to the cardinal influence of infant mortality in determining a city's place in the scale of mortality. Infant mortality was not only a major component of the general death rate, but it also accounted for much of the difference in local rates. In the *Supplement to the Twenty-fifth Annual Report* Farr showed that the deaths of children under five years of age accounted for 80 percent of the difference in the general mortality rates between the Healthy Districts and the thirty large towns.[76] Such findings justified the warning about the dangers of neglecting age differences. They also suggested the possibility of using infant mortality itself as a measure of salubrity. In the supplement for the years 1861–1870, he did in fact illustrate the "death-tax which the great city populations of England now pay," by comparing infant mortality of Liverpool with the healthy district standard.[77]

There was no effective response to the use of the standarized death rates, but one urban spokesman, the Manchester industrialist William

Lucas Sargant, attempted to discredit Farr's conclusions about infant mortality rates in cities.[78] In a critique of the registration system and the census, one that echoed the criticism of other urban critics, Sargant tried to show that because of defects in registering births and in the census returns of ages in the 1861 census, infant mortality of large cities was grossly overstated. Farr wrote an ungracious response in which he called Sargant the "sage soothsayer of Birmingham."[79] He pointed to Sargant's errors on details of the G.R.O.'s procedures and attempted to account for the discrepancies Sargant found between the birth registers and the census returns of ages by pointing to the role of immigration and to confusion about returning young ages in the census. Farr silenced Sargant's criticism (his explanation however, has not satisfied the contemporary demographer D. V. Glass).[80]

In his later studies of the health of towns Farr returned several times to a problem we have seen him broach in the first five *Annual Reports*, the relation between population density and mortality. During the early 1850s he supplemented these studies with additional data.[81] It was in the report of the 1851 census that he seems to have first modified his approach to this problem by considering not only population density but also mean proximity between people.[82] Farr considered the problem of human crowding in two dimensions only. If a district's population were equally distributed over its surface area, then the proximity could be defined as the mean distance between residents and the density as the number of residents per square mile. The census report offered a geometrical illustration.[83] (See fig. 9.) Two circular areas represented the degree of human crowding in England and Wales in 1801 and 1851. Density was represented by the number of intersections of two series of perpendicular parallel line segments. The distance between adjacent points of intersection represented the proximity.

In the 1851 census Farr merely listed the mean proximity for the metropolis and for the other ten registration divisions. The following decade, in the *Supplement to the Twenty-fifth Annual Report*, he began to consider more systematically the proximity of districts.[84] He ranked the 631 registration districts of England and Wales according to their average annual mortality, expressed as a whole number of deaths per 1,000, calculated from the deaths registered from 1851 to 1860. The figures ranged from fourteen in the first group to a high between twenty-eight and thirty-three in the fifteenth group. Farr's summary table showed that as the mortality increased, population density also increased and mean proximity declined. The figures confirmed the same sort of relationship Farr had claimed to have found two decades earlier. Now, however, he did not offer a numerical law.

The goal of finding such a numerical law remained, however. In the

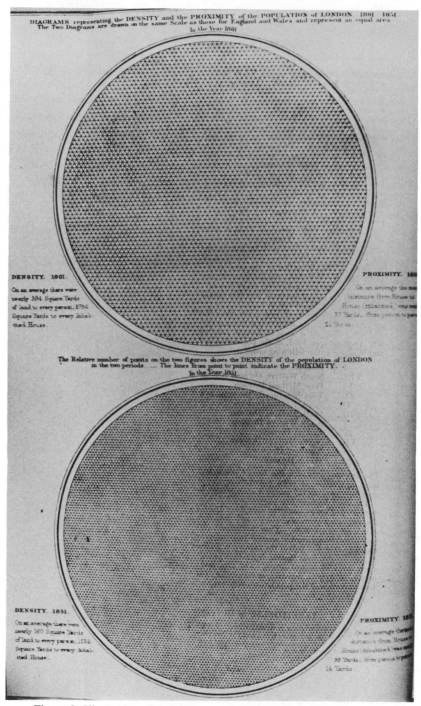

Figure 9. Illustrations for density and proximity of the English population, 1801 and 1851, from 1851 census. Census of England and Wales for 1851, populations tables [PP, 1852-53, LXXXV, facing p. 1].

Supplement to the Thirty-fifth Annual Report he once again ranked the nation's registration districts (excluding those of the metropolis) by mortality, and obtained similar qualitative results.[85] In keeping with this report's emphasis on the role of age, Farr pointed out that density had different effects on various age groups. We can see his continued interest in a numerical law when he recalled the formula he had published three decades earlier in the *Fifth Annual Report* and in a tentative suggestion he now made about general mortality's variance with population density.[86]

Only in the last several years of his career did Farr succeed in finding the type of numerical or statistical law he wanted for his more recent data.[87] In the census report for 1871 and again in two papers presented in the late 1870s he considered the role of proximity. Proximity was now represented geometrically by the distance between the centers of coterminous regular hexagons, each hexagon equal in area to the allotment each person would be given if all the land of his district were equally divided among its residents. Using simple trigonometry, Farr arrived at an expression for proximity in terms of the area allotted to each person. He assumed regular hexagonal areas, but shortly thereafter Professor Tait provided a general solution for an area of any shape. Using the registration materials for the decade 1861–1870, Farr arrived at a formula for the relationship between proximity and mean lifetime, which he believed held for all England and Wales except the metropolis.[88] Fig. 10 is Farr's geometrical representation for this, his last major statistical law. In arriving at his formula Farr used an approximation for the mean lifetime based on the death rate and the birth rate, an approximation which, he claimed, life tables showed was usually valid.[89]

In this respect at least Farr ended his career at the G.R.O. as he had started it, demonstrating with a formula that human life was shortened in a predictable manner as more people crowded into urban areas. The later studies, like the first, were predicated on a disease theory which emphasized the importance of adequate ventilation to remove airborne organic material. In fact, this notion undoubtedly underlay Farr's interest in the whole question of population density. As he gradually came to accept the doctrine of *contagium vivum* he did not reject his belief in the role of air purity or the string of sanitary reforms which it justified. Despite the changes in his disease theory, which were most pronounced in the case of cholera, Farr's understanding of the causes and remedies for excess mortality remained remarkably unchanged. In the *Fifth Annual Report* his density law appeared in the midst of one of his earliest and most extensive discussions of his disease theory, and it was accompanied by various recommendations for sanitary reform.[90] Although the discussion was more guarded thirty-five years later, it is clear that Farr's basic interest in the question was the same. In fact, both the *Fifth* and the *Fortieth Annual*

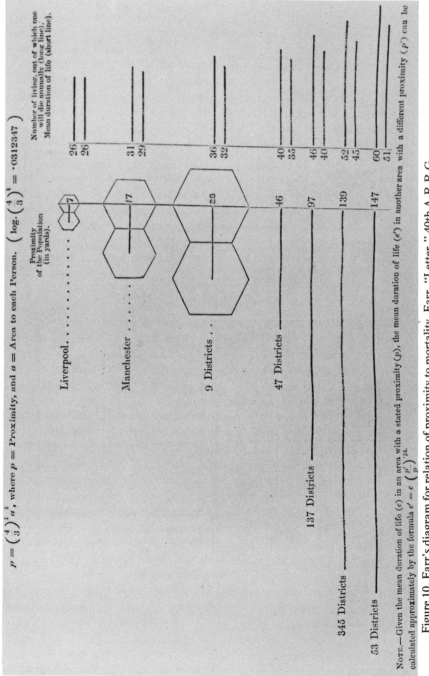

Figure 10. Farr's diagram for relation of proximity to mortality. Farr, "Letter," 40th A.R.R.G., p. 237 [PP, 1878-79, XIX].

Reports employed the same geometrical illustration to explain the means by which density or proximity affects health.[91] In keeping with Farr's zymotic theory the crucial element in preserving human health was access to air uncontaminated with organic waste. Using a large square divided into smaller equal squares, Farr showed in both discussions that the ratio of exterior to interior squares decreased rapidly as the number of smaller squares increased. If the smaller squares were taken to represent city houses, we can see how Farr conceived of the problem. Only the houses on the edge of town or those bordering open places had adequate access to ventilation. Characteristically, in both reports Farr commented on current provisions for parks and open spaces and on plans for increasing such areas and for using street building to reduce crowding in rookeries.[92]

The topic was a timely one, and Farr's pronouncements attracted the attention of many advocates of preventive medicine and sanitary science.[93] By 1891 Arthur Newsholme was critical of the fact that Farr's conclusions on the effects of density on mortality had become "almost axiomatic."[94] In this paper Newsholme used statistics of apartment complexes provided on philanthropic principles for London working class families. Rents were low in these block dwellings, but population density measured in terms of occupied surface area was very high. According to the form of the density law Farr proposed in the *Supplement to the Thirty-fifth Annual Report*, the mortality in these housing projects ought to have been 24.21 per 1,000, whereas it was only 16.49 per 1,000.[95] The density law seemed to fail in a very important case. Newsholme suggested why. Although he believed that there was "no causal relationship between density of population *per se* and a high mortality,"[96] Newsholme did not question the notion that human crowding exercised a pernicious influence on health. The crucial circumstance, however, was not the number of inhabitants per unit of surface area but rather the number of inhabitants per room.

Farr's density law was not quickly abandoned by Victorian statisticians. As the questions and comments on Newsholme's paper showed, the law was considered to express a relationship too fundamental to be overturned by one counter-example.[97] Even medical officers of health like Newsholme were not free from its fascination. As late as the second third of the twentieth century, Newsholme included a discussion of Farr's density law in a chapter on population density in his *Fifty Years of Public Health*.[98] He summarized his 1891 paper and offered comments more in keeping with modern medical science.

The density law could have received pessimistic interpretations. If mortality increased with population density, then cities would be inherently unhealthy. Sanitary reform and the efforts of the housing trusts would both be in vain. Farr never interpreted his findings this way. He did not regard his density or proximity laws as invariable, although in the *Fifth Annual Report* he suggested the density law held with sufficient certainty that it could be used to eliminate the role of density in comparing the mortality of two areas.[99] He believed instead that because there was danger in high density, extraordinary measures were needed to protect health and life. If such means were taken, cities could be made nearly as healthy as less populous areas. In his first letter to the registrar general he pointed out that occasionally densely populated districts had mortality rates nearly as low as the more sparsely populated districts.

The necessary deduction from the double series of facts, then, is that the mortality has a tendency to increase as the density of the population increases, but that the unhealthful tendency can be counteracted by artificial agencies. In other terms, the mortality of cities in England and Wales is high, but it may be immeasurably reduced. A good, general system of sewers; the intersection of the dense, crowded districts of the metropolis by a few spacious streets; and a park in the East end of London would probably diminish the annual deaths by several thousands, prevent many years of sickness, and add several years to the lives of the entire population.[100]

Writing in 1865 when he had begun to acknowledge a greater role for contagion, he explained:

there can be no doubt that mere proximity of the dwellings of the people does not necessarily involve a high rate of mortality. When any zymotic matter, such as varioline, scarlatinine, or typhine finds its way into a village or street, it is more likely to pass from house to house than it is where the people are brought less frequently into contact. The exhalations into the air are thicker. But if an adequate water supply, and sufficient arrangements for drainage and cleansing are secured, as they can be by combination in towns, the evils which now make dense districts so fatal may be mitigated. Indeed some of the dense districts of cities are in the present day comparatively salubrious.[101]

In the paper on the proximity law he read to the Social Science Association, he pointed out that recent registration demonstrated that the effect of density was not an iron-clad law.[102] Although the population had increased during the nearly forty years of civil registration, the general mortality rate had remained quite stationary. Hygienic improvements had kept at bay the harm resulting from higher population density.

Farr's reform optimism then was not tarnished by his demonstration of the dependence of mortality on density. Nor was it weakened by objections various cities raised to the sanitary campaign. There were of course constitutional and economic objections. Farr acknowledged that personal and property rights were abridged by state action to promote health. As he put it, "all 'improvements' disturb property, and injure individual interests; they are therefore not only attended by expense, but open to positive objections, over which it can only be shown that the advantages preponderate."[103] He went on to argue that for all the human and financial costs of the Great Fire of London, it was a small price to pay for the elimination of the plague. More to the point, he had already claimed that although the more affluent classes were being asked to finance projects that would benefit primarily the lower classes, the former would also benefit from sanitary reform.[104] The more prosperous districts would be protected from epidemics originating in poorer neighborhoods. Furthermore, the required improvements would increase both property values and rents. He had no doubt that men would willingly pay more to live in healthier circumstances.

Housing reform posed special monetary problems. Farr discussed two of these in the *Fifth Annual Report*. The first was the problem of distributing the financial burden of urban improvements equitably.[105] As the rich and poor of London often lived in different parishes and each parish supported its own poor, the burden of providing the social services for the poor often fell most heavily on those least able to pay. Farr suggested that the metropolis should be treated as one poor law union for tax purposes, and claimed that the rich had no right to complain if for some extraordinary sanitary improvement, all property should be taxed equally. The second problem was more fundamental. Farr conceded that the former residents of poor districts were often unable to afford living in the new improved neighborhoods. Improvements then seemed merely to displace the population they were designed to assist. For the idle and unemployed of these redeveloped areas Farr had no sympathy. "It is, undoubtedly, much easier to displace than to regenerate such a population—the sediment of vast cities which sinks into these obscure receptacles . . . The people dispersed, if they obtain money, obtain houses; or they return, like the Irish, home."[106] The case was different in Farr's mind with hard-working but poor artisans threatened with increased rents. Farr asked whether model artisans' dwellings might not be built on some of London's new streets, and believed if the changes were undertaken gradually the rents would not increase beyond the capacities of the working class. Thirty years later the problem remained. Increased city rents drove the more affluent to the suburbs while the working poor were forced to crowd together in old houses. By this time Farr was willing to call upon cities to acquire large tracts of residential city land so that they could regulate the kind of housing built and, through the rents charged, relieve the property tax and still improve social services.[107] Farr, like other Victorian liberal reformers, was slowly led to advance state action as a remedy for social evils. His arguments were, of course, not unique. Other sanitarians also argued that the limits of individual freedom were passed when public health was threatened.[108] Air and water were public trusts which no man might own or abuse.

Farr on the Population Question

A second major group of criticisms of the sanitary campaign was based upon the principle of population. Malthusians claimed that a genuine improvement in the life of the mass of the people was impossible because, in the absence of prudential restraint or vice, population growth would outstrip the means of subsistence, bringing social misery and a high death rate. Quetelet joined Malthus in issuing a related biological challenge.[109] Human effort to prevent epidemics was wasted, they claimed, because if deaths from one disease were reduced, mortality from other causes would increase proportionately. These challenges were fundamental and demanded a response from the proponents of health reform.

Eversley has pointed out that to a certain degree all nineteenth-century liberals were Malthusian, although they might modify Malthus's original doctrine somewhat.[110] This generalization is true of Farr, at least to the extent that he accepted the population question in the terms Malthus posed. Farr believed the major incentives for limiting population growth were economic, and he accepted the rate and the age of marriage as the proper means of control.[111] He, of course, reached different conclusions about the causes and probable consequences of population growth. Malthus, Farr insisted, had reasoned improperly and had used unreliable data. Malthus had offered the United States as a case in which a population had doubled itself in twenty-five years. This example Farr rejected.[112] Malthus had overlooked the high American immigration rate. Farr offered as a counter-example the British peerage. Although placed in the most favorable economic circumstances, circumstances which therefore ought not to have restrained their numbers, the peerage nevertheless did not increase with abnormal rapidity, and in fact suffered the extinction of family lines.

Here, as in certain other cases, Farr outlined his basic position in the early 1840s.[113] When he returned to answer the Malthusian criticisms in later decades, he used the more extensive census and registration materials to add weight to the answers he had already proposed. Farr put forward two basic objections to Malthus's gloomy forecast: first, Malthus had seriously underestimated the potential for growth in the means of subsistence; and second, Malthus had failed to notice that population growth, far from being uncontrolled, was in fact already subject to a highly effective form of regulation and responded to economic conditions and national need. The first objection was argued more frequently in the sixties and seventies.[114] Farr pointed out repeatedly that the means of subsistence was capable of increasing as a geometrical series, not merely arithmetically as Malthus claimed, and that the means of subsistence actually could increase faster than the population. The plants and animals upon which man feeds increase according to the same law as mankind, but, in addition, human creativity and labor give mankind a greater advantage. Unlike wild animals, whose population is limited to the means of subsistence they can find, mankind has the capacity to increase immeasurably the means of subsistence at its disposal. While no one had measured the extent to which humans had multiplied their means of subsistence, Farr offered several examples to suggest that this increase had been great. The growth of capital at compound interest was a favorite. Another was the increase in wheat production, in the value of livestock, and in the acres of improved land in the United States accompanying its great population increase from 1850 to 1870. The American experience illustrated to Farr that the means of subsistence became more rather than less accessible as the population of skilled laborers increased. He apparently did not consider the possibility that the agricultural development of a virgin continent was an inappropriate example. He also argued that industrial nations had an advantage over economically undeveloped ones. A nation like England was not strictly limited by its small land area since it could exchange the products of one of its acres for the produce of several thousand agricultural acres.

This portion of Farr's argument was hardly original. While he cited Sir James Steuart and Adolphe Quetelet for the importance of man's capacity for production, he might have mentioned the writings of political economists such as Nassau Senior and John Stuart Mill or even those of Edwin Chadwick.[115] Nor was his first objection based to any significant degree on the evidence of vital statistics. But in arguing that the rate of population growth was subject to instinctive yet effective control, Farr attempted to use national vital statistics. At several periods of his career he used the census and the registration materials to calculate the percentage of the population married, the average age at marriage, and the average fertility of English marriages.[116] He was able to demonstrate that the English birth rate was well below what was physiologically possible. He concluded as early as 1842 that "the facts prove, beyond all question, that the population of the country is susceptible of an immense expansion; that it is voluntarily repressed, and always has been repressed, to an extent which has not been clearly conceived or stated; and that the means in the hands of nature, and of society, for increasing and diminishing the population are simple, efficient, and quite compatible with our ideas of the benevolence of the divine government of the world."[117] Those means of increasing or diminishing the population were the individual decisions of prudent men about marriage. Population growth was controlled, Farr maintained, because the time of marriage was delayed by most Englishmen and marriage was foregone entirely by many. He suggested in this same report that the population of England could be made stationary if either one-half, not one-fifth, of its women did not marry, or if no women under twenty-three married and the mean age of females who married were raised from twenty-four to thirty years, assuming the maintenance of the rates of fertility and mortality of the period 1839 to 1842.[118]

Farr eventually came to suspect that there was a connection between birth rate and death rate. In the *Supplement to the Thirty-fifth Annual Report* he ranked the registration districts of England and Wales by general mortality rate and observed that both population density and birth rate increased with mortality.[119] He did not draw the same conclusion from such information as some Victorian critics of Malthus who argued that the solution to the threat of overpopulation was to raise the standard of living, giving men an economic stake in society and hence cause for prudence in reproduction.[120] Farr observed instead that until the death rate climbed to 26 per 1,000 the annual excess of births over deaths remained almost constant, about 13 per 1,000. This observation suggested to him that the prospect of a reduced death rate should not raise the specter of overpopulation. His figures indicated that a district's birth rate should drop with its death rate. The healthy districts, for example, had not only the lowest death rates but also the lowest birth rates.

Thus there is no inevitable connection between the gradual reduction of the mortality of the whole kingdom to the rate of 17 per 1,000 and the more rapid increase of population; because the birth-rate may of itself fall to the level of that now prevailing in the healthiest districts and leave the increase of population as it was. Statesmen are not then, by alarming cries of increase of population in a faster geometrical progression, to be deterred from the noblest work in which they can engage [sanitary reform]; for it is certain that population as it improves in England will not increase faster than the requirements of industry in all its forms at home or the new openings of colonial enterprise abroad.[121]

There was no reason to fear that efforts to reduce the death rate would be followed by misery and pestilence. Furthermore the reliance on disasters to control population was both inhuman and unwise. Zymotic diseases, Farr pointed out, disabled and maimed the bodies and minds of more people than they killed.[122] As a means of population control disease was wasteful and harmful to society. He used the example of Paris in the thirties to show that not only did births not quickly compensate for epidemic casualties, but society suffered additionally because its new members were helpless infants, not productive adults.[123] By contrast, sanitary reform extended the average length of life and hence period of productivity of most citizens.[124] To lower the death rate with the prospect of a fall in the birth rate was clearly wiser than to rely on misery and disease to carry off excess population.

To dread, therefore, any ill consequences from arresting epidemics, or to argue on *a priori* grounds that it is impossible in opposition to nature to save life, to prolong life, to strengthen, and in every respect to improve the English race, is illogical; for give them health, and if the increased numbers cannot be sustained on subsistence by their industry within the shores of those islands, the births will naturally decline; but the natural remedies are increased industry to command produce from abroad, and emigration to seek after subsistence on the vast trans-oceanic territories.[125]

Like most of his contemporaries Farr assumed that voluntary control of marriage was the manner in which the birth rate would be lowered.[126] Farr added to typical moral objections to contraception fears for the nation or race. He was fond of comparing poor France with its multitudes of peasants practicing birth control in order to survive on their little plots of land with the greatness of industrial England, its cities teeming with people.[127] He had no doubt that England's population policy contributed to her greatness. The topic inspired a burst of oratorical eloquence in the 1871 census report that is undeniably Farr's.

If the French parent asks how many of his children have a chance of a livelihood on a parcel of the dear land he loves so well, and regulates his family accordingly, he appears to have the sanction of the school of economists founded by an Englishman: while on the English side we contend, with the facts revealed by the Census in our hands, that the English people have instinctively pursued a great and wise policy: they have increased at variable rates; by increasing rapidly since the last century they have exalted England to a height overtopped by no other power; they have peopled colonies; they have planted wide in perpetuity the English race; and they have exercised a great part in the government of the finest regions of the earth. That they have done under great discouragements and at great sacrifices. Malthus told them at the beginning of the century that by the principle of population they were increasing in geometrical progression; that they were thus perpetually pressing upon the means of subsistence, which increased in arithmetical progression; [and] that this was the inevitable cause of misery. . . .[128]

National eminence sprang from a heroic struggle.

But greatness was opening on the country; so in the midst of struggling poverty, in spite of difficulties, in the face of death itself, the nation, conscious of its energy, fought on through the conflict, led by the same daring spirit as animated its fathers at the cry of the king:

"Once more unto the breach, dear friends, once more;
Or close the wall up with our English dead!"

Thousands perished in the strife, but millions survived with all the vigour of their breed.[129]

The nationalist feeling expressed so clearly here was reflected often in Farr's attitudes toward the population question. Not only did he think that the threat of overpopulation was a chimera, an unreal threat to reform; but that the rate of population growth was controlled by national needs: economic, military, or imperial. For these reasons, he, like eighteenth-century mercantilists or physiocrats, often viewed a high birth rate not as a warning of impending disaster, but as a sign of national vigor and as a potential economic advantage.[130] The birth rate reflected the manpower needs of nations. "Thus, England has an increasing industry and a vast colonial empire to people, so the births are numerous . . . France had no colonial demand for population, and so the population was not depressed by a high death-rate but by a low birth-rate."[131] He condemned only the means by which the French birth rate was suppressed and not the fact of its suppression. The French experience simply confirmed the extent to which population growth was responsive to national needs.

Farr's Eugenic Ideas

In Farr's pronouncements on the population question one discovers frequent evidence of hereditarian or racial concerns. The issue was more than incidental. It was one Farr considered repeatedly. Although the well-known cynicism of eugenicists about sanitary reform might lead one to suspect otherwise, Farr and later advocates of eugenics shared a number of hereditarian ideas.[132] As Victor Hilts has recently pointed out, the sanitary reform program and Farr, especially, articulated concern for both nature and nurture, for the role of heredity as well as for the environment in determining human nature.[133]

Farr's concern with the role of inheritance is expressed in his earliest writings, decades before the appearance of Darwinism. Farr was, after all, heir to a medical tradition which recognized that men were not biologically identical. Even crudely constructed family medical histories revealed that certain diseases seemed to be especially prevalent in some families. In his early reports Farr explained that different families seemed to suffer different ailments, even when living in the same environment. He concluded men were born with hereditary predispositions to disease, and furthermore he suspected that the races of mankind differed in this regard.[134] He came to acknowledge heredity as one of the most important factors in determining an individual's prospects of future health. In the 1870s, in writing of the possibility of mass health insurance in the face of acknowledged human differences, he explained that although it was impossible to select the persons out of a given number who would die of a given disease, say consumption, one could, by studying "ancestral descent, temperament, premonitory symptoms . . . select a class apart, having what is technically called a consumptive tendency, . . . whose mortality would approximate to that of the persons actually dying of consumption."[135]

Farr not only acknowledged the biological differences between men, but he also shared in the nineteenth-century passion to make them a subject of study. According to one account he measured the heads of cretins while visiting Switzerland during his student days.[136] During the sixties and seventies, when anthropometry was especially popular in Western Europe and the United States, Farr took an active interest in the subject.[137] He suggested in his paper on sanitary statistics at the London meeting of the International Statistical Congress of 1860 that an international effort be made to measure the population of various European countries, and mentioned the necessity of collecting data not only on stature, weight, and strength, but also on intelligence.[138] Six years later he proposed that there be established in England a national register of sickness and physical disabilities, and that such a register include the results of tests of strength and the capacity for physical or mental work.[139]

During the last five years of his career Farr was chairman of the Anthropometric Committee of the British Association.[140] The committee collected returns on age, sex, race, height, weight, hair color, girth of chest, strength of arm, and eyesight for people of the British Isles, mainly soldiers, students, and civil servants. It supplied researchers who would agree to cooperate with several sets of instructions, a scale, an apparatus for measuring lung capacity, a spring balance for measuring strength of arm, tinted paper for reporting hair color, and a chart of dots for testing eyesight. The committee also made some attempt to collect photographs of human types. Apparently the committee had assigned itself two major tasks: to collect information on and to characterize the physical differences of the races of the British empire, and to weigh the influence of class upon physique. The first enterprise largely failed, although an attempt was made to compare the measurements of the height and weight of the British population which the committee had collected with the measurements of Americans, data accumulated by Bowditch, and of Belgians, data reported by Quetelet. To evaluate the effects of social class the committee identified four classes: a professional class composed of upper and middle class persons whose nurture was "very good," a commercial class composed of the lower middle class whose nurture was "good," a laboring class having "imperfect" nurture, and an industrial class whose nurture was "bad." The physical characteristics of the professional class were first given and used as a standard to judge the influence of the social environment on other classes.[141]

One reason why sanitary reformers such as Farr and Florence Nightingale took an interest in anthropometry was their fear that racial degeneration would occur in unhealthy environments.[142] Farr used the idea of race to denote not only physical differences between Western and non-Western peoples, such as skin color, but also to indicate both the tribal origin of the inhabitants of Great Britain and the differences among the classes in British society.[143] Although he lacked facts to substantiate his idea about environmentally induced degeneration, Farr had no doubts about its validity. Urban life was his primary concern, and he believed that children who lived in city districts with high mortality rates were likely to be crippled or weakened.[144] Such disabilities affected future generations, and so the results were cumulative.

To illustrate his ideas Farr pointed to colonial experience and ancient history to suggest that even healthy, vigorous stock degenerated in tropical climates. Low land seemed especially pernicious.

The people bred on marshy coasts and low river margins, where pestilence is generated, live sordidly, without liberty, without poetry, without virtue, without science. They neither invent nor practise the arts; they possess neither hospitals, nor castles, nor habitations fit to dwell in; neither farms, freeholds, nor workshops. They are conquered and oppressed by successive tribes of the stronger races, and appear to be incapable of any form of society except that in which they are slaves. Strangers no sooner set foot or attempt to settle on the soil than the endemic terror attacks them as if to bid them begone; and if they remain, their institutions, palaces, and monuments, fall into ruins, as the generations degenerate.[145]

In the most crowded parts of industrial towns and seaports physical and mental enfeeblement and degeneration seemed inevitable. Epidemic disease was a warning of impending racial disaster.

All analogy, however, proves that no extensive or permanent degeneration of a race can be accomplished in less than two or three generations. The great change is as slow and insidious as it is certain. It is rarely perceived by its victims; who remain rooted and benumbed on the spot unless they and the community are aroused by sudden and terrible catastrophes. That angel which, it would seem, it has pleased the Almighty Creator and Preserver of Mankind to charge with this dread mission is the Pestilence. Wherever the human race, yielding to ignorance, indolence, or accident, is in such a situation as to be liable to lose its strength, courage, liberty, wisdom, lofty emotions—the plague, the fever, or the cholera comes; not committing havoc perpetually, but turning men to destruction, and then suddenly ceasing, that they may consider. As the lost father speaks to the family and the slight epidemic to the city, so the pestilence speaks to nations in order that greater calamities than the untimely death of the population may be averted. For to a nation of good and noble men Death is a less evil than Degradation of Race.[146]

It was the great cholera epidemic of 1848–1849 that engendered these outbursts, but the demand which followed, that mankind take control of his biological future, was one Farr had made a decade earlier. In his first published article, Farr called for a hygienic policy which had as its aim to "increase the *sum of vitality* by extending individual life to its full term (averting death); by obviating sickness; and by increasing the energy of all vital forces, whether nutritive, formative, locomotive, or sensitive and intellectual."[147] He used as examples the selective breeding of animals, the rejuvenation of the Hebrew people under the Mosaic hygienic law, and the population control of Sparta by infanticide to illustrate that the organic progress of man was subject to human control. Modern governments, he argued in the 1830s, should revive these ancient concerns. A wise national legislature "deems the physical perfection of the people the sole basis of their moral and intellectual greatness."[148] Not only was inactivity in the face of conditions that caused preventable disease and premature death cruel and profligate, but it also threatened more lasting and less easily remedied consequences.

There was, however, a fundamental problem in Farr's position. The weak and disabled who would be spared the rigors of a hostile environment would live to reproduce. Would not this fact pose an even greater threat to the future of the race than the unhealthy environment itself? Farr recognized the dilemma.

In his first paper, in discussing Spartan infanticide, he considered the effect of sparing 800 normally sacrificed Spartan children.[149] He concluded that most would probably have been killed by the severities of that society, but if they had lived to reproduce they would have produced a great proportion of unfit persons. He raised the problem again in his article on vital statistics in McCulloch's statistical digest. He suggested that as the infant death rate declined, more weak persons would be introduced into the population "and that, unless proper means . . . [were] taken to fortify the constitution in manhood, the relative vigour . . . [would] not increase in the same ratio as the population."[150]

The solution was not to be found in infanticide, either direct as in ancient Sparta or indirect via disease, as in modern cities. Both methods were blind, and took not only the weak and undesirable but also the weak and promising.[151] Both Newton and D'Alembert would have been lost in Sparta. The wiser course was to reduce mortality so that many could live, and then, if necessary, to prohibit the reproduction of the least desirable types.

Even before the publication of Darwin's *Origin of Species*, Farr had been impressed with the importance of artificial selection in modifying domestic species. "It is known to everybody that all the species of cultivated plants, and all the breeds of domestic animals, have been greatly improved in Europe. The improvement is partly due to the favorable conditions in which each kind has been placed. It is mainly due, however, to the constant elimination of imperfect types, and to the skillful selection of the finest individuals out of each successive generation."[152] He concluded that environmental reform by itself was not enough. He told the British Medical Association's Section on State Medicine, "How, out of the existing seed, to raise races of men to a divine perfection, is the final problem of Public Medicine."[153]

Human reproduction, Farr concluded, should be controlled for social ends. He argued on one occasion that soldiers ought to be allowed and encouraged to marry both as a means of suppressing vice and the high mortality of illegitimate children, and because "valour is transmissible" and the present generation of soldiers ought to breed the next one.[154] More in keeping with the ideas of later eugenics advocates, Farr spoke for the permanent custody of the criminal and the insane. Writing in 1852 he singled out two trends which were dangerous to the race: the movement of population to lower elevations, and the freedom given to criminals, the insane, and persons with hereditary diseases to reproduce.[155] The problem of hereditary insanity, Farr believed, was particularly serious in the aristocracy, which tried to keep its presence a secret. Such knowledge, he claimed, should be made public so that the "peerage should be purified, and not corrupted still further by inter-marriage," and he suggested in 1837 that a list of all insane in Britain possessing property, along with individual case histories, be submitted annually to Parliament.[156] The confirmed criminal also should be discouraged from reproducing. Such criminals were in his opinion separate degenerate human types. "The State alone has the power to deal with criminals and lunatics; by wise reformatories in the first instance, and in confirmed criminals, who breed and educate successive waves of degenerate men, by humane but eternal seclusion."[157] Whereas Galton after him would direct human evolution primarily by encouraging marriage and reproduction by the socially desirable, Farr would act primarily by prohibiting the reproduction of the unfit.[158]

Farr welcomed racial competition between Europeans and the "unsettled unproductive savages"[159] who populated parts of the world. An enthusiasm for this conflict, which chills the contemporary reader, swallowed up fears of overpopulation and provided an answer to those who viewed with suspicion the saving of infant life by sanitary improvement.

What have we to say when we are told that Europe will be over-run with population if fewer children are destroyed in infancy? England answers for me: over-run the world. There is room for all the European types in the other quarters of the globe, and Europe itself is still only half peopled.

It is certainly in conformity with Darwin's law, that in the struggle for existence, out of which the improvement of species springs, the race which breeds and educates the greatest number of vigorous, intelligent children, has the best chance of winning and of holding its own. Let all Europe, then, strive for the prize: the English race in these islands, in the northern provinces of America, as well as in the United States, has a firm hold on the earth, and welcomes them as generous rivals in common efforts for the elevation and development of humanity.[160]

Thus the third world would stand as insurance against the West's dilemma of progress.

SEVEN

FARR, FLORENCE NIGHTINGALE, AND MEDICAL SERVICES

A Sanitary and Statistical Pact

William Farr met Florence Nightingale at a dinner party in the autumn of 1856.[1] She had just returned from the Crimea a national heroine and was about to begin her campaign to reform the Army Medical Department. As she listened to Farr, Nightingale realized he possessed knowledge and experience that would be of great value to her cause. They began a correspondence, and by February 1857 had made a pact: he would help her promote the health of the army in return for her help with the campaign to reduce civilian mortality.[2] Thus in 1856 began a collaboration that lasted nearly two decades and left some four hundred letters as testimony to its scope and vitality.[3]

The two sanitarians shared many interests, and, at least at first, were in agreement on the proper means of reaching their shared goals. Their alliance was based on complementary abilities and opportunities. From Farr, Nightingale obtained expert statistical and actuarial advice. He had the practical bent, the reform sympathies, and the experience with certain statistical problems that made his counsel invaluable. He had access, moreover, to unpublished vital records and commanded a staff of trained clerks whose services she employed in completing her books and papers.[4] For his part Farr obtained a certain amount of information, on the nursing practices of major hospitals and on child-raising customs in Europe, for example. But most important, through Florence Nightingale, Farr gained a more direct hearing among the politically influential: Sidney Herbert, Sir Charles Wood, Lord Palmerstone, Lord Stanley, and other ministers whom Nightingale had either bullied or enticed into cooperation.

The collaboration led to a warm friendship. The surviving letters are witnesses both to personal favors exchanged and to mutual respect and affection. Farr often wrote, enquiring about her health and recommending periods of rest in his Healthy Districts.[5] He sometimes urged her to present papers at the Social Science Association or at the International Statistical Congress and helped see to their presentation and reception.[6] It was he who proposed her as a member of the Statistical Society of London in

1858.[7] As we shall see he also defended her from attacks in the medical press. By the middle sixties they were addressing each other as beloved co-workers. He frequently wrote a note during the holiday season wishing her a happy New Year and reflecting on the importance of her labors. It was a time for extravagant compliments. In 1865 he called her the "great leader in the good cause," and in 1869 he asked that "God grant that you may live long a martyr truly—a witness—an angel—a messenger—but also an apostle 'that has labored more than them all'—in advancing His Truth—His Mission of Healing the World."[8]

Nightingale came to value Farr as one of her most trusted friends. She referred to him as one of her best friends, as her "Patron Saint," and at his death as "my beloved friend Dr. Farr, one of the truest benefactors to the world that has lived."[9] During his life she took an active interest in his affairs and reputation. We find her writing to him in 1860 to warn him of forthcoming attacks by his medical critics from industrial cities and again in 1871 to urge him to answer an attack on the registrar general's reports in the medical press.[10] She herself apparently even undertook to counter criticisms by Alfred Aspland and Henry Rumsey in 1859 when she sensed he lacked her enthusiasm for a fight.[11] With his concurrence she sought to secure his election as foreign member in the Institute de France to replace J. R. McCulloch. When her correspondent in Paris informed her that Farr's case was doubtful because "they choose flashy people, of the Broughamite class, mostly hollow drums who in their time have made a great noise. . . ." and, later, that it was hopeless because Gladstone, J. S. Mill, and Whewell had been proposed, and Gladstone was sure to be named, she expressed grave disappointment; but she pushed for his election, this time successfully, as corresponding member.[12]

Her support was purchased at a high price. She expected untiring effort from her associates. John Sutherland, her closest medical adviser, tolerated demands and withstood criticism that would have made most professional men rebell.[13] While Farr was a regular collaborator during the decade following their meeting, and though at times he worked very hard for her, he maintained an unusual independence for a member of her inner circle. She treated him with deference, relying most often on flattery to secure his cooperation. She wrote to him, for example, in 1858 to say that she was coming to sit at his feet for a few more favors.[14] In 1871 she said that she felt like a small boy writing to Aristotle when she sought his statistical advice.[15] When such gentle tactics did not secure the promptness she expected, she wrote to embarrass him for the trouble he caused her, and on rare occasions, she could be mildly sarcastic, as when she addressed him as she would a pope in pleading for the delivery of a bull.[16]

Why should Farr, a co-worker without political influence, receive special treatment at her hands? Much of the reason must certainly lie in the fact that Florence Nightingale attached extraordinary value to statistics. Statistics had the power to gain attention and sway opinion. They formed therefore an important part of her tracts and of the Blue Books prepared under her shadow. She had a flair for devising graphic methods, her famous "coxcombs," for popularizing numerical data.[17] Such "statistical aesthetics," she told Farr, lagged behind the progress of numerical statistics and languished in a state like that of the fine arts before Cimabue.[18] But Nightingale's commitment to statistics was even more complete. She regarded them both as a master science of human affairs and as a substitute religion. These twin ideas are reflected in a letter she wrote Farr on Quetelet's death.[19] "I cannot tell you how the death of our old friend touches me: the founder of the most important science in the whole world, for upon it depends the practical application of every other: the Science essential to all Political & Social Administration, all Education & Organization based on experience, for *it only* gives exact results of our experience." She continued by explaining she had in hand an unfinished essay dedicated to Quetelet, elucidating "the application of his discoveries to explaining the plan of God in teaching us by these results the laws of our moral progress: to explaining, in short, the path on which we must go if we are to discover the laws of the Divine Government of the Moral World."

The study of statistics was then a moral imperative, a religious duty. It was the surest way of learning the divine plan of the world and directing human action in accordance with it.[20] Perhaps for this reason she took delight in even the dullest statistical compilations. When during the deliberations of the Indian Sanitary Commission Farr promised her a New Year's gift of tables, she wrote that she was "exceedingly anxious, as you may suppose, to see your charming New Year's gifts."[21] She chided an unnamed correspondent, perhaps T. Graham Balfour, for the quality of the first volume of Army statistics. "We want facts. 'Facta, facta, facta' is the motto which ought to stand at the head of all statistical work. If we cannot have all the facts, let us at all events have all the reliable facts we can." She objected to his including discussion of causes in his statistical report, even if exclusion made the report dry. "The dryer the better. Statistics should be the dryest of all reading."[22] Ironically, her writing, like Farr's, was anything but a dry compilation of facts. They were both passionate statisticians impatient for sanitary reform.[23]

Army Statistics and Hygiene

Their first common project was the Army Sanitary Commission of 1857, the establishment and management of which owed a large debt to Nightingale's personal campaign.[24] The commission followed on the medical scandals of the Crimean War and in the wake of royal and popular fascination with Florence Nightingale's military nursing. The commission was given broad powers of investigation and reported on the sanitary condition of the army in Britain and on the conduct of the Army Medical Department. Nightingale had a large say in choosing the members of the commission. She had originally wanted Farr to be a member, but during the negotiations he was dropped in favor of an examining lawyer, Sir Thomas Phillips. Nevertheless Farr promised to work for the commission informally. Behind the scenes he helped Nightingale through all stages of the commission's work.

The investigation was carefully managed by a sanitary clique: Sir Sidney Herbert, chairman, commission members Dr. John Sutherland and Dr. James Martin, and Florence Nightingale, nonmember but guiding force. She relied on Farr for the analysis of the army returns of death and disease and for some of the tactics of using mortality statistics argumentatively. Their letters from May to September are full of the commission's statistical affairs.[25] He asked for information on troop strength and age composition of military units. He offered suggestions for displaying information in tables and helped design questionnaires to demonstrate the causes of high mortality in military camps and hospitals. He also reviewed some of the material she prepared, sometimes complimenting, at other times offering lengthy criticism. He even suggested questions to ask witnesses.

Farr appeared as an expert witness before the commission. He answered questions on his proposal to register deaths of soldiers abroad with the General Register Office, defended the G.R.O.'s nosology, and in Appendix 70 compared the mortality of soldiers with that of English civilians in various trades.[26] He reserved his major points, however, for Appendix 72, in which he analyzed the army mortality and morbidity returns.[27] If, as Sir Edward Cook suggested, the strength of the commission's argument rested upon the differences in mortality rates between soldiers and men of military age in civilian life,[28] it was Farr who made the case.

The purpose of Appendix 72 was to provide convincing and easily understood evidence to prove that the mortality of soldiers, even in peace time, was excessive, and to demonstrate that such excess mortality could be prevented. In doing this Farr used methods he had developed to describe the mortality of the civilian population. In fact his whole approach in this and subsequent investigations seems to have been to try to bring military sanitary statistics within the civilian fold. He measured the health of soldiers against three civilian standards: the mortality of men of military age in all of England and Wales, the mortality for the same group in the Healthy Districts, and again in Manchester, one of the least healthy cities. These were, of course, the populations he had used several times previously to represent average, good, and poor health. He proceeded by comparing the mortality of these groups, corrected for differences in age. He computed age group mortality rates for troops and compared them with similar rates for these civilians. He then calculated how many lives would be saved if soldiers in peacetime experienced the same risks of dying as civilians of the same ages. Finally he constructed a life table for English troops at home and compared it to the English life table and to the healthy district life table.

In making this comparison Farr reminded his reader that the mortality of the troops in peacetime ought to be lower than that of civilians.[29] First of all, there was a process of selection involved. Soldiers were "picked lives." They had passed a medical examination at the time of recruitment, while those who failed remained in the general population. Furthermore, men who developed chronic diseases in the army were discharged and reappeared in the civilian ranks. Second, soldiers, at least in peacetime, ought to have added advantages over their civilian counterparts. Troops were subject to a strict discipline and their material wants were provided at considerable expense to the nation. But despite his apparent advantages the English soldier, by Farr's calculations, had poorer health than any of his civilian contemporaries.[30] For the years 1839 to 1853 the mortality of troops at home and abroad averaged 33.0 per 1,000 while at the same ages it was only 7.7 per 1,000 for males of military age in the Healthy Districts and 9.2 per 1,000 for those in all of England and Wales. Even those soldiers stationed in England died at a much faster rate than other Englishmen at the same age. This was true for all age groups. The difference was greatest among recruits ages twenty to twenty-five who suffered a mortality rate of 17 per 1,000 annually, while their counterparts in civilian life experienced a rate of only 8.4 per 1,000.

Farr was not content merely to demonstrate the net effect of differing degrees of health. He wanted to demonstrate the causes of the excess mortality. In order to do this he rearranged the Army returns of the causes of death and the case records of the military hospitals in the Crimean War according to his nosology. He found that two classes of disease were responsible for most of the difference in mortality between soldiers and civilians: zymotic diseases, and chest and tubercular diseases.[31] He found, for example, that among the infantry of the line serving at home from 1837 to 1846 diseases of these two groups accounted for seven-ninths of all deaths. Such diseases alone produced a higher mortality among these troops than similarly aged civilians experienced from all causes. Furthermore, although among English civilians of these ages chest and tubercular diseases were very serious, causing each year twice as many deaths as the zymotic diseases, the chest and tubercular diseases were more than twice as fatal among the troops. Among the troops the zymotic diseases caused nearly as many deaths as the chest and tubercular diseases caused among the civilians of military age. While these two groups of disease seemed to be primarily responsible for the poor health of soldiers in peacetime, a similar analysis of the mortality returns showed that it was the zymotic diseases that were responsible for the medical disasters of the Crimean War.[32]

The analysis of the causes of sickness and death was a prelude to a discussion of prevention. Farr's writing here was stripped of subtlety and qualification. The sanitarians' analysis and recommendation appeared in simple, unequivocal form. "Consumption and diseases of that class are the result of breathing foul air contaminated by the breath of other people."[33] Overcrowding and filth, it was explained, were the major deterrents to health. But there were grounds for optimism. The fact that mortality in the military hospitals during the Crimean War had dropped in the spring of 1855 illustrated, Farr suggested, that great improvement was possible.[34] He saw no reason why men in the Army at home ought not to be as healthy as men of military age in the civil population, and he calculated that 1,500 lives would be saved in a force of 100,000 Guards at home, if the soldiers' mortality were no higher than that of civilian males of military age.[35]

One of the striking differences between this paper and most others by Farr is the extensive use of diagrams and other visual aids. We may perhaps see here Nightingale's concern with impressing the commission's statistical findings on minds unused to perusing life tables. Farr of course had used some diagrams before, but in Appendix 72 to the *Report of the Army Sanitary Commission* he threw his entire visual armament at the reader.[36] There were bar graphs showing the mortality of soldiers and the mortality of male civilians in individual years and at various periods of life, as well as the mortality from various causes of death at all ages. There were diagrams, like the ones in his *Fifth Annual Report*, illustrating what Farr called the decrement of life from life tables of English soldiers, Englishmen, and Englishmen in healthy districts.[37] In these three diagrams (see fig. 11) a straight line divided a rectangle by intersecting its lower left corner, forming, in each case, a triangle on the rectangle's base. The rectangle illustrated twenty years of service of 10,000 recruits at age twenty. Years of life were represented along the horizontal axis and numbers of troops on the vertical axis. The area below the intersecting line portrayed the dead and the area above, the number living. The slope of the intersecting line represented the law of mortality for each life table.

Farr then produced similar diagrams to illustrate the losses over a twenty year career from both death and invaliding for the Army stationed in England. (See fig. 12.) In this case the rectangle representing years of life was intersected at the upper left corner by two lines to form two adja-

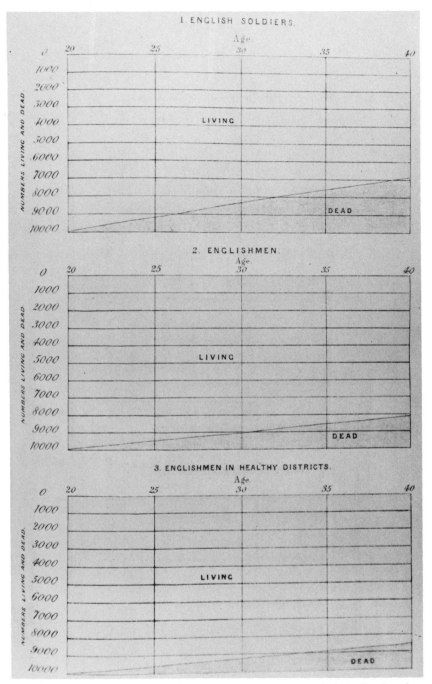

Figure 11. Farr's diagram E for the Army Sanitary Commission, showing the fate of a cohort of English soldiers, English males, and English males in the healthy districts. *Report of the Commissioners,* App. 72, diagram E [PP, 1857–58, XVIII, following p. 526].

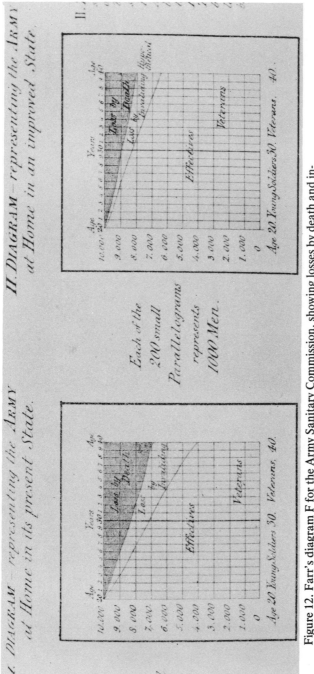

Figure 12. Farr's diagram F for the Army Sanitary Commission, showing losses by death and invaling for a cohort of recruits in the present state of health and in an improved state. *Report of the Commissioners*, App. 72, diagram F [PP, 1857–58, XVIII, following p. 526].

cent triangles. The black triangle represented the dead, and the yellow triangle portrayed the invalids. One such rectangle was for the home Army at present. Another represented the losses the Army would experience if its health were improved to equal the state of English male civilians at the same ages. This second table was based on the English Life Table for ages 20 to 40 and on the ratio of invalids to dead then prevailing in the home Army. The diagrams were intended to illustrate the loss of effective troop strength caused by disease and the gain in manpower that could be expected to follow even moderate sanitary reform.

Farr offered several comments to emphasize the point. The statistics showed, he claimed, that in the present state of health, 10,000 annual recruits who, if they lived, would serve twenty years, could maintain an effective force of only 141,764. Under the state of health enjoyed by Englishmen of military age, the same number of annual recruits would maintain an effective force of 166,910, a net gain of 25,146 soldiers. He suggested that the gain to the nation from the sanitary reform of the Army would probably be even greater than his mode of calculating indicated, because he considered in this case only the troops stationed in England, ignoring completely the high mortality experienced abroad. In addition it was reasonable to expect that the ratio of invaliding to deaths would decrease as the mortality fell. In the text of this appendix he had already set the stage for this argument about losses of effective troop strength by maintaining that all deaths among soldiers above the rate prevailing among males of military age in the Healthy Districts of England ought to be computed as a direct financial loss to the Nation.[38]

Diagrams I & K are circular graphs representing deaths in hospitals during the Crimean War. They resemble the ones he prepared for his report on the 1848–1849 cholera epidemic to illustrate the fluctuation in cholera mortality during the epidemic, and they may have been inspired by charts of meteorological observations kept at the Greenwich Observatory.[39] In both of the diagrams for the Army there were two main circular graphs, the first for mortality between April 1854 and March 1855, and the second for the following twelve months.

In Diagram I (fig. 13) the annual rate of mortality per 1,000 in the hospitals of the Army of the East was portrayed. The enormous losses from August 1854 to March 1855 were dramatically shown by a black area Farr called "a great bat's wing," which extended well outside the concentric circles of the graph. During January 1855, a peak was reached of 1,174 deaths per 1,000 annually, a rate, Farr explained in a note, that was higher than London experienced during the Plague of 1665. As we will soon see, this enormous rate was due in part to the way Farr calculated hospital mortality. There is a third circle in diagram I, given to provide a standard of comparison. Farr portrayed here the mortality that would

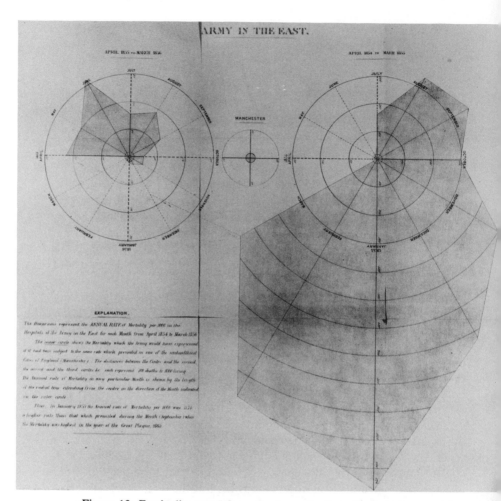

Figure 13. Farr's diagram I from the Army Sanitary Commission, showing hospital mortality in the Crimean campaign, April 1854 to March 1856. *Report of the Commissioners*, App. 72, diagram I [PP, 1857-58, XVIII, following p. 526].

have occurred in the Army hospitals if their rate of mortality were no higher than the general rate of mortality in one of his favorite standards of poor health, Manchester.

Diagram K, (fig. 14) illustrated the mortality in the Army hospitals in three classes: deaths caused by wounds, deaths caused by zymotic disease, and deaths from all other causes. While mortality from all three classes varied considerably over time, it was unquestionably the zymotic diseases that accounted for the disastrous experiences in the fall and

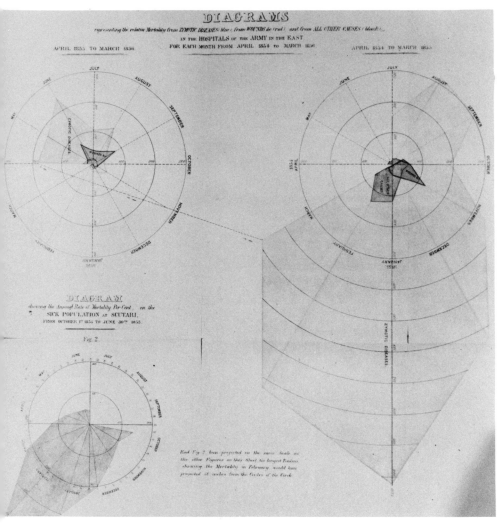

Figure 14. Farr's diagram K for the Army Sanitary Commission, showing the components of the mortality in figure 11. *Report of the Commissioners,* App. 72, diagram K [PP, 1857–58, XVIII, following p. 526].

winter of 1854–1855. This revelation was a poignant sanitary indictment because, according to the reformers, the zymotic diseases could be prevented by well-known measures.

The third circular graph in diagram K illustrated the annual case fatality percent from October 1854 through June 1855 at the Scutari Hospital, where Florence Nightingale had labored so industriously. The mor-

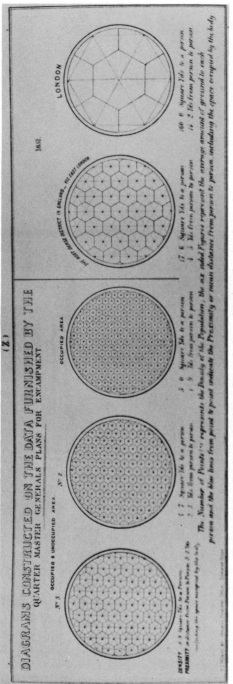
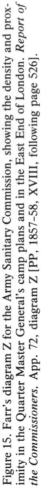

Figure 15. Farr's diagram Z for the Army Sanitary Commission, showing the density and proximity in the Quarter Master General's camp plans and in the East End of London. *Report of the Commissioners*, App. 72, diagram Z [PP, 1857–58, XVIII, following page 526].

tality was extremely high, reaching a peak of 415 percent per annum in February 1855. At such a rate, Farr explained, the entire population of the military hospitals in the war zone would have perished four times. In explaining this diagram, Farr preached a short sanitary sermon which ended with a plea for military hygiene by appealing to imperial and racial fears.

The question of military hygiene is rapidly becoming a question of vital importance to the interests of the empire. Upon the British race alone the integrity of that empire at this moment appears to depend. The conquering race must retain possession. Experience has shown that without special information and skillful application of the resources of science in preserving health, the drain on our home population must exhaust our means. The introduction, therefore, of a proper sanitary system into the British army is of essential importance to the public interests.[40]

Farr's final diagram, Z, explored the problem of crowding. (See fig. 15.) It was the same type of illustration he used in the report for the 1851 Census to represent the density and average proximity of inhabitants of districts by arrays of intersecting lines.[41] The purpose of the illustration and Farr's discussion was to criticize the Army's method of laying out its field encampments. By means of these diagrams Farr portrayed the density and proximity that resulted from the camp plans proposed by the Quartermaster General. For comparison he made similar constructions for the metropolis and for the most densely peopled district in England, East London. The least crowded camp plan gave each soldier only one-twentieth of the area allotted to each resident of the metropolis and one-half the area of the inhabitants of East London. Reversing the comparison and using the most crowded camp plan, Farr explained that if the metropolis were as densely populated, it would have to contain eighty-one million people.[42] Could any but disastrous consequences be expected to follow?

Farr provided the Army Sanitary Commission with the type of analysis and testimony Florence Nightingale wanted. She clearly was pleased with his work and saw to it that he was on one of four succeeding committees appointed to draw up specific proposals for enacting the commission's recommendations. He was one of three members on the Committee of Army Medical Statistics.[43] The others were Sidney Herbert and Colonel Alexander Tulloch. The committee's brief report of 1861 had as its aim a reordering of the Army's vital statistics.[44] One major theme dominated the report: the Army should establish a comprehensive system of mortality and morbidity statistics and that scheme should be modeled as closely as possible after the one administered in England by the registrar general. The recommendations were sweeping. The Army Medical Department's forms and tables should resemble those of the G.R.O., and the reports for the vital statistics of the military should appear at the same intervals as those for the civilian population: weekly, quarterly, and annually. The committee wanted deaths of soldiers abroad registered with the Registrar General. It also recommended that the Army adopt in its recruitment records the classification of occupations Farr developed for the census.

Finally, the Army was to adopt Farr's nosology and nomenclature of diseases subject to any modifications which might be suggested by a committee of the Royal College of Physicians.[45]

Farr was having his way with the committee. Through Nightingale's circle he worked closely with Sidney Herbert, the chairman. The third committee member, Colonel Tulloch, India officer and longtime student of army statistics, resented Farr's domination.[46] It was not that he was antagonistic to a rationalization of the Army medical branch or to Farr's goals; he did object, however, to the wholesale adoption of the civilian system of vital statistics. He registered his objections in a brief memorandum addressed to Herbert which was published at the end of the report.[47] Tulloch believed the majority report was much too rigid, allowing too little room for medical officers to modify procedures in the face of practical difficulties. He objected particularly to the recommended nosology, which he implied was theoretical and impractical and offered no real advantages over the nomenclature the Army doctors had developed over the last twenty-five years. There may have been a certain justice in Tulloch's reservations. Farr's reaction is not recorded, although Sidney Herbert's perfunctory response may have echoed Farr's insistence that the committee had made both useful and reasonable suggestions. We do know, however, that Farr was anxious about the response the War Office would give this report. We find him writing to Nightingale in May of 1861, asking her to use her influence to see that the committee's report appear as a Blue Book; otherwise "some essential parts of our scheme will be shelved—or pigeonholed."[48] Judging from the reports issued by the Army Medical Department over the next few years, the committee's recommendations had an impact on Army practices.

With a reform program launched for the Army in England, Nightingale turned her attention to the Army in India. The aftermath of the India Mutiny gave her an opportunity. Once again through politically influential friends she got a royal commission appointed and had a hand in both its staffing and management.[49] This was a period of considerable political influence for her. During the commission's deliberations she was able to work through her friends among its members, Sidney Herbert, the first Chairman, and his successor Lord Stanley, as well as her old associates Sutherland, Martin, Alexander, and Farr. After the commission reported, she found a very important collaborator in the newly appointed viceroy, Sir John Lawrence.[50]

The warrant for the Indian Sanitary Commission was issued in May

1859, but the report did not appear until May 1863. The delay was due in part to the difficulties in the statistical work of the commission. Forms were sent to India for information on troop strength, sickness, and death for the previous ten years. Responses were often late or imperfect. In addition, Farr, the commission's statistician, was concurrently occupied with several major projects besides the routine work at the G.R.O. and the deliberations of the Committee of Army Medical Statistics. The work of the royal commission coincided with the planning and convening of the London meeting of the International Statistical Congress and with the taking of the 1861 census. Farr was heavily involved with the work of both.

In their extensive correspondence during these four years Nightingale complained to Farr about delays in receiving returns from India and about the quality of the responses. As the commission's report was beginning to take shape, she pleaded with him to prepare the statistical section of the text so that the body of the report could appear at a politically opportune time.[51] Indian sanitary reform, she said, rested in his hands. Statistical details could go into the appendix. He responded in characteristic fashion:

I am working at the Indian statistics—a most treacherous & troublesome field. And I devote all the time I can spare from the office & the Census work to it.

The importance of the subject—& the fact that I shall draw conclusions from the information—differing from those of previous writers—render it necessary that I should go into the whole of this vast heap of material around me & sift it as well as I can—gathering hints everywhere. The history, geography, meteorology, have all to be considered—as we have not only to satisfy ourselves—in itself no easy matter—but to satisfy others—by decisive demonstrations.[52]

Farr was both a commission member and its paid actuarial consultant. His official duties included the collection and analysis of data. For this tedious work the Treasury provided him with four clerks.[53] In addition he was heavily involved in behind-the-scenes management of the commission's work. He was in frequent correspondence with Florence Nightingale and met regularly with the members of her cabal. They discussed questions to be asked, and Farr reported to Nightingale on the performances of several of the witnesses.[54] Unbeknownst to Lord Stanley, Farr routed all returns from India to her. He also wrote the questions she answered in her written testimony and offered suggestions on her evidence.[55] He entered into her spirit of campaign. One of her pieces for the Commission's report brought the following response.

Thanks for your admirable paper.

It is the sort of cavalry charge that is required—to scatter the mares of Indian imbecillity [sic]. I only add. More, More[.] Do not be afraid of saying—proving—or reproving—too much.

When I can read calmly—I will make any marks that occur to me.[56]

Farr was responsible for the statistical section of the report.[57] The types of evidence and the tabular illustrations were similar to those he prepared for the Army Sanitary Commission. But in this case the actuary work was more comprehensive. He compared general and age group mortality and morbidity rates for soldiers in India and English civilians in various situations, and he prepared life tables and compared life expectancies at various ages. But he also extended the analysis to other groups of people (native Indian troops, Indian civilians, English civil servants, English officers, English wives, widows, and children, and pensioned or retired former Indian troops or officers) and found other ways of illustrating relative risks (by comparing life insurance premiums or the value of annuities for the various groups studied). In assessing the health of the Army he tried to weigh the effects of both age and length of service in India. He explained to Florence Nightingale what is apparent in his arrangement of evidence: the purpose of his statistical section was to prove that "it is not the climate that sweeps away our soldiers."[58] The high mortality of the English troops in India was not inevitable. The fact that English officers and civil servants in India had much lower rates demonstrated, Farr argued, that the manner in which the troops lived and the provisions made for protecting their health were grossly deficient. He blamed sanitation and life style, not climate or racial differences, for the fact that mortality was higher among English troops in India than among native Indian troops.[59]

This conclusion marked a change in Farr's opinion. He had paid only limited attention to the mortality of the Army and Navy in his early statistical writings, for the most part merely digesting the work of previous writers.[60] He had become convinced, however, in the later 1830s that the tropics were inherently unhealthy to Europeans.[61] In his article in McCulloch's *Statistical Account of the British Empire* he concluded the mortality of an English soldier increased with each step he took from his native climate, until in the West Indies a soldier twenty-eight years of age stood as great a risk of dying as an Englishman of eighty living at home.[62] Farr's work for the two royal commissions had forced him to consider this subject again in more detail. In a series of papers he summarized the commission's findings for the Statistical Society and for the London and Berlin meetings of the International Statistical Congress.[63]

His study of the Army returns and his experiences in dealing with Nightingale's circle caused him to abandon his pessimism about military service in the tropics. As he explained to Florence Nightingale in February 1863 when he sent her his part of the Indian Sanitary Commission Report, "I entered upon the subject in gloom; but the air brightened on the way, & I now leave it with gladness—as I see that the evils which we dreaded might be dissipated—that the English army may live in health in India— that the blessings of health may be conferred upon the people—& that the

English race may be established around its ancient seats in the tropics."[64]

The commission echoed such optimism and recommended a series of reforms in sanitation, barracks and hospital construction, diet and water supply, site selection, and discipline, and the formation in each presidency of a regional sanitary commission.[65] Farr told Nightingale that they would do some good in India if a national system of medical relief were established for all cases and casts, and if good annual sanitary reports for India brought the state of health in India routinely under the eyes, or perhaps, he punned, under the nose, of the Secretary of State.[66] In the face of stiff criticism from India, Farr stood by his recommendation for regular and complete statistical reporting, including weekly reports for large cities "on the London plan" and concluded, "I want the thing started all over Europe—& America."[67]

Rumors of an attack by the Indian authorities had reached Nightingale's ears by November of 1863. She wrote Farr to warn him to be prepared to defend his statistics. For nearly two years their correspondence was full of the problems of defending the commission's report and encouraging the implementation of its recommendations. In the face of this criticism Farr counseled calmness. "Let us wait, & keep our powder dry," he told her November 24, 1863.

We are not going to fire in the air—like people frightened out of their wits.

Let them point out our "mistakes," & if they are mistakes—we will admit them freely: but shake our foundations—or blow down our walls—the fellows cannot.[68]

With prompting from Nightingale, Farr eventually prepared an answer to the Indian government's criticism of the commission's statistics to assist the home government in answering questions in Parliament.[69] The Indian officials argued the present rate of general mortality among the Indian troops was more nearly 20 per 1,000 rather than 69 per 1,000 as the commission had reported. They argued that the period for which the commission gathered its data, 1816–1856, included extraordinary events, warfare and cholera pandemics, which ought to have been excluded. Farr and his defenders replied that the low rate the Indian government reported was for a single year, 1863, and that during the following year the mortality had climbed to its more ordinary level. Even if one excluded the deaths in years of epidemics or war, the mortality of the Army was much in excess of what it should be for such a group of men.

The Mortality of Hospitals: Farr, Nightingale, and the Medical Establishment

Farr and his associates were able to vindicate the conclusions of the Indian Sanitary Commission. He had much more difficulty with another, nearly contemporary, controversy which resulted from his collaboration with Florence Nightingale. This dispute coalesced around the third edition of her *Notes on Hospitals* (1863). In the course of the ensuing discussion Farr was brought, much to his disadvantage, into battle against the London hospital surgeons and John Simon's colleagues.

Unlike army mortality, which had drawn little of his attention prior to his cooperation with Nightingale, the mortality of hospitals was a topic Farr had dealt with several times before. As editor of the *British Medical Almanack* he prepared, from materials collected by others, an article in 1836 on hospital statistics.[70] Besides pointing out the value of accurate hospital statistics to the profession and to the public and urging hospital staffs to keep accurate records on a uniform scheme, Farr showed how existing hospital records could be tabulated and what ratios might be profitably calculated. In view of the controversy in 1864 it is of considerable interest to review Farr's approach nearly thirty years earlier. His interest in 1836 was in both mortality and patient costs. In discussing hospital mortality he used three major rates: the percentage of deaths out of the average patient population during a period of 36.5 days, case fatality as a percentage, and days of sickness per death. The first rate is comparable to the one that was so highly disputed in 1864. Not only had Farr used other rates as early as 1836, but he recognized that a number of factors besides the physical environment might contribute to the higher mortality of the large urban hospitals. Among these were forces which selected more severe cases for urban hospitals. The figures for the average number of days of sickness per death suggested to Farr that provincial city hospitals such as Leeds, Manchester, and Birmingham accepted more serious cases than the county infirmaries. He explicitly denied that hospital mortality was a complete measure of utility. "Let it not for a moment be supposed that those are always the most useful institutions in which the mortality is lowest; the contrary is often the case."[71] He did state, however, his belief that the metropolitan hospitals were inferior, as institutions of healing, to the best managed hospitals in the provincial cities.

We have already seen that Farr's first independent statistical articles were based upon a combing of hospital and asylum records.[72] In these 1837 articles he showed that such records could be used to produce sickness or survivorship tables, and he suggested that such tables might be used to assess the effectiveness of therapy. He also tried, without great success, to determine the quality of care of the insane in the English county asylums by comparing figures for mortality and average duration of confinement. These studies had made him aware of the inadequacies of the record keeping of British hospitals. Through his work on the Statistical Society's Committee on Hospital Statistics (1840–1844) he tried to initiate improvements.[73] The committee campaigned for the keeping of hospital statistics on a uniform scheme which would permit comparative studies. It made recommendations and tried to initiate change by taking two censuses of the patient population of the London hospitals.

The reports of the Statistical Society Committee reflect two axioms about hospital statistics that would become fundamental in the statistical work of Farr and subsequently of Nightingale. First, the classification of diseases and deaths recommended for hospital statistics was based on the official nosology Farr had drawn up for the registrar general. Second, the rate of mortality for hospitals was calculated not on the number of cases treated but on the average patient population. The reason for the first position is not difficult to surmise. Farr consistently recommended the G.R.O. nosology for all works in vital statistics. This demand appeared in discussions of widely ranging subjects from international statistical cooperation to the reports of the British Army. He believed this nosology was the best available for statistical purposes. In addition, since it was being successfully used for the mortality statistics of English civilians, any extension of its use would facilitate easy comparison. The Committee on Hospital Statistics did in fact use the official nosology to report the cases enumerated in the London hospitals.[74]

The second principle, the calculation of hospital mortality on the average patient population, marks a narrowing of Farr's perspective. In understanding this change, we must recall that at this time Farr was studying vital statistics and actuary principles and was formulating a number of his basic ideas. By 1837 he seems to have decided that hospital mortality must be calculated by means consistent with those used to determine the mortality of the general population. We have already described how he understood the rate of mortality.[75] In explaining how mortality was calculated, he was careful to insist that mortality was not the ratio of deaths to lives but rather the ratio of deaths to years of life. The amount of life at risk was the proper denominator, and this value depended on both the number of lives and the time. He typically asked his reader to imagine a group of people living in isolation in such conditions that each person who died or left was immediately replaced. In such a case it was easy to see that the denominator for the rate of mortality would be the number of persons constantly in the group, that is to say the average population, and not the total number of individuals who had been for some time group members. The Statistical Society's committee used similar illustrations in explaining how it calculated the mortality for diseases in the London hospitals.[76] The reader was to imagine separate hospitals for each disease in which a new case immediately replaced each death. The hospital for consumption would have to have ninety-five beds (the number constantly sick from consumption according to the hospital census) and would experience 342 deaths during a year (the number of deaths from consumption occurring in the London hospitals as recorded in the Registrar General's *Third Annual Report*.) Simple division produced a rate of mortality for consumption in the London hospitals of 360 percent. For all diseases the London hospital mortality was 91 percent. Such figures were produced by computations strictly analogous to those used to compute the mortality for the civil population. That fact offered little comfort, however, to hospital governors or staff members confronted with such enormous figures, figures consistently higher than rates computed on cases treated.

This is not to suggest that the medical profession or even those members on hospital staffs were uniformly opposed to the approach Farr proposed. One London physician, Robert Barnes, published a record of cases of the London and the Metropolitan Free hospitals gathered during August 1855.[77] Barnes used Farr's nosology for classifying cases and was as insistent as Farr on the importance of hospitals keeping and publishing statistics of their cases on a uniform plan. He made no mention of the way Farr proposed to calculate hospital mortality, but the general tone of the article is one of admiration for the statistical endeavors of Farr and his staff.

We see then that by the time Farr met Florence Nightingale, he had experience with and decided opinions about the manner in which hospital statistics should be gathered and that his views were familiar to at least some members of the London medical profession. Their correspondence shows that Farr and Nightingale discussed the problem early in 1857. He sent tables and prepared a memorandum for her on January 5, 1857, which showed the extent to which the mortality in London hospitals exceeded that of hospitals in less populous districts.[78] A month later Farr sent her copies of some of his past work: the two volumes of the *Journal of the Statistical Society of London* containing the reports of the Committee of Hospital Statistics, and the fourth edition of his chapter "Vital Statistics" in McCulloch's volume. We can safely assume that by the spring of that year, Florence Nightingale was well versed in Farr's statistical methods.

Her early inquiries about hospital mortality were made while she was formulating the views eventually published in 1859 as her *Notes on Hospitals*.[79] The work was popular with general audiences, presumably because of its clear, concise style, its air of practical common sense, and the esteem in which its author was held. Sanitation, ward arrangement and management, and hospital construction were the focus of the book. While her views on ward ventilation and her commitment to the sprawling pavilion design were extreme, they were within the mainstream of British opinion at the time.[80] Although she alluded to the importance of good hospital statistics and the defects of existing hospital records, she made very little use of statistics in this first edition. She neither recommended statistical forms or procedures, nor advocated the use of mortality as a test of hospital management. There was no significant criticism from the medical profession.

By 1859 she began to deal more directly with the defects she perceived in hospital statistics and began a campaign for the adoption of a common system of reporting case records and hospital mortality. With Farr's advice she drew up model forms employing the G.R.O.'s nosology to classify cases. Several London hospitals tried these forms, and the spring of 1860 found Nightingale, Sutherland, and Farr going over the returns and discussing improvements in the system.[81] Farr helped advance the project by making her proposals a central topic in the program for the Sanitary Section of the London meeting of the International Statistical Congress July, 1860.[82] The Congress endorsed her plan with slight modifications and directed that forms and recommendations be sent to all member nations. With this advantage she continued to pressure the London hospitals to comply, issuing another popular appeal to the Social Science Association in 1861.[83] For several years the major London hospitals did publish uniform returns.[84] Nightingale's group was especially pleased with the reports issued by St. Bartholomew's with the cooperation of Sir James Paget.[85]

But all was not smooth sailing. Following the congress, the *Medical Times and Gazette* carried strong criticisms of the scheme by John W. Tripe, medical officer of health for Hackney, and by William H. Stone, a registrar in Aberdeenshire.[86] Both authors claimed to support the goals of Nightingale's plan but they found her scheme impractical and faulty on two counts: the length and complexity of the forms, and the use of Farr's nosology. Stone was especially severe on this nosology, which he claimed was too elaborate, and based upon a speculative disease theory. He believed its numerous subdivisions would give a false impression of precision. In addition, his letter was cynical about the value of statistics in medicine and of the principle of classifying diseases. He referred, for example, to the "alluring but illusive phantom of a scientific terminology" and warned against trying to build upon a foundation so confused or idiosyncratic as medical terminology.[87]

Farr defended Nightingale's plan and his nosologies in two letters to the editor.[88] He could point to the experiences of the G.R.O. to illustrate that the proposed forms and classification were practical, and he offered hospital registrars the opportunity to observe their use at his office. He estimated that two men, presumably the registrar and a medical student, could enter 300 cases per hour. While he admitted his nosology was not perfect, he suggested Florence Nightingale had wisely chosen it because it was the best available for sanitary purposes. The recording schemes for the hospitals which these critics favored because of their brevity Farr called confusing, and he reminded his readers that at present English hospitals followed no uniform plan. Stone's cynicism about the principle of classification was answered by an analogy to the natural sciences. Although these sciences study phenomena as complex and resistant to tidy subdivision as human diseases, they are still founded upon systems of classification. He concluded his first letter with a militant call for joining Nightingale, suggesting the critics were raising useless quibbles.

Her arrangements are made, her forms are ready, her troops are at their posts, and she is ready to do battle with the enemy, when her zealous friend boldly asserts that all her positions are bad, that her order of battle is "cumbrous," that, indeed, any scientific classification of an army is worse than useless; besides, he hints, it is perfectly notorious that men in firing do not hit an enemy one time in a hundred—not oftener, in fact, than Doctors hit the truth in their diagnoses, that, consequently, it is perfectly useless to fire at all. . . .[89]

Nightingale dismissed Stone as a "quack" who condemned Farr's nosology without having a better one to put in its place. The objection that the plan would entail too much trouble and labor, she suggested, was merely symptomatic of the reason why the hospitals of England had never issued satisfactory statistics.[90]

Farr effectively answered these critics with analogy and example. Four years later, however, more effective rivals appeared whom Farr could not so easily vanquish. Once again it was his contributions to a Nightingale project that bore the brunt of medical attack. In a letter of November 15, 1862, Nightingale told Farr that she was "sadly & unwillingly" preparing a new, a third, edition of her *Notes on Hospitals*.[91] This reticence, we must presume, grew only from the press of other work. The third edition was longer, more explicit in recommendation, and more critical of existing hospitals. Design, construction, management, and discipline were discussed at length. New in this edition—besides the greater wealth of detail on the physical facilities of hospitals—was the increased attention paid to statistics. Chapter Nine was devoted to statistics. In it Nightingale presented her plan which the Statistical Congress had endorsed as well as forms she had more recently drawn up for recording surgical cases.[92] It was, however, a table she presented in the first chapter that became the focus of the next battle. The table showed the mortality for 106 English hospitals.[93]

This table was drawn from the registrar general's *Twenty-fourth Annual Report* and was part of a study Farr undertook of the mortality in public institutions.[94] It used the census and registration figures for 1861, assuming that the population in an institution on the census day was its mean daily population throughout the year. Mortality rates were calculated on the mean inmate population for all institutions including hospitals. According to this table the mortality of hospitals varied enormously with location. Twenty-four London hospitals had a combined mortality rate of 90.84 percent, twelve hospitals in other large towns had a rate of 83.16 percent, while the rate for twenty-five hospitals in the counties or in provincial towns was only 39.41 percent. "However the great differences in the death rate may be explained," she surmised, "it cannot be denied that the most unhealthy hospitals are those situated within the vast circuit of the metropolis . . . and that by far the most healthy hospitals are those of the smaller country towns."[95]

This conclusion was qualified by several succeeding paragraphs retained from the first edition, in which she explained that mortality by itself was not a reliable measure of the relative sanitary state of hospitals for a variety of reasons, among which were differences in the severity of cases accepted by different hospitals.[96] Some authorities, she conceded, preferred to rely on prevalence of hospital infections. Other experienced observers could detect subtle changes in the condition of patients which revealed that the laws of health were being violated. Despite such disclaimers, the fact remained she had used mortality as a criterion for judging hospitals and had concluded that the hospitals of the metropolis were the most unhealthy in the land.

The critical reaction which followed could have been predicted. The first volley began January 30, 1864, with an anonymous review of abrasive tone in the *Medical Times and Gazette*.[97] It was followed on February 13 by Farr's reply and the editor's comments.[98] In the lead editorial two weeks later the *Lancet* joined the discussion.[99] These writers criticized both Farr's statistics and Nightingale's conclusions. Round two began when the editor of the *Lancet* sent the third edition to Timothy Holmes, assistant surgeon at St. George's Hospital, for comment. Holmes harshly criticized Farr's statistics in two articles, and a bitter controversy ensued in the pages of the *Lancet* and the *Medical Times* in March and April.[100] Farr's statistics had by then become the issue.

The reviewers dealt very carefully with Florence Nightingale. She had a formidable popular reputation and enviable social connections. Farr, of course, had no such advantages. No critic disparaged either her experience or her motives. The journal editors even welcomed her pointed insistence on sanitation, ventilation, and site selection, which they interpreted as a vindication of informed medical opinion, strong enough to jolt lethargic hospital governors.

Nightingale was criticized on two counts: her dogmatic anticontagionist stance, and her use of Farr's hospital statistics. In the third edition, as in the first, she not only produced the standard anticontagionist illustrations, but also ridiculed the very idea of contagion, a belief she suggested was ignorant and superstitious.[101] She was cynical of the practice of isolating so-called "infectious" diseases. These, she claimed, might be safely mingled in well-arranged wards. By the early 1860s such views were becoming dated. The *Medical Times* reviewer merely said such views "if not promulgated by a lady, would require rough treatment."[102] The *Lancet* more coyly marveled how Nightingale could hold such views and compared her to a brave soldier who refused to think about, and who even scorned, the dangers he had passed unharmed.[103] The editor found her comments neither convincing nor worthy of further discussion. His counterpart at the *Medical Times* branded her opinions as "just that half-view of the truth which characterizes the old anti-contagionists."[104] He argued for a more contemporary position, a compromise between contagionism and anticontagionism.

Despite its length, the dispute over Farr's statistics rested on only a few points of difference. First, the critics, for the most part members of the medical or surgical staffs of the London hospitals, denied that the mortality of the metropolitan hospitals could fairly be compared to that of the provincial hospitals. Selection processes were at work, much to the disadvantage of the London institutions. Metropolitan hospitals, they argued, were filled with more serious cases, had a faster turnover of patients, and served a population in poorer general health than did the provincial hospitals. Holmes was delighted when J. Burney Yeo, a surgeon at the Hampshire County Hospital wrote in support of this argument.[105] Nightingale had anticipated this objection. William Augustus Guy had lately used selection in explaining the increased mortality at King's College Hospital in recent years. Graduates, he claimed, referred their most difficult cases to the hospital with the result that "the rate of mortality of an hospital is mainly determined by the reputation of its hospital staff amongst the public at large and amongst its own pupils."[106] In her third edition Nightingale responded in characteristic form. The claim had "no other practical meaning than this:—that a greater number of people go there to die next year, because so many have died there this year, a principle equally applicable in private practice, and according to which, the physician or surgeon who loses the largest percentage of cases is the man most worthy of confidence."[107] Her reply, the *Medical Times* reviewer claimed, was "incorrect, illogical, and impulsive" and made sarcasm stand in place of argument.[108] The editor, more politely, suggested her work contained mistakes and was "written in haste and left uncorrected."[109]

The second major point of controversy over Farr's statistics was his method of calculating hospital mortality. It brought wholesale denials. The *Medical Times* reviewer compared it to the division of 100 apples by 15 red herrings.[110] He denied that mortality could teach anything about the way hospitals were managed. Holmes, in the *Lancet*, claimed Farr's conclusions about the relative salubrity of large and small institutions were patently absurd. "No one who has any practical knowledge of the institutions comprised in his list [Farr's table of hospital mortality which Nightingale used] can fail to see that there must be a fallacy somewhere."[111] That fallacy lay, he argued, in using as the denominator for hospital death rates the average daily patient population and not the number of patients treated during the year. He offered as counter-examples pairs of hospitals in various locations in which the case fatality rate was higher in the smaller institution than in the larger. Applying Farr's procedure to individual wards of a hypothetical hospital, Holmes argued that if Farr's method were used the surgical or accident ward would invariably have a higher mortality than the cancer ward, even though cancer was usually fatal. The reason lay in the fact that many more cases were treated in the surgical ward. He denied completely the validity of Farr's statistics in judging existing hospitals. "I regard Dr. Farr's statistics as being utterly delusive; and if these are the whole foundation for the assertion that hospitals do harm instead of good, I should not hesitate to characterize that assertion as reckless, and inconsistent with the facts."[112]

The vehemence of the critics and the anger of Farr's replies can best be understood if this skirmish is seen as a reflection of a larger conflict within the medical world of London. Farr was a known critic of large urban hospitals, and he shared with Florence Nightingale extreme views on hospital construction and management and a nagging suspicion that most patients would be better off at home.[113] Any critical comparison he made of hospitals was likely to be regarded as an attack.

In interpreting his tables of mortality for public institutions in the *Twenty-fourth Annual Report* he made just such a comparison. His tables for prisons, workhouses, lunatic asylums, and hospitals were drawn up ostensibly to permit the correction of local mortality rates for deaths in these institutions. The plan was an important adjunct to his studies of the mortality in urban districts, and his mode of computing the death rate was reasonable for this purpose. What the critics seized upon was the conclusion of his letter, in which he suggested that at present the large hospitals were less healthy than smaller ones. Most of them ignored his final paragraph.

In the meantime it is evident from the Tables that the mortality of the sick who are treated in the large general hospitals of large towns is twice as great as the mortality of the sick who are treated in small hospitals in small towns.

It remains to be seen whether the mortality in small hospitals is not twice as great as the mortality of the same diseases in patients who are treated in clean cottages.

Should this turn out to be the case, the means of realizing the advantages of the *hospital system*, without its disadvantages, will then be sought and probably found, as the problem is not insoluble.[114]

The issue of the health of the metropolitan hospitals had recently become particularly sensitive, as the debate over the relocating of St. Thomas's Hospital brought sanitarians and the London hospital staff members to loggerheads. The same issues of the *Medical Times* that carried the discussion of Farr's hospital mortality rates also printed a lengthy exchange between the medical sanitarian Benjamin Ward Richardson, who had used mortality figures to argue that lithotomy was more safely carried out in the Norwich Infirmary than in the metropolitan hospitals, and the London surgeons Holmes and Henry Thompson.[115] In this dispute Holmes pointed out that Richardson had used his evidence in testimony before the Court of Chancery in relation to the selection of a new site for St. Thomas's; hence, Holmes claimed, it was of immediate practical importance to clarify Richardson's claims of the relative health of hospitals.[116]

Nightingale was deeply interested in the St. Thomas's affair. She was in this decade advising various charities on hospital design. Moreover her ties to St. Thomas's were especially close. She had considerable influence among the hospital governors and actively supported the idea of building a completely new hospital when the new London Bridge Railway Station threatened the environs of the old. She and Farr both wanted to see a surburban site chosen, and they criticized the location that was selected, the southern bank of the Thames, opposite the Houses of Parliament.[117]

But in this affair Nightingale had an able opponent in John Simon, medical officer of the Privy Council, former surgeon and present lecturer on pathology at St. Thomas's. Simon waged a masterful campaign in the press and behind the scenes to obtain the central London site and to influence the plans, other than the architecture, of the new hospital.[118] In the wake of this controversy Simon appointed Dr. John Seyer Bristowe of St. Thomas's and Holmes to make a major report on British and continental hospitals.[119] There appeared suddenly a second authority on hospitals, a rival to Nightingale and her sanitary junta.

She disliked and distrusted Simon and viewed Holmes and Bristowe as his henchmen. When she caught wind of their investigation she warned Farr that according to her sources the report then still unpublished was to contain many serious errors, that it would reach conclusions opposite to those drawn from Farr's statistics, and that Bristowe and Holmes were novices in investigations of this type.[120] When these "novices" dared not only disagree with the conclusions Nightengale's group had reached but criticized Farr's statistics, one of the group's primary sources of evidence, strong response was called for. Farr came to believe a conspiracy was at work. He wrote to Florence Nightingale April 9, 1864, sending her Holmes's two "fierce epistles" and his own reply. He explained that Holmes was put up to the job by Simon with a view to prepare the way for the forthcoming report on hospitals. He condemned what he regarded as Simon's shabby dealings.

> The employment of such men—for such a purpose—& the use made of the infor-
> mation so collected—is altogether disgraceful.
>
> Our purpose must go to prevent them stopping the improvements in Hospi-
> tals—which we may expect to arise—from your Book & from the progress of
> General Hygiene.[121]

Farr's response in the *Lancet* was angry and haughty.[122] He accused Simon, Holmes, and Bristowe of using the reviews of Nightingale's book and Holmes's attack on his statistics to influence opinion in the St. Thomas's affair and to discredit or minimize concern for hospital sanita-tion. He criticized the conduct of the campaign, which he compared to picking one's cards from several packs to which one's opponents had no access. He was referring to the use of selected examples from the report in discussions with authorities, while the full report was still unpublished. He argued that Holmes's examples were incorrect or irrelevant. The com-parison of the two wards in the same hospital was rejected since his figures were for groups of general hospitals only. In that case such differences in the types of cases involved would not arise. He answered Holmes with some examples of his own, described his opponent as incompetent in sta-tistics and ignorant of the principles of hygiene, and in a one-sentence postscript declined any further controversy with Holmes on statistics.

Both Holmes and Bristowe wrote to the *Lancet* to protest the tone of Farr's letter.[123] They claimed a desire only for scholarly discussion and denied that their study was undertaken to prove foregone conclusions or that any collusion had occurred in the St. Thomas's affair. The contro-versy in the *Lancet* ended with Farr's reply, in which he said he would be glad to end the proposed controversy and to elaborate on his methods at a future time when he was less busy.[124] Bristowe fired the closing shot in a letter of judgment and able example. He cleverly showed that if Farr had reversed his perspective and had calculated hospital recovery rates by his method, the figures would range from 899 percent to 953 percent.[125]

Farr had left himself open to much of this criticism by his glib com-ment in the registrar general's *Twenty-fourth Annual Report* and by his too comprehensive defense of Nightingale's sanitary pronouncements. He proved to be no match in controversy to Holmes or Bristowe, who may have had Simon's coaching. Recent historians have been impressed by the cogency of Holmes's and Bristowe's criticism.[126] They have tended to adopt implicitly the bias of Farr's opponents, to misread Farr's purposes, and to miss the fact that his method, if subject to question in this applica-tion, was part of a reasonable approach of broader dimensions. This is a point Bristowe himself conceded.[127]

The St. Thomas's affair aside, the substantial differences between the two camps can be reduced to the question: What, precisely, should hospital mortality statistics measure? Farr's critics were members of medical or surgical staffs of the London hospitals. They were disturbed by his imputing excessively high rates of mortality to their institutions. The method of computation they favored calculated the mortality on the number of cases treated. Not only did this method give for the London hospitals rates drastically lower than Farr's, but it also measured that aspect of hospital life they found most interesting, the success or failure of therapy.

Farr certainly understood the objections raised against his approach. As we have seen, he calculated hospital mortality rates in 1836 by using both cases treated annually and average patient population as denominators. He also pointed out that certain processes of selection worked to raise the mortality rates of urban hospitals. Nothing he said in 1864 indicates that he denied either the role of selection or that he minimized the importance of the knowledge and skill of the medical staff. He argued, however, that these factors had limited effect. He reminded his readers that few patients actually died on the operating table and that surgeons commonly refused to operate on the most hopeless cases.[128] Sanitarian that he was, Farr looked to the hospital environment, especially to the atmosphere of the wards, in explaining great differences in mortality. To measure the salubrity of the hospital as an environment for treatment and recovery, he needed to know the number of lives constantly exposed to its hazards. From his perspective, one hospital stay of twelve months was statistically equivalent to twelve cases of one month each. In either case one year of life was at risk. Clearly the proper mortality rate for this purpose, leaving aside for the moment the question of whether this be the purpose we might choose today, was a rate which had as its denominator the mean population at risk over the year. Farr's method was, in fact, perfectly correct for the purposes he had in mind.

But such purposes change, and when that happens a stubborn champion of a former goal can appear a ludicrous figure. In the early twentieth century some of the Farr's admirers in the British medical profession were embarrassed by his collaboration with Florence Nightingale and his spirited defense of her views on hospitals. Sir Arthur Newsholme felt obliged to remind his audience of the horrible conditions of hospitals before Lister in explaining how Nightingale could insist that people were better treated at home than in most hospitals, or how Farr "like other able men of her generation was commandeered to provide the necessary data for her active and persistent advocacy of reform in hospitals as elsewhere."[129]

The opposing sides in the 1864 controversy were divided over more than simply the condition of hospitals. During these years medical advocates of preventive medicine were wrenching control of the public health movement from the older lay and medical sanitarians. The new leaders, led by John Simon, were skeptical of the narrow sanitary program and placed greater faith in the value of curative medicine and in specific medical or scientific measures, such as vaccination and, eventually, the microscopic and chemical examination of drinking water.

In the early 1860s Farr's position was equivocal. His stance in the hospital debate was tempered not only by his sincere support of the type of reforms Florence Nightingale advocated, but also by his pique at Simon's success as leader of English public health. Farr complained in August of 1858 that his liberal cooperation with Simon and his associates, who were just beginning their epidemiological research, had been illiberally repaid.[130] It was Farr who had suggested the water field study in South London during the 1854 cholera epidemic, yet it was Simon who got all the credit. More vexing was the fact that Greenhow used with scant acknowledgment in his *Papers Relating to the Sanitary Condition of the People of England* the occupational figures Farr had been collecting for a major study. Not only did this work not measure up to Farr's standards, but its author had the poor taste to say jokingly to Farr that he was going to take the wind out of his sails. Farr told Nightingale this confidentially, adding he believed Greenhow meant well and that it was not unnatural for men to overrate their own and to underrate others' work. Over a decade later he complained of the tender way in which his critics treated Simon and the coverage the medical press gave those critics.[131]

Farr had no doubts about Simon's ability. Quite early in their correspondence, Farr answered Nightingale's criticism of Simon by reminding her that although he had not yet done much to improve public health, Simon was nonetheless a man of ability, from whom better things could be expected in the future.[132] Judging from Nightingale's comments about Simon to Farr, the gulf between Farr and Simon began to narrow in the later sixties. There is evidence to suggest that the two men met cordially to discuss private affairs after Simon's retirement from his medical officership.[133]

Nightingale was suspicious of curative medicine and medical science.[134] She shared none of Farr's respect for Simon. She wrote to Farr in 1866 when she sensed that her colleague was increasingly impressed with the medical officer.[135] She was "entirely recalcitrant" about Simon's merits. "Mr. Simon is an arrangement of the Privy Council for making the bigger Body, which is a big quack, appear (to the lesser Bodies, who are little quacks,) to know something." He and other doctors were bringing medicine down from a profession to a trade with a product to sell. "Now you will say I am a Nuisance—& come under the Nuisances Removal Act. And Mr. Simon, if you write to him, will gladly put it in force against me.

But I shall have been the only nuisance Mr. Simon will ever have removed."[136]

She was not content merely to complain. It is well known that she plotted against her rival. She arranged to have Sutherland appointed to the commission for the London meeting of the Statistical Congress "in order to hedge Simon."[137] During the dispute over the moving of St. Thomas's Hospital she wrote to Robert Lowe, and tried unsuccessfully to undermine Simon.[138] Eleven years later, in 1871, when the central health agency was remodeled, Nightingale and Edwin Chadwick waged another campaign against Simon and poured out their complaints against theoretical medicine and the recent innovations in the state health program into the ear of James Stansfield, president of the Local Government Board.[139] While Farr approved of the appointment of Sutherland, it is extremely unlikely he would have approved of covert activity against Simon.[140]

The evolution of Farr's ideas was, if anything, serving to divide him from Nightingale's inner circle, and it probably made him more sympathetic to Simon. The crucial change most likely did not occur until the 1866 cholera epidemic, by which time Farr, as we have seen, had become a convert to contagionism and was fast becoming sympathetic to a germ theory of disease. But even prior to that date he expressed ideas antithetical to some of Nightingale's. He recognized that human biology imposed limits on sanitary reform.[141] His letter prompted her to add a cryptic note, "He has given it up." Although he agreed with her that quarantine was unjustified, he had by the time he met her come to assign a fairly large role to contagion.[142] Their differences over disease theory are nicely illustrated in a pair of letters. In discussing quarantine Farr denied completely its ability to keep zymotic disease out of a country which had neglected sanitation, but he had become convinced that for certain diseases a "leaven is generated which *under certain conditions* will leaven the whole lump."[143] He called both the contagionists and the anticontagionists "fanatics of the most desperate description," and he asked her not to "Chadwickize" and to try to be scientific. She would have none of his moderation and compromise:

Either your "contagionists" are in the right & then they are not fanatical—or your "non-contagionists" are in the right & *they* are not fanatical—*Both* cannot be fanatical any more than both can be in the right.

Quarantine follows logically & inevitably on "contagion"—as Sanitary measures on non-contagion—

Farther than this, I do not venture to argue with you—because, as you say, I am not scientific. Neither do I quote the opinion of those men (whom you think I worship) such as Chadwick, for the same reason—he is not scientific—I only modestly & *really* humbly say, I never saw a fact adduced in favor of contagion which would bear scientific enquiry. And I could name to you men whom *you* would acknowledge as scientific who place "contagion" on the same footing as witch-craft & other superstitions—[144]

Farr never wavered in his commitment to sanitary reform, but as he accepted an increasing body of new ideas about etiology and pathology, agreement with Florence Nightingale must have become more difficult. She never modified her rigid stance on this matter.[145] Judging from their correspondence, the collaboration between Farr and Nightingale reached a peak in 1864 or 1865 and tapered off rapidly thereafter with a brief revival in 1871, centered on childbirth mortality statistics and her book *Introductory Notes on Lying-in Institutions*. There were probably other reasons for this waning of cooperation than theoretical disagreement. Farr was increasingly preoccupied with issues that did not so immediately concern her, such as the reform of taxation and the pursuit of anthropometry. Also, in the early 1870s his health began to fail.

They continued on friendly terms and exchanged letters until his death. She did not forget her old friend. In the bitter disappointment in his bid to become registrar general, she offered him support.[146] She wrote a warm letter of sympathy to Florence Farr, her namesake, at his death.

I mourned for you, & our loss, & rejoiced for your Father, & our friend, who is now set free to bless new worlds.
How much he must enjoy! I could write so much about him.[147]

EIGHT

FARR AND THE LEDGERS OF DEATH

ASSESSMENTS OF HIS USE OF MORTALITY DATA

William Farr resigned his post at the General Register Office in January 1880 and retired completely from public life. He left in bitter disappointment, for he had been passed over in the filling of the vacancy left by George Graham's retirement the year before. Formal tributes followed in due course.[1] The Council of the Statistical Society of London voted Farr special thanks for his contributions to the society and to the government. The British Medical Association presented its gold medal, and the government awarded him the decoration, Companion of the Bath.

Farr was superannuated at £800 per year, which was his base salary, less the £300 personal allowance he had been granted by the government since 1874, and less the £30 annual fee from London University.[2] His investment losses had caused him some financial anxiety, and he was especially worried about the security of his three unmarried daughters.[3] To mark their appreciation for his work and to ease his financial plight Farr's friends organized a testimonial fund in his behalf in March 1880.[4] Donations were collected from prominent figures in public life and from members of the medical and scientific communities. After his death and following two large donations from the government and from Florence Nightingale the fund was closed at £1724. As Farr had requested, the funds were used to support Farr's daughters.

At the time of Farr's retirement and even recently the government has been castigated for not appointing Farr registrar general. In 1965 M. W. Flinn believed "it is to the discredit of Victorian governments that he [Farr] was never appointed to the nominal headship of the department that owed everything to his genius. . . ."[5] While rules of fair play might lead one to this conclusion, long established practices worked against it. Graham's successor, the man appointed in place of Farr, was Sir Brydges Henniker, an ex-captain of the Royal Horse Guards, a brother-in-law of a cabinet member, and by birth, marriage, and life-style a member of the British landed gentry without medical or statistical qualifications.[6] Posts such as registrar general had traditionally been given as political spoils.

While by the last third of the century the patronage system was giving way to more competitive appointment schemes, technical experts were not major beneficiaries. The British government preferred professional civil servants, a preference reflected in the choice of registrars general well into the twentieth century.[7] Farr's status as an expert on vital statistics did not therefore automatically recommend him for the position.

Farr's poor health was the reason the government gave for passing him by. It was an answer to criticism, but it had substance. Farr was then seventy-two years old and his health was beginning to fail. Soon after his retirement both his physical and mental faculties declined rapidly. He lived as an invalid for another three years, until April 14, 1883. But even given robust health, Farr may not have been an ideal candidate for a major administrative post. "He was a student, somewhat forgetful and absent-minded, rather than a man of business talents," concluded his biographer in the *Dictionary of National Biography*.[8] To this we might add that Farr was stubborn and could be argumentative. He wrote often in an emotionally charged style. The arts of compromise and conciliation might well have been beyond him.

While Farr's pension was not especially generous, the government had in no way mistreated him. His salary had been raised above the statutory limit during his last years in the G.R.O. At the time he retired he was earning £1130 annually, only £70 less than his chief. While at his retirement John Simon was earning the substantial salary of £2,000, Simon's permanent medical inspectors, men who admittedly might have other sources of professional income, received a government salary of only £800 annually.[9] Farr's salary was certainly not out of line with those of other medical men employed in the civil service. Furthermore, the decoration "C.B." was an acknowledgment of special services. It was a recognition denied George Graham.[10]

It seems then as if Farr could not possibly be portrayed as a martyr to official callousness and ingratitude. But this is precisely what the spokesmen of organized medicine attempted to do. For a brief period in 1880 his retirement became a *cause célèbre* in the profession. Medical journals complained first of his being passed over, next about the delay in awarding him a pension, and finally about the size of that pension. On January 10, Ernest Hart, editor of the *British Medical Journal* and militant champion of the profession, called for resolutions on Farr's behalf from every medical society and corporation in the country.[11] Numerous societies responded. The medical press recorded the action, and the resolutions were forwarded to Farr and to the government.[12] The profession also found spokesmen in Parliament, among them Lyon Playfair, who brought Farr's case to the attention of both houses in February.[13]

As it became clear that the government was prepared to act no more swiftly and generously in this matter than law and custom demanded, medical assessments of Farr's worth swelled to enormous proportions. Alfred Carpenter, president of the Council of the British Medical Association outdid all others. There was "no other single person" Carpenter proclaimed,"—not even Lord Beaconsfield [the Prime Minister]—who had done so much good for the world at large as Dr. Farr. . . . Had he been in any political position, he would have been called to the House of Lords as a matter of course; but no medical man was ever called to the House of Lords, and it was not likely that he would be."[14] Nor was the title "Companion of the Bath" sufficient recognition. The medical journalists claimed, "We are no more grateful for the acknowledgment than for the ugly hall-marking sometimes graciously bestowed on pure gold."[15]

The reaction of the profession was grossly exaggerated and out of all proportion to events. Farr had been, it is true, an active supporter of the B.M.A. and had served as president of its Section on State Medicine. But he was somewhat outside the mainstream of the profession by 1880, and he had quarreled more than once with both local health officers and with the central medical authorities. Generous editorials in the leading medical journals might have sufficed to mark the occasion of his retirement.

His retirement was seized as a convenient means for voicing larger complaints against the government. At issue in particular was the policy of the Local Government Board. Since the administrative reorganization of 1871–1872, Simon's office and the G.R.O. had been placed under the supervision of the new Local Government Board. As a result of the merger and the Board's internal policies, Simon lost much of his old autonomy, and the medical profession some of its initiative in public policy.[16] After several years of struggle with the Poor Law administrators who were now his superiors, Simon resigned in 1876. He and other public-minded medical men believed the Poor Law authorities were hostile to medicine and were intent on dismantling the nascent apparatus of state medicine.

The case of William Farr seemed particularly offensive to the doctors because until the time of his appointment Henniker had been the private secretary to George Sclater-Booth, second president of the Local Government Board. The first articles on this topic in the medical journals pointed out most clearly Henniker's connections with the rival authority, and saw the appointment as "further evidence of the singular fatality which appears to have attended the ill-starred connection between Poor-law and Public-health administration" and of the "repressive policy adopted towards the sanitary and medical department by the central authorities of Poor-law administration."[17]

This conflict of organized medicine with the Local Government Board is reason for caution in reviewing contemporaries' assessments of Farr at the time of his retirement. But even making ample allowance for extravagant claims born of this campaign for recognition, it is clear that Farr's professional colleagues accepted him as the leading authority on vital statistics and as a prominent member of the public health enterprise. Leoni Levi spoke for the Statistical Society at Farr's death. He ranked Farr with Quetelet and termed them the "foremost lights" of the International Statistical Congress.[18] William T. Gairdner, professor of medicine at Glasgow, repeated before the Sanitary Institute the assessment of Farr that he had made in lectures to medical students on sanitary science in 1861.[19] He believed Farr's work was as important to sanitary science and preventive medicine as Harvey's had been to physiology or Lavoisier's to chemistry. In its obituary *The British Medical Journal* claimed that Farr was one of the major forces in the public health movement. "It is not too much to say that the figures collected by him, the principles which he deduced from them, and the accomplished skill with which he impressed the doctrines of sanitary law upon statesmen and upon the public mind, have done more to forward the progress of sanitation throughout the world than the labours, perhaps, of any other man who could be named. Farr and John Simon stand side by side as the foremost figures of their time among the heroes of preventive medicine. . ."[20]

Despite the fact that Farr's methods and conclusions were widely emulated and became, in fact, an intimate part of Victorian health policy, there wss an undercurrent of criticism that is historically significant. In the early years of civil registration criticism dwelt on details. As we have observed, organized medicine supported the passage of civil registration in the thirties and believed that valuable information could be derived from the returns of the causes of death. The criticisms that were raised concerned the defects in the registration system and details of Farr's nosology. Farr not only acknowledged the problems of collecting vital statistics, but he took part in the efforts that led to modest reforms in the system. The zymotic class was the focus of the medical criticism of the official nosology. While this classification and Farr's remarks about the cause of disease which accompanied it offered a reasonable synthesis of known information and a rational basis for health reform, some doctors found it both too speculative in concept and impractical in application. The more critical also recognized that statistics based on such a broad category might obscure important differences among the zymotic diseases. The investigations John Simon either sponsored or encouraged typically used mortality rates calculated for single diseases or for a small group of diseases similar in their clinical course or morbid anatomy. Edward Headlam Greenhow's famous mortality study of 1856 foreshadowed the change in approach the Privy Council doctors would adopt in using the registration materials.[21]

This change in approach suggests the maturing of public medicine in Britain. Simon's administration gave much fuller reign to medical expertise. At the local level medical officers of health had increased both in number and in self confidence. By the late fifties some of these officers from resort towns or industrial cities began to challenge the official interpretation of death rates. They were soon joined by the staff members of the London hospitals. Both groups were agitated by the ranking, according to mortality, of their districts or institutions in works intended for the public: the daily press and Florence Nightingale's works on hospitals. These medical critics made the most of the flaws in the methods of gathering the official figures. They also raised several important methodological problems, the most important of which was the role of selection in determining the rates for urban districts or large city hospitals.

Such objections were not new to Farr. In some cases he had tried to come to terms with them some two decades before his critics spoke. Perhaps the most striking examples are found in the *Fifth Annual Report*, and in the *Supplements* to the *Twenty-fifth* and to the *Thirty-fifth Annual Reports*. In these volumes Farr illustrated how life tables and life-table death rates could be used to compare correctly the mortality and the longevity of difference populations. He dealt with less difficult objections as well. He warned repeatedly that municipal and registration district boundaries did not coincide. For that reason the death rates for districts with town names might not represent accurately the mortality of those towns. He also tried to take account of the disturbance caused by hospitals and other welfare institutions. As early as 1849 Farr explained how to correct the crude mortality rates of the London districts for deaths which occurred in hospitals and work houses.[22] His investigation of the mortality of public institutions fifteen years later, the study from which Florence Nightingale derived her ranking of hospitals, was undertaken to permit this correction of urban death rates.[23] In discussing the relationship of density to mortality in the seventies, Farr excluded the metropolitan districts precisely because of the disturbance caused by deaths in these public institutions.[24] There is certainly justice to Noel Humphreys's claim of 1874 that these urban critics of the official mortality rates were latecomers who had only begun to perceive problems more experienced statisticians had come to terms with years earlier.[25]

Farr did not deal as effectively with the objections raised by the hospital staff members. His association with Florence Nightingale in this case was to his disadvantage and made him the brunt of the doctor's attack on external critics. But more was at stake than a dispute over the health of urban hospitals, a dispute sharpened by the plans to relocate St. Thomas's. Behind the debate over how hospital mortality should be computed lay more fundamental differences in attitudes about hospital management and about the causes of high mortality rates. Farr adopted the older position of the sanitary reformers whose major interest was the effects on human health of the physical environment. For this purpose his statistical approach was very reasonable. His method had the added advantage of producing rates which could be easily used to correct mortality figures for urban districts. His critics assumed a more clinical perspective, emphasizing the role of therapy over that of the environment. It seems, then, that although the parties in this controversy argued over means, they really differed over goals. For that reason some criticism of Farr's hospital statistics was really wide of the mark.

To appreciate Farr's work, especially his ability to exercise reasonable judgment while using data he knew was imperfect, one need only notice the recommendations or approaches offered by his critics. Some of these men let the discovery of a single objection to the G.R.O.'s statistics lead them to use methods that ignored other, equally serious, pitfalls. Greenhow's 1858 investigation used a more sensitive classification of the causes of death, but it ignored differences in the age composition of the districts compared, and it assumed that the entire population of a district was engaged in the district's predominant occupation.[26] Farr pointed out these weaknesses in a letter to Florence Nightingale, and he claimed his planned study of occupational mortality, for which he had been collecting the data Greenhow used, would have taken account of differences in age compositions.[27] Other critics were led onto even less solid ground. The cogency of Rumsey's critiques comes into question when one reads beyond the criticism to his specific recommendations. His attitudes begin to seem like stubborn and simple faith in raw facts, when he expresses suspicion of all methods of extrapolation and when he fails to appreciate the statistical advantages of a life table. In 1866 he offered the impractical suggestion of holding an annual national census and suggested that in comparing the health of districts investigators should return to the use of the mean age at death, a thoroughly discredited index of salubrity.[28] Rumsey probably exaggerated the consequences of the defects in registration, at least as practiced in the 1860s. Farr complained, with some justice, of the "exaggerations & rash assertions on subject which he [Rumsey] ought to understand."[29]

Despite what this criticism suggests about the development of social medicine, its importance as a criterion for judging Farr's work can be overemphasized. The appropriateness of Farr's methods can be judged from the respect they have commanded from twentieth-century experts in public health and epidemiology. Those working in the early part of this century regarded themselves as Farr's heirs. Sir Arthur Newsholme recalled that, when he first became a local medical officer of health, he turned to Farr's reports to learn the nature of vital statistics and from this study grew his own book, *Elements of Vital Statistics*, of 1889.[30] Newsholme went on to become an expert on infant mortality and on the epidemiology of tuberculosis and to serve as medical officer of the Local Government Board. Newsholme's enthusiasm for Farr never waned. He praised Farr's humanity and reformist stance, called him a chief architect of public health administration, and repeated the comparison of Farr's work with Harvey's in physiology and Lavoisier's in Chemistry.[31] Major Greenwood, the prominent twentieth-century epidemiologist, was only slightly less enthusiastic. He considered Farr one of Britain's four greatest statisticians, and described the methods Farr devised for using vital data as "the most valuable single instrument of social-medical research our national armoury contains."[32] A third prominent early twentieth-century technical expert who had profound respect for Farr's work was John Brownlee, director of statistics of Britain's Medical Research Council. It was he who rediscovered Farr's study of the cattle plague and evaluated Farr's method of predicting the course of that epidemic.[33] Some of his warmest praise came in a publication in which he dealt with a problem that had drawn criticism during Farr's career, the use of mortality rates in measuring health.[34] He admired especially Farr's *Supplement to the Thirty-fifth Annual Report* in which he found represented every major method since deemed useful in health statistics.[35] Experts in social medicine like Newsholme, Greenwood, and Brownlee discovered in Farr the beginning of the research tradition in which they worked. They were pleased especially with his studies of occupational mortality, his recognition of laws of epidemics, his interest in comparing the mortality of various places with a view to raising problems for local investigation, and his interest in the relationship between population density and mortality.

Their admiration is continued by contemporary epidemiologists who find in Farr's work anticipations of concepts and methods still employed in studying health and disease in a complex social or environmental setting.[36] He has recently been called "a founder, even the founder of epidemiology in its modern form," and the study of his methods of employing death rates in research has been recommended to modern health experts.[37] It seems clear then that on most points of contention during Farr's lifetime, posterity has decided in his favor. A noticeable exception is hospital mortality.

From a purely technical point of view it is possible to trace the evolution of Farr's statistical methods to the middle 1830s. Although his initial interest in hygiene and medical statistics may owe a good deal to the influence of the Paris medical school, his statistical methods were inspired by the British actuary tradition, especially by the work of Thomas Rowe Edmonds. In Edmonds's work Farr discovered a model for a statistical law, Edmonds's law of mortality, as well as important suggestions for ways in which census and mortality data might be used to study health and welfare. Farr developed these techniques beyond anything Edmonds had anticipated, but it is possible to find in Edmonds's influence a continuity to Farr's work. The statistical goal of his most ambitious studies was the discovery of a statistical law of the form he first encountered in Edmonds's publications. Such a law showed how mortality figures changed with time or circumstance. The law itself was a numerical expression, often an exponential function discovered by subtracting orders of differences of logarithms, which would permit the computation of a series of figures which approximated the observed series. Farr, like Edmonds, often displayed both series side by side. This approach Farr used again and again: in his laws of recovery and death in smallpox (1837), in his elevation law for cholera mortality in London (1852), in his prediction of the course of the cattle plague (1866), and in his density law (1879). Such laws, Farr believed, demonstrated both that health and disease were orderly processes and that numerical analysis had the power to unlock their secrets.

In analyzing the causes of disease and premature death Farr worked by comparing death rates of people living in different circumstances. Crude mortality rates were the most frequently used. But he also employed with increasing frequency more specialized rates, those calculated according to age, sex, or cause. From an early period of his career he recognized the importance of establishing standard populations whose mortality experience could serve as criteria for evaluating the health of other people. He settled on several such standards. The most commonly employed was the entire population of England and Wales and the population of the Healthy Districts, those places whose crude mortality rates were below 17 per 1,000. Occasionally he also used the population of the metropolis and of either Liverpool or Manchester. Using these rates he could show how much excess mortality might be attributed to the peculiar circumstances in which certain people lived. This approach often gave striking results as when he calculated the "degrees of insalubrity" for British cities or compared the mortality of British miners or soldiers with that of the civil population. This was an avenue of approach which led him eventually to compare mortality rates standarized for age and sex, an innovation which has drawn the praise of modern epidemiologists.[38]

But as important as Farr's work was for the development of scientific fields such as epidemiology or vital statistics or for the functioning of Victorian health administration, his writings have other historical interest as well. Statistics were for Farr always a means to an end, a tool in a greater reform campaign. This fact is seen most forcefully in his early works, in the first five *Annual Reports* for example, but evidence for it can be found repeatedly throughout his career. "And what are figures worth," he asked Florence Nightingale in 1864, "if they do no good to men's bodies or souls[?]"[39] At times he showed greater interest in getting results that would startle than in the precision of the figures on which those conclusions were based. In responding to the threatened attack on the statistical section of the Indian Sanitary Commission's report, he began: "My position is (1) that the mortality of the British soldiers in India should not exceed 10 in 1,000; (2) that it has exceeded that figure hitherto—by never mind how much—but to a terrific extent—cook the figures as they will—by leaving out cholera years, & crimean campaigns in a small way; (3) that it is time the destruction of life—& efficiency should be put an end to—by displacing the incapables if necessary."[40]

We have examined Farr's social and medical ideas in some detail. There is little need to repeat observations made in earlier chapters. There is one generalization, however, which should be made. Farr's example illustrates in a forceful manner the remarkable correspondence and interplay of ideas about society, medicine, and social science possible in early Victorian England. The 1830s emerge as a period of incubation for a set of related socio-medical attitudes common among public-minded Victorians who flourished at mid-century. The wellspring of this attitude was the agitation and anxieties surrounding the reform of English government and institutions begun in the thirties. The reform campaign not only heightened discontent in the lower ranks of the medical profession with traditional means of controlling professional affairs; more important is the fact that middle class preoccupations with unrest among the urban poor served to awaken medical interests in hygiene and public health. There is also reason to believe that economic and political notions congenial to newly enfranchised commercial and professional men may have helped modify medical ideas. The rapid decline of the traditional theory of contagion is a case in point.[41] Such a theory already in doubt on medical grounds which had been used to justify unpopular policies such as quarantine was a likely target for reform-minded medical men.

But the influences were not all in one direction. Medical expertise played a role in establishing reform policy and had an effect on men in public affairs outside the medical profession. The environmental theory of disease identified local conditions, manners of living, as the cause of illness and premature death. This understanding of disease helped assign meaning to human misery and to establish the sphere of human responsibility for illness. It became possible to argue that the sick individual was a victim of circumstances beyond his personal control. This was an important point because it helped to minimize a powerful objection to any social amelioration, the claim that the miserable were responsible for their own condition. Epidemic diseases annually carried off thousands of innocent lives, the new-born among them.

The same understanding of illness, however, could be used to argue that mankind collectively was responsible for disease. Modern man had created conditions which endangered health, but he also had at his disposal the means to save lives and preserve health. Farr's impassioned plea for action in his 1840 letter to *The Lancet* in which he compared the victims of smallpox to infants deliberately thrown from London Bridge,[42] or his likening the infants killed in large cities through ignorance or neglect to children sacrificed by an "idolatrous tribe"[43] combined both sides of the argument to form a powerful indictment of the *status quo*. If human welfare were accepted as a social goal, then such a disease theory opened the door for the use of disease and premature death as instruments of social criticism and valuable weapons in reform agitation.[44] The tactic was common among social activists in the nineteenth-century medical profession. Farr was simply one of the more articulate in claiming preventable disease and premature death were signs of fundamental social or political ills. "No variation in the health of the states of Europe," he wrote, "is the result of chance; it is the direct result of the physical and political conditions in which nations live."[45] When combined with calculations of monetary losses due to preventable disease, this line of reasoning in the hands of Chadwick, Farr, and others could be very compelling.

Contemporary disease theory both aided in establishing a case for intervention and helped determine and justify the nature of that intervention. Particularly in its common miasmatic form, the dominant understanding of disease in the thirties and forties called for measures that were politically acceptable: sanitation and other modifications to the urban landscape which for the most part left the rights of property and the relationship between employer and employee untouched. In its initial phases the public health campaign succeeded not only because it had convinced the nation that some public action was necessary, but also because the intervention most loudly touted, public sanitation, interfered least with cherished political values. The fate of measures which stepped beyond the bounds of political acceptability, such as Chadwick's plan to nationalize the metropolitan burial grounds or the compulsory vaccination laws, illustrates how strong constitutional objections to health measures could be.[46]

Particularly in the thirties many reform-minded professional men turned to statistics as an ally. As understood by its British proponents of that decade, statistics was a science, a social science, perhaps the only science of society. It was an empirical science whose purpose was to discover the principles of legislation and administration. In the extravagant claims of both objectivity and utility issued by the early statistical societies we can see a popular vision of science and a reflection of the social and political concerns of the founders.

These first statisticians, Farr among them, hoped to bring the power and certainty of the scientific method to bear on policy issues where uncertainty and disagreement reigned. By promising to construct a positive science of the state, the statistician claimed special authority in the public arena. While abjuring direct participation in the governing process, he nevertheless expected to help guide social change by supplying irrefutable facts and knowledge of first principles. It is not difficult to see in the activities of the statistical societies in the first years thinly veiled political activity. Many of their studies were anything but objective, and the statistical program appears in retrospect to have been a way of disarming political opponents and of obtaining a hearing for reform demands.[47]

Statistics had special appeal to certain members of the medical profession. Not only did these men share the political and social concerns of their colleagues in the statistical societies, but they also had a special interest in statistics as well. To a vocal minority statistics seemed the key for improving medical knowledge. In articles written in the mid-thirties British medical spokesmen argued that medicine was backward precisely because physicians had not yet begun to follow physical scientists in using quantitative methods.[48] If they would only do so, these spokesmen claimed, medicine would achieve greater precision and certainty, and might gain that enviable power of the physical sciences, the power of prediction. To medical men such as Farr, interested in hygiene, the use of statistics seemed invaluable. Statistics offered itself as the only likely instrument for sorting out and weighing the host of environmental determinants of health and disease. The evolution of Farr's own ideas, in fact, suggests that his initial concern was hygiene or public health, and that slightly later he turned to statistics as a tool for its advancement.

Farr's works, then, reveal the interplay of three ideas cherished among prominent Victorian professional men: political liberalism, an environmental approach to the understanding of human misery, and a belief that social progress would follow the construction of a positive science of statecraft. The combination was not the product of chance or caprice. Its components were interrelated and mutually supporting. This complex of notions not only helps explain Farr's particular ideas and interpretations, it also partially accounts for a feature of his work that recent observers have found so puzzling, the enormous breadth of his interests, which transcends any contemporary scheme of disciplinary boundaries.[49] Farr moved from life insurance to hospital mortality, from estimates of human capital to studies of Asiatic cholera, from discussions of population growth to improvements in nosology with perfect ease, because he regarded them as part of the same enterprise: the construction of a numerical science of health and human progress.

Farr knew of profound objections to his self-confident perspective. He denied the gloomy prognosis of the Malthusians, preferring to adopt the older view, which saw population growth as a sign of national health rather than a premonition of demographic disaster. He turned neo-eugenic worries about racial degeneration from an indictment to a plea for intervention. In essence Farr was an optimist. Improvement in human welfare was not only possible; it was already under way. From the uncertainties of the thirties, faith in the reality of this vision expanded so that by the sixties, when the means of controlling cholera and smallpox seemed at hand, when the number of healthy districts was growing, and when it seemed possible to end the waste of life in the Army and in medical institutions, his reform proclamations sounded like trumpets. "I entered upon the subject [the Indian Sanitary Commission] in gloom; but the air brightened on the way, & I now leave it with gladness—as I see that the evils which we dreaded might be dissipated. . . ."[50]

The perspective Farr represented could not be maintained long after his death. The germ theory of disease redefined the environment's role in disease causation and made immediate appeals from deaths to social engineering more difficult. The older vision of statistics was also dissolved. The two irreconcilable components of the statistical movement of the thirties finally went their separate ways.[51] Increasingly, social and policy concerns were either cultivated by the newer social sciences, or represented directly in party politics. The computational activities became the preserve of mathematicians and scientists who constructed a methodology which excluded untrained social reformers in search of a science of the state. Statistics lost its status as an independent science, yet it gained scientific respectability. Finally, the political and economic balance so carefully preserved through most of Victoria's reign began to shift. The decline of Victorian liberalism made solutions to social and economic problems such as Farr's seem increasingly antique.

But for all that, the attitudes Farr represents (may we call them Victorian socio-medical liberalism?) had a remarkable longevity. They coalesced into a recognizable complex in the 1830s and could still be found intact half a century later. They were an influential force in Victorian social policy, in public health especially. Today their documentary remains permit us to observe the Victorian mind at work on complicated problems of human welfare, public responsibility, and the application of scientific knowledge.

ABBREVIATIONS

A.R.R.G.   *Annual Report of the Registrar-General of Births, Deaths, and Marriages in England.* [Title varies. Citation following in square brackets is the location in the Parliamentary Papers. Note that the contents and pagination of the separate volumes and of the versions in the Parliamentary Papers are not identical for the early reports.]

B.M. Add. Mss.   British Library [British Museum] Additional Manuscript.

Br. Ann. Med.   *British Annals of Medicine, Pharmacy, Vital Statistics, and General Science.*

Br. Med. Almanack   *British Medical Almanack.* [Title varies.]

D.N.B.   *Dictionary of National Biography.*

G.R.O.   General Register Office [recently named Office of Population Censuses and Surveys].

J. Statist. Soc. Lond.   *Journal of the Statistical Society of London.*

L.S.E. Farr Collection   London School of Economics, Farr Papers.

PP   Parliamentary Papers.

Report, B.A.A.S.   *Report. . . of the British Association for the Advancement of Science.*

Trans. Epidem. Soc. Lond.   *Transactions of the Epidemiological Society of London.*

Trans. Manchr. Statist. Soc.   *Transactions of the Manchester Statistical Society.*

Trans. N.A.P.S.S.   *Transactions of the National Association for the Promotion of Social Science [Social Science Association]*

NOTES

Chapter One

1. The standard biographical account of Farr is that of Noel A. Humphreys, "Biographical Sketch of William Farr," in William Farr, *Vital Statistics: A Memorial Volume of Selections from the Reports and Writings of William Farr, M.D., D.C.L., C.B., F.R.S.*, ed. Noel A. Humphreys (London, 1885), pp. vii–xxiv. Hereafter cited as Humphreys in Farr, *Vital Statistics*. Also useful among the early accounts is F. A. C. Hare's *William Farr, F.S.S., M.D., F.R.S., C.B., etc., etc.* (London, 1883). The copy of this pamphlet I have seen is a galley proof in L. S. E. Farr Collection, XI, item 30. Citations are to that version. Presumably because of its criticism of some of Farr's statistical and actuary practices and its candor about his humble social origins, Hare's account raised objections from Farr's friends, who blocked its publication in *J. Statist. Soc. Lond.* See W. J. H. Whittall's note, L. S. E. Farr Collection, XI, item 32. Whittall was Farr's brother-in-law, executor of his estate, and donor of Farr's papers to the London School of Economics.

2. Salop Record Office, Condover Parish Records 1977/7/1882. Thanks here is due to Mrs. M. Halford, County Archivist, Shrewsbury, for her help in locating and interpreting this information.

3. The education of Thomas Wakley in the previous decade provides a useful comparison. Wakley was successively apprentice to an apothecary, apprentice to a surgeon, assistant to a provincial physician, and student at the United Schools of St. Thomas's and Guy's Hospitals, London. See S. Squire Sprigge, *The Life and Times of Thomas Wakley* (London, New York, and Bombay, 1899), pp. 6–7.

4. W[illiam] Farr, "Mortality in Hospitals," *Lancet*, 1864, i, 420.

5. Farr, "Letter," *25th A.R.R.G.*, p. 179n. [PP, 1864, XVII].

6. Farr, "Letter," *Suppl. 35th A.R.R.G.*, p. xxxiii [PP, 1875, XVIII, pt. 2].

7. Richard H. Shryock, "The History of Quantification in Medical Science," *Isis* 52 (1961): 231; George Rosen, "Problems in the Application of Statistical Analysis to Questions of Health: 1700–1880," *Bull. Hist. Med.* 29 (1955): 38–39.

8. "Illustration, William Farr, F.R.S.," *Midland Medical Miscellany and Provincial Medical Journal* 2 (Aug. 1, 1883): 225; Humphreys in Farr, *Vital Statistics*, p. x; Sir Arthur Newsholme, "The Measurement of Progress in Public Health with Special Reference to the Life and Work of William Farr," *Economica* 3 (1923): 189; and Richard H. Shryock, *The Development of Modern Medicine: An Interpretation of the Social and Scientific Factors Involved,* [1947] (Philadelphia and London; 1969), p. 226.

9. Humphreys reports Farr attended the lectures of "Grant, Carswill, Jenner, Elliotson," Humphreys in Farr, *Vital Statistics*, p. xi. The statement is puzzling. While Robert Edmond Grant and John Elliotson were on the faculty in these years, William Jenner did not join the faculty until 1849. Carswill is probably Sir Robert Carswell, Professor of Morbid Anatomy, See: *D.N.B.*, 7: 403; Ibid., 6: 683; Ibid., 22, suppl.: 909; and Fielding H. Garrison and Leslie T. Morton, *A Medical Bibliography*, 3rd ed. (London, 1970), p. 272.

10. His diploma is dated March 29, 1832, and is preserved in L. S. E. Farr Collection, XIV, item 1.

11. A good short summary is M. Jeanne Peterson, *The Medical Profession in Mid-Victorian London* (Berkeley, Los Angeles, and London, 1978), pp. 5–39. See also S. W. F. Holloway, "The Apothecaries' Act, 1815: A Reinterpretation. Part II: The Consequences of the Act," *Med. Hist.* 10 (1966): 221–36; and S. W. F. Holloway, "Medical Education in England, 1830–1858: A Sociological Analysis," *History* 49 (1964): 306–14.

12. By 1837 Farr was listed as the editor, *Br. Med. Almanack* (1837), title page.

13. No editor is named in the journal. Hare, *William Farr*, p. 3, claims Farr was the editor, and this seems very plausible, both from the circumstances of Farr's life and the con-

tents of the journal. Farr was also identified as editor in M[ichael] J. Cullen, *The Statistical Movement in Early Victorian Britain: The Foundations of Empirical Social Research* (New York, 1975), p. 54.

14. "Contribution to the Natural History of Quackery," *Br. Ann. Med.* 1 (1837): 314-15; and "The State of Medical Science," Ibid., pp. 22-26.

15. "On a Method of Determining the Danger and the Duration of Diseases at Every Period of Their Progress. Article I," Ibid. 1 (1837): 72-79; "On the Law of Recovery and Dying in Small-Pox. Article II.," Ibid., pp. 134-43; "Vital Statistics," Ibid., pp. 353-60; and "Statistics of Insanity—County Lunatic Asylums," Ibid. 1 (1837): 648-53, 679-83, 744-48, 811-14.

16. W[illiam] F[arr], "History of the Medical Profession, and Its Influence on Public Health, in England," *The Medical Annual, or, British Medical Almanack*, suppl. (1839), p. 113.

17. "Address," *Br. Med. Almanack* (1835), p. 5.

18. Farr endorsed the objects of this body in a short account of its purposes and history: "The Rise and Progress of the Provincial Medical and Surgical Association," Ibid. (1837), pp. 121-30.

19. Peterson, *The Medical Profession*, pp. 19-28.

20. For information on this reform society see: Ernest Muirhead Little, *History of the British Medical Association: 1832-1932* (London, [1932]), pp. 32-34. Farr delivered a reform oration to this group see: William Farr, "Medical Reform. An Oration Delivered at the Last Anniversary Meeting of the British Medical Association," *Lancet*, 1839-40, i, p. 106.

21. It has been observed that the reforms of the thirties, especially Parliamentary reform and Poor Law reform, stimulated reform efforts within the medical profession. See W. H. McMenemey, "Education and the Medical Reform Movement," in *The Evolution of Medical Education in Britain*, ed. F. N. L. Poynter (London, 1966), pp. 135-54.

22. [William Farr], "Progress of the Medical Profession—Obstructions in the Way," *Br. Ann. Med.* 1 (1837): 630.

23. Ibid.

24. [William Farr], "Medical Reform: Representative Bodies v. the Corporations," Ibid., 563.

25. [William Farr], "Medical Competition," Ibid. 2 (1837): 116.

26. "The College of Physicians v. Scotch Graduates," Ibid. 1 (1837): 662-63.

27. "Apothecaries' Company an Anomaly—Necessity for Its Reform, and Conversion into a College of Pharmacy," Ibid., pp. 340-43;. "Apothecaries' Hall," Ibid. 2 (1837): 248-49; and "Concours—Trial of Mr. Nice—Practical Knowledge not Indentures the Passport to Practise," Ibid. 1 (1837): 468-70.

28. [William Farr], "Curricula," Ibid. 1 (1837): 430.

29. Ibid.

30. [William Farr], "Progress of the Medical Profession—Obstructions in the Way," Ibid., p. 631.

31. [Farr], "Curricula," pp. 431-32.

32. [William Farr], "Observation," *Br. Ann. Med.* 1 (1837): 692-95.

33. [William Farr], "Physiology—Mode of Studying It," Ibid., pp. 727-28.

34. "The Provincial Medical and Surgical Association," Ibid. 2 (1837): 61.

35. "Lecture Introductory to a Course on Hygiene, or the Preservation of the Public Health," *Lancet*, 1835-36, i, 240-45; and "Lecture on the History of Hygiene," Ibid., pp. 773-80.

36. Farr, "Lecture Introductory to a Course on Hygiene," p. 241.

37. Farr, "Lecture on the History of Hygiene," pp. 779-80.

38. William Farr, testimony, *Report of the Commissioners Appointed to Inquire into the Regulations Affecting the Sanitary Condition of the Army, the Organization of Military Hospitals, and the Treatment of the Sick and Wounded*, PP, 1857-58, XVIII, 246; and Farr, "Letter," *Suppl. 35th A.R.R.G.*, p. lxxix [PP, 1875, XVIII, pt. 2].

39. Farr, "Lecture on the History of Hygiene," p. 779.

40. Ibid.

41. Hare, *William Farr*, p. 3, records the testimony of a surgeon who lodged with Farr in these years and helped him study statistics.

42. Farr, "Lecture on the History of Hygiene," p. 776.

43. The most important are: "On a Method of Determining the Danger and the Duration of Diseases at Every Period of Their Progress, Article I," *Br. Ann. Med.* 1 (1837): 72-79; "On the Law of Recovery and Dying in Small-Pox. Article II," Ibid, pp. 134-43; and "On Prognosis," *Br. Med. Almanack* (1838), pp. 199-216. We will discuss these important articles in detail in Chapter Five.

44. "The State of Medical Science," *Br. Ann. Med.* 1 (1837): 25.

45. [William Farr], "Vital Statistics; or, the Statistics of Health, Sickness, Diseases, and Death," in *A Statistical Account of the British Empire: Exhibiting its Extent, Physical Capacities, Population, Industry, and Civil and Religious Institutions,* ed. J[ohn] R[amsay] McCulloch (London, 1837), 2: 567-601. Hereafter cited as Farr, "Vital Statistics," in McCulloch, 1st ed., vol. 2.

46. Humphreys in Farr, *Vital Statistics,* p. xii.

47. We will discuss Edmond's methods in Chapter Four.

48. Farr, "Vital Statistics," in McCulloch, 1st ed., 2: 573 and 594.

49. Farr was apparently in charge of the G.R.O.'s statistical department even before he joined the permanent staff on July 10, 1839. Humphreys in Farr, *Vital Statistics,* p. xii; and M. J. Cullen, *The Statistical Movement,* p. 29.

50. Farr, "Letter," *2nd A.R.R.G.,* app., p. 95 [PP, 1840, XVII, 18] See also George Rosen, "Jacob Henle and William Farr," *Bull. Hist. Med.* 9 (1941): 585-89.

51. *5th A.R.R.G.,* p. 388 [PP, 1843, XXI, 189] Holmes repaid the compliment by citing Farr in a later edition of his essay. Oliver Wendell Holmes, "The Contagiousness of Puerperal Fever," in *Medical Essays, 1842-1882* (Boston and New York, 1892), p. 104.

52. *Report on the Cholera Epidemic of 1866 in England, Suppl. 29th A.R.R.G.* [PP. 1867-68, XXXVII, xiii-xv and lxv-lxxii].

53. For Farr's appreciation of his British predecessors, especially Sydenham, see: Farr, "History of the Medical Profession," p. 178; Farr, "On a Method of Determining the Danger," p. 72; Farr, "On the Law of Recovery," p. 134; Farr, "Letter," *1st A.R.R.G.,* pp. 86-88 [PP, 1839, XVI, 63-64]; and Wm. Farr, "On the Modes of Calculating the Death-Rate of a Population," *Lancet,* 1862, i, 568.

54. See, for example, his sections on occupational mortality, syphilis, and hygiene in Farr, "Letter," *Suppl. 35th A.R.R.G.,* pp. lii-liii, lxvii-lxx, and lxxix-lxxxii [PP, 1875, XVIII, pt. 2].

55. "Statistical Nosology," *4th A.R.R.G.,* pp. 147-216 [PP, 1842, XIX, 93-127].

56. See the following editorials: "Medical Relief of Paupers," *Br. Ann. Med.* 1 (1837): 243-45; "On Some Points Connected with the Inquiry into the Present State of the Poor," Ibid., 455-62; and "Remuneration of Medical Men. Pay of Surgeons in the Army Contrasted with the Pay of Surgeons in the Unions," Ibid, 553-55. For the medical opposition to the treatment of medical men by the Poor Law authorities and the role that opposition played in encouraging ordinary practitioners to unite see McMenemey, "Education," p. 144; William H. McMenemey, *The Life and Times of Sir Charles Hastings: Founder of the British Medical Association* (Edinburgh and London, 1959), pp. 235-36; and M. J. Cullen, "The Making of the Civil Registration Act of 1836," *J. Ecclesiastical Hist.* 25 (1974): 57-59.

57. "The Assistant Registrar-General on Medical Coroners," *Lancet,* 1862, i, 677. Two drafts of this letter and Dr. Edwin Lankester's letter of thanks are preserved in L. S. E. Farr Collection, I, items 31, 32, and 65. See also evidence of his intervention in the selection of a medical officer for Marylebone, *Lancet,* 1856, i, 19.

58. [William Farr], "Coroners' Inquests," *Br. Ann. Med.* 1 (1837): 182-84; and "Medical Reform," *Lancet,* 1839-40, i, 106. For Wakley's ideas and activities see Sprigge, *The Life and Times,* pp. 353-427.

59. Farr's presidential address is preserved. See William Farr, "An Address Delivered in the Section of State Medicine, at the Annual Meeting of the British Medical Association, in Leeds, July 1869," *Br. Med. J.,* 1869, ii, 265-67.

60. For a summary of the joint committee's activities see *Br. Med. J.,* 1868, i, 33, 489, and 541-43; and Ibid., 1868, ii, 194-95. Basic information on the work of the Royal Sanitary Commission may be found in Jeanne L. Brand, *Doctors and the State: The British Medical Profession and Government Action in Public Health, 1870-1912* (Baltimore, 1965), pp. 8-21; and Sir John Simon, *English Sanitary Institutions, Reviewed in Their Course of*

Development, and in Some of Their Political and Social Relations (London, 1890), pp. 322-52.

61. N. Arnott, et. al., *Report of the Committee for Scientific Inquiries in Relation to the Cholera-Epidemic of 1854,* PP, 1854-55, XXI.

62. L. S. E. Farr Collection, XIII, items 6-8. For the establishment of these examinations see Roy M. MacLeod, "The Anatomy of State Medicine: Concept and Application," in *Medicine and Science in the 1860s: Proceedings of the Sixth British Congress on the History of Medicine,* ed. F. N. L. Poynter (London, 1968), pp. 221-24.

Chapter Two

1. G. M. Young, *Victorian England: Portrait of an Age*, 2nd ed. (London, 1963), p. 32.

2. The most comprehensive discussions of the statistical movement are found in Cullen, *The Statistical Movement*. See also Victor L. Hilts, "Aliis exterendum, or, the Origins of the Statistical Society of London," *Isis* 69 (1978): 21-43; Philip Abrams, *The Origins of British Sociology: 1834-1914.* (Chicago and London, 1968), pp. 13-30; and Harald Westergaard, *Contributions to the History of Statistics* [1932] (New York, 1968), pp. 136-71.

3. Recent studies of the Manchester Statistical Society include: David Elesh, "The Manchester Statistical Society: A Case Study of a Discontinuity in the History of Empirical Social Research," *J. Hist. Behavioral Sci.* 8 (1972): 280-301 and 407-17; Cullen, *The Statistical Movement*, pp. 105-17. The older standard account is T. S. Ashton, *Economic and Social Investigations in Manchester, 1833-1933: A Centenary History of the Manchester Statistical Society* (London, 1934).

4. Elesh, "The Manchester Statistical Society," pp. 411-12, see also pp. 281-87.

5. Cullen, *The Statistical Movement*, pp. 79-82.

6. Fully half of the 72 papers read to the society between 1841 and 1850 were written by seven of the new activists, Ibid., p. 103.

7. "Dr. William Farr, C.B., D.C.L., etc.," *J. Statist. Soc. Lond.* 46 (1883): 350.

8. Farr foresaw the creation of chairs of politics and statistics in British universities: William Farr, "Inaugural Address," *J. Statist. Soc. Lond.* 34 (1871): 410-11. Both he and Florence Nightingale had hoped to see a professorship in statistics established at Oxford. Nightingale tried but failed to interest Francis Galton in the project in 1891. Karl Pearson, *The Life, Letters and Labours of Francis Galton* (Cambridge, 1924), 2: 416-24. The first university home for statistics was probably the research fellowship and the professorship in eugenics Galton established at University College, London in 1904 and 1911, respectively. The first British chair of statistics was established at the same institution in 1933.

9. *Report B.A.A.S.* 3 (1833): 492-95; *J. Statist. Soc. Lond.* 1 (1838): 1-5; and Ibid. 3 (1840), 1-13.

10. *J. Statist. Soc. Lond.* 3 (1840): 1-2.

11. Ibid. 1 (1838): 3.

12. *Report, B.A.A.S.* 3 (1840): 492.

13. *J. Statist. Soc. Lond.* 1 (1833): 1.

14. Ibid. 3 (1840): 6-7.

15. Ibid. 1 (1838): 2-3.

16. Ibid. 3 (1840): 2.

17. Cullen, *The Statistical Movement*, pp. 94-101, 111-15, 119-33, and 136-42; and Elesh, "The Manchester Statistical Society," pp. 291-300.

18. *Annals of the Royal Statistical Society, 1834-1934* (London, 1934), p. 59.

19. Ashton, *Economic and Social Investigations,* p. 45.

20. Another but probably less important source of interest in statistics came from the peculiar needs of the insurance business. Brief suggestions of its importance to the movement are found in Young, *Victorian England*, p. 32 and M. W. Flinn, *Public Health Reform in Britain* (New York, 1968), pp. 21-22.

21. O. R. McGregor, "Social Research and Social Policy in the Nineteenth Century," *Br. J. Sociology* 8 (1957): 147-48.

22. This point is argued at length in Hilts, "Aliis exterendum," pp. 21-43.

23. Standard sources for the following summary are: V. John, "The term 'Statistics.' Translated from a Work by Dr. V. John, Professor of the University of Berne, entitled 'Der Name Statistik—Eine Etymologisch-historische Skizze,' Berne: Verlag von K. J. Weiss, 1883," *J. Statist. Soc. Lond.* 46 (1883): 656-79; and August Meitzen, *History, Theory, and Technique of Statistics*, trans. Roland P. Falkner (Philadelphia, 1891), pp. 18-53. More recent discussions include: Paul F. Lazarsfeld, "Notes on the History of Quantification in Sociology—Trends, Sources and Problems," *Isis* 52 (1961): 279-94; and Frank Lorimer, "The Development of Demography," in *The Study of Population: An Inventory and Appraisal*, eds. Philip M. Hauser and Otis Dudley Duncan (Chicago, 1959), pp. 124-31.

24. *J. Statist. Soc. Lond.* 1 (1838): 1.

25. Graunt's *Natural and Political Observations upon the Bills of Mortality* was translated into German in 1702, John, "The Term 'Statistics,'" p. 663. For the differences and conflict of these two traditions see Ibid., pp. 669-72; and Lazarsfeld, "Notes," pp. 283-85.

26. A recent treatment of this revival is Harold Stolerman, "Francis Bacon and the Victorians, 1830-1885," (Ph.D. diss., New York University, 1969).

27. *Edinburgh Rev.* 65 (July, 1837): 1-104.

28. Stolerman, "Francis Bacon," pp. 683-84, and also 127-29, 213-14, 295-312, 687-89.

29. "On the Original and Acquired Meaning of the Term 'Statistics,' and on the Proper Functions of a Statistical Society: also on the Question Whether There Be a Science of Statistics; and, if so, What Are Its Nature and Objects, and What Is Its Relation to Political Economy and 'Social Science,'" *J. Statist. Soc. Lond.* 28 (1865): 491.

30. Stolerman, "Francis Bacon," pp. 220-24.

31. Mary P. Mack, *Jeremy Bentham: An Odyssey of Ideas 1748-1792* (London, Melbourne, Toronto, 1962), pp. 115-16. For this aspect of Bentham's thought see also Ibid., pp. 235-40.

32. Bentham cited in Mack, *Jeremy Bentham*, p. 240.

33. Mack, *Jeremy Bentham*, pp. 3, 244-45, and 269-70.

34. "Sixth Annual Report of the Council . . . ," *J. Statist. Soc. Lond.* 3 (1840): 6.

35. W. R. Deverell, "Statistics of the Population of Saxony . . . ," *J. Statist. Soc. Lond.* 2 (1839): 104.

36. Mack, *Jeremy Bentham*, pp. 237-40.

37. Ibid., pp. 237 and 239.

38. Young, *Victorian England*, p. 32.

39. Elesh, "The Manchester Statistical Society," pp. 412-13.

40. See in particular Abrams, *The Origins*, p. 19, and Cullen, *The Statistical Movement*, p. 144.

41. See especially pp. 106-10 and 135-47.

42. Cullen, *The Statistical Movement*, p. 137.

43. See especially pp. 8-15, 17-18, 21, and 35-37.

44. Abrams, *The Origins*, p. 12.

45. Ibid., pp. 23-30.

46. McGregor, "Social Research," p. 154.

47. "Causes of the High Mortality in Town Districts," *5th A.R.R.G.*, app., pp. 433-34 [PP, 1843, XXI, 214-15].

48. Cullen, *The Statistical Movement*, p. 36.

49. Farr, "Vital Statistics," in McCulloch, 1st ed., 2: 572.

50. Farr, "Letter," *Suppl. 35th A.R.R.G.*, p. lxxi [PP, 1875, XVIII, pt. 2].

51. [William Farr], "Medical Relief of Paupers," *Br. Ann. Med.* 1 (1837): 244.

52. Ibid.

53. William Farr, "On Some Doctrines of Population. A Paper Read in Section F of the British Association, at Plymouth, in August Last," *J. Statist. Soc. Lond.* 40 (1877): 577.

54. "Poor Law—Steam-boiler Explosions—Coroners' Inquests," *Br. Ann. Med.* 1 (1837): 790.

55. Cullen, *The Statistical Movement*, p. 35; and Major Greenwood, *Some British Pioneers of Social Medicine* (London, New York, Toronto, 1948), p. 62.

56. William Farr, letter to T. H. Lister, Registrar General, March 17, 1840, in D. V.

Glass, *Numbering the People: The Eighteenth-Century Population Controversy and the Development of Census and Vital Statistics in Britain* (Farnborough, Hants, 1973), p. 163.

57. "Causes of the High Mortality," p. 434 [215].

58. This correspondence originally was published in the Poor Law Commissioners' *Official Circulars*. It has been republished with comment in Glass, *Numbering the People*, pp. 146–47 and 150–67.

59. Farr, "Vital Statistics," in McCulloch, 1st ed., 2: 577; Farr, "Letter," *1st A.R.R.G.*, pp. 108–13 [PP, 1839, XVI, 76–80]; and Farr, "Causes of the High Mortality," pp. 410–11 [202–3].

60. [Farr], "Causes of the High Mortality," p. 433 [214].

61. "Note on the Present Epidemic of Small-Pox and on the Necessity of Arresting Its Ravages," *Lancet*, 1840–41, i, 353.

62. For the National Association for the Promotion of Social Science see: Brian Rodgers, "The Social Science Association, 1857–1886," *Manchester School of Economic and Social Studies* 20 (1952): 283–310; Abrams, *The Origins*, pp. 44–52; and McGregor, "Social Research," pp. 152–54. Farr's participation in its inception is mentioned in S. E. Finer, *The Life and Times of Sir Edwin Chadwick* (London, 1952), p. 488.

63. *J. Statist. Soc.* 35 (1872): 417.

64. "Report to the Registrar-General on the International Statistical Congress held at Paris in 1855," *16th A.R.R.G.*, p. 111 and "[Presidential] Address [to Section F]," *Report, B.A.A.S.* 34 (1864): 151.

65. Francis Galton, "Considerations Adverse to the Maintenance of Section F. (Economic Science and Statistics), submitted by Mr. Francis Galton to the Committee Appointed by the Council to Consider and Report on the Possibility of Excluding Unscientific or Otherwise Unsuitable Papers and Discussions from the Sectional Proceedings of the Association," *J. Statist. Soc. Lond.* 40 (1877): 468–73; and W[illiam] Farr, "Considerations, in the Form of a Draft Report, Submitted to Committee, Favourable to the Maintenance of Section F," Ibid., pp. 473–76. See also Karl Pearson, *The Life*, 2: 348.

66. Farr had apparently written to Chadwick about the proposed amendment of Section F, and Chadwick's reply was similar to Farr's views, Edwin Chadwick, letter to William Farr, July 12, 1877, L. S. E. Farr Collection, I, item 19.

67. *Report, B.A.A.S.* 46 (1876): 266; Ibid. 47 (1877): 231–32; Ibid. 48 (1878): 152–53; Ibid. 49 (1879): 175–209; and Ibid. 50 (1880): 120–59.

68. Ibid. 51 (1881): 245–49.

69. William Farr, "[Presidential] Address [to Section F]," *Report B.A.A.S.* 34 (1864): 158.

70. "Observation," *Br. Ann. Med.* 1 (1837): 693.

71. Ibid., and "[Presidential] Address [to Section F]," *Report, B.A.A.S.* 34 (1864): 158.

72. *J. Statist. Soc. Lond.* 35 (1872): 427.

73. In the London society 28 of the 72 papers read between 1841 and 1850 dealt with vital or medical statistics. During the same years only 7 papers were read on problems of crime and education. Cullen, *The Statistical Movement*, p. 103.

74. Ibid., pp. 136–37.

75. There has been no major study of this important subject. Suggestions may be found in: Charles Creighton, *A History of Epidemics in Britain* (Cambridge, 1894), 2: 133–51; M. Dorothy George, *London Life in the Eighteenth Century* [1925] (New York and Evanston, 1965), pp. 50–55; G. Talbot Griffith, *Population Problems of the Age of Malthus*, 2nd ed. (London, 1967), pp. 224–34; and George Rosen, "John Ferriar's Advice to the Poor,'" *Bull. Hist. Med.* 11 (1942): 222–27.

76. During an epidemic of typhus in Edinburgh James Phillips Kay had been clinical assistant to W. P. Alison, professor of the institutes of medicine. Alison was both a contagionist and a vocal proponent of the view that privation is responsible for the prevalence of disease. He was also a strong advocate of the reform of the Scottish Poor Law. See, for example, William Pulteney Alison, *Observations on the Epidemic of Fever of MDCCCXLIII in Scotland, and Its Connection with the Destitute Condition of the Poor* (Edinburgh, 1844). For the teaching of medical police in Edinburgh see George Rosen, "The Fate of the Concept

of Medical Police 1780-1890," *Centaurus* 5 (1957): 107-8; and John Roberton, *A Treatise on Medical Police* . . . (Edinburgh, 1809).

77. Quoted in Frank Smith, *The Life and Work of Sir James Kay-Shuttleworth* (London, 1923), p. 28.

78. *Elements of Medical Statistics* . . . (London, 1829), pp. 2-3.

79. William Augustus Guy, "On the Value of the Numerical Method as Applied to Science, but Especially to Physiology and Medicine," *J. Statist. Soc. Lond.* 2 (1839): 25-47; and Daniel Griffin and William Griffin, *Observations on the Application of Mathematics to the Science of Medicine* (London, 1843).

80. Griffin and Griffin, *Observations*, pp. 28-29.

81. Guy, "On the Value of the Numerical Method," pp. 36-38.

82. Ibid., p. 38.

83. In Chapter Four we will discuss this study by Farr. Although Guy referred to "On Prognosis," *Br. Med. Almanack* (1838), pp. 199-216; the original version is in two articles: "On a Method of Determining," pp. 72-79; and "On the Law of Recovery," pp. 134-43.

84. Farr, "Vital Statistics," in McCulloch, 1st ed., 2: 581; and Farr, "On the Law of Recovery," p. 137.

85. Farr, "Letter," *Suppl. 35th A.R.R.G.*, p. xxviii [PP, 1875, XVIII, pt. 2].

86. Farr, "Vital Statistics," in McCulloch, 1st ed., 2: 567.

87. William Farr, "Inaugural Address," *J. Statist. Soc. Lond.* 35 (1872): 417.

88. "On Benevolent Funds and Life Assurance in Health and Sickness," *Lancet*, 1837-38, i, 703.

89. Farr, "On the Law of Recovery," p. 143.

90. [William Farr], "Vital Statistics of Sweden," *Br. Med. Almanack, Suppl.*, (1838), p. 216.

91. Farr, "Letter," *Suppl. 35th A.R.R.G.*, p. v [PP, 1875, XVIII, pt. 2].

92. [William Farr], "Vital Statistics," *Br. Ann. Med.*, 1 (1837): 353-54.

93. Farr, "Letter," *31st A.R.R.G.*, p. 198 [PP, 1870, XVI.

94. William Farr, "The Influence of Scarcities and of the High Prices of Wheat on the Mortality of the People of England," *J. Statist. Soc. Lond.* 9 (1846): 163.

95. Farr, "Letter," *40th A.R.R.G.*, p. 235 [PP, 1878-79, XIX]; and William Farr, "Density or Proximity of Population: Its Advantages and Disadvantages," *Trans., N.A.P.S.S.* (Cheltenham, 1878), p. 532.

96. Farr, "On Prognosis," p. 200.

97. Cullen, *The Statistical Movement*, p. 148.

98. See for example the following letters to Farr in L. S. E. Farr Collection, I, items: 5, W. H. Archer (Australia): 10, F. T. Berg (Sweden); 12, L. Bodio (Italy?); 21, W. C. B. Eatwell (Calcutta); and 81 and 82, A. Quetelet (Belgium).

99. "Report of Dr. Farr on the Progress of Government Statistics in Great Britain," *J. Statist. Soc. Lond.* 21 (1858): 13-16; "Reports of the Official Delegates from England at the Meeting of the International Statistical Congress, Berlin, September 1863," *J. Statist. Soc. Lond.* 26 (1863): 412-16; "Report to the Registrar-General on the International Statistical Congress held at Paris in 1855," *16th A.R.R.G.*, App., pp. 106-15 [not found in PP]; "Report to the Registrar General on the International Statistical Congress at Vienna," *19th A.R.R.G.*, App., 206-22 [PP, 1857-58, XXIII].

100. *J. Statist. Soc. Lond.* 21 (1858): 16-17.

101. Harriet H. Shoen, "Prince Albert and the Application of Statistics to Problems of Government," *Osiris* 5 (1935): 295; and William Farr, letters of May 29 and June 11, 1860, to Henry Lord Brougham, Brougham Mss., University College, London University.

102. See, for example, his summary of the 1872 congress at St. Petersburg in Farr, "Inaugural Address—1872," pp. 418-27.

103. Farr, "Report of Paris Congress," p. 106.

104. William Farr, "Report on the Nomenclature and Statistical Classification of Diseases, for Statistical Returns," *16th A.R.R.G.*, pp. 71-96 [not in PP].

105. Farr, "Report of Paris Congress," pp. 109-10.

106. Ibid., pp. 111-14; Farr "Address," *Report, B.A.A.S.* 34 (1864): 155; and Farr, "Inaugural Address—1872," p. 427.

107. Farr, "Address," *Report, B.A.A.S.* 34 (1864): 160.
108. [William] Farr, "The Great Powers," *Assurance Mag. and J. Institute Actuaries* 6 (1857): 147-59, or in *16th A.R.R.G.*, App., pp. 116-25 [not in PP].
109. Farr, "Report of Paris Congress," pp. 106-7.
110. William Farr, "On Some Doctrines of Population," p. 568.
111. Farr, "Inaugural Address—1872," p. 425.

Chapter Three

1. The best treatment of these activities is in Cullen, *The Statistical Movement,* pp. 19-74.
2. The early history of registration has been quite thoroughly studied. The best short summaries are probably D. V. Glass, "The population Controversy in Eighteenth-Century England. Part I. The Background," *Population Studies* 6 (1952): 71-82; a revised edition is found in Glass, *Numbering the People,* pp. 12-21; J. T. Krause, "The Changing Adequacy of English Registration, 1690-1837," in *Population in History: Essays in Historical Demography,* eds. D. V. Glass and D. E. C. Eversley, (Chicago, 1965), pp. 379-93.
3. Krause, "The Changing Adequacy," esp. pp. 385-93.
4. Ibid., 382 and 384-85.
5. Frank Lorimer, "The Development of Demography," in *The Study of Population: An Inventory and Appraisal,* eds. Philip M. Hauser and Otis Dudley Duncan (Chicago, 1959), p. 124; and [William Farr], "Vital Statistics" in J[ohn] R[amsay] McCulloch (ed.), *A Descriptive and Statistical Account of the British Empire . . .,* 4th ed. (London, 1854) 2:601. For a pleasant account of the keeping of the bills of mortality in one London parish and a discussion of what those records reveal about London life see Thomas Rogers Forbes, *Chronicle from Aldgate: Life and Death in Shakespeare's London* (New Haven and London, 1971).
6. For a discussion of the recognition of these inadequacies and recommendations for improvement see Glass, "Population Controversy," p. 76 in the version in *Population Studies* (see above, n.2), p. 16 in *Numbering the People;* James H. Cassedy, *Demography in Early America: Beginnings of the Statistical Mind, 1600-1800* (Cambridge, Mass., 1969), pp. 277 and 280-81; and George Rosen, "Problems in the Application," p. 34.
7. Quoted in Glass, "Population Controversy," pp. 80-81 in *Population Studies* (see above, n. 2), pp. 19-20 in *Numbering the People.*
8. Ibid., 77 and 17, respectively.
9. The best treatment of this subject is Glass, *Numbering the People,* pp. 21-26 and 47-67, part of which is also found in his "Population Controversy," *Population Studies,* pp. 82-91 (see above, n. 2).
10. Cullen, *The Statistical Movement,* pp. 12-13; and Glass, *Numbering the People,* pp. 96-98, n. 8.
11. For Rickman's suggestion and appointment see: Orlo Williams, *Lamb's Friend the Census-Taker: Life and Letters of John Rickman* (London, 1911), pp. 40-41; and Cullen, *The Statistical Movement,* pp. 12-13. For more complete discussion of the early enumerations see: Glass, *Numbering the People,* pp. 90-105; *General Report,* Census of 1851, PP, 1852-53, LXXXV, ix-xviii; A. J. Taylor, "The Taking of the Census, 1801-1951," *Br. Med. J.,* 1951, i, 715-18; and W. A. Armstrong, "Social Structure from the Early Census Returns: An Analysis of Enumerators' Books for Censuses after 1841," in *An Introduction to English Historical Demography from the Sixteenth to the Nineteenth Century,* ed. E. A. Wrigley (London, 1966), pp. 209-10.
12. Glass, *Numbering the People,* pp. 93 and 100-1, n. 20.
13. Rickman is quoted in Taylor, "The Taking of the Census," p. 716.
14. Glass, *Numbering the People,* p. 95.
15. "Census of the Population—Law of Mortality, &c.," *Edinburgh Review* 49 (1829): 1-34.
16. Quoted in Williams, *Lamb's Friend,* p. 261. See also Glass, *Numbering the People,* p. 94.
17. Glass, *Numbering the People,* p. 94; Armstrong, pp. 211-13; and Taylor, pp. 716-19.

18. Cullen, *The Statistical Movement,* pp. 66 and 96–97.

19. Notes Farr made in planning the 1851 census have been preserved in L. S. E. Farr Collection, II, items 15–17, ff. 186–205.

20. Humphreys in Farr, *Vital Statistics,* p. 5. See also Joseph Whittall's comments on his chronological list of Farr's works in L. S. E. Farr Collection, X, f. 3. A more popular appreciation of Farr's contribution to the census reports is found in "Sketch of Dr. William Farr," *Popular Science Monthly* 23 (July, 1883): 405.

21. W. P. D. Logan, "Medical Significance of the Census," *Br. Med. J.,* 1951, i, 721.

22. See the general reports of the 1861 and 1871 censuses: PP 1863, LIII, pt. 1: 42–65 and 68–69; and PP, 1873, LXXI, pt. 2, pp. liv–lxvii.

23. *Census of 1851, Ages, Civil Condition, Occupations and Birth-Place of the People,* PP, 1852–53, LXXXVIII, pt. 1: lxxxii–c.

24. For this new scheme see William Farr, "The New Classification of the People According to their Employments," [app. to the *General Report,* Census of 1861] PP, 1863, LIII, pt. 1: pp. 225–48. See also pp. 27–39 of the general report in the same volume and the General Report of the 1871 census, PP, 1873, LXXI, pt. 2, xl–liv.

25. T. A. Welton, "On the Classification of the People by Occupations; and on Other Subjects Connected with Population Statistics of England," *J. Statist. Soc. Lond.* 32 (1869): 271–87.

26. "Report of the Fifth Section, on the Census and on the Occupations of the People," *Report of the Proceedings of the Fourth Session of the International Statistical Congress, Held in London July 16th, 1860, and the Five Following Days* (London, 1861), p. 150.

27. *Suppl. 25th A.R.R.G.,* pp. xxxv–xxxvi and 439–554 [PP, 1865, XIII]; and *Suppl. 35th A.R.R.G.,* pp. lii–lviii and 447–514 [PP, 1875, XVIII, pt. 2].

28. PP, 1833, XIV. Glass, *Numbering the People,* pp. 119 and 126–29; and Cullen, "The Making," pp. 45–46.

29. This point is demonstrated very well in Cullen, "The Making," pp. 39–50.

30. Ibid., pp. 45–46.

31. "Parochial Registration with Reference to Medical Statistics," *London Medical Gazette* 14 (1834): 102–6; Glass, *Numbering the People,* pp. 137–38, n. 41 and 46; and Cullen, "The Making," pp. 49–50.

32. For the enactment of the Registration Act see Cullen, "The Making," pp. 50–59.

33. Cullen, *The Statistical Movement,* p. 31; and D. V. Glass, "A Note on the Under-Registration of Births in Britain in the Nineteenth Century," *Population Studies* 5 (1952): 70.

34. Great Britain, *Statutes at Large,* 6 and 7 Wm. IV, c. 85 (1836), and 6 and 7 Wm. IV, c. 86 (1836).

35. *Regulations for the Duties of Superintendent Registrars* (London, 1838). I am indebted to Professor Saul Benison for a copy of this publication.

36. Humphreys in Farr, *Vital Statistics,* p. 8.

37. For Scotland see 17 and 18 Vict. c. 80 (1854); and 18 and 19 Vict. c. 29 (1854–55). For Ireland see 26 and 27 Vict. c. 11 (1863); and 26 and 27 Vict. c. 27 (1863).

38. P. Granville Edge, "Vital Registration in Europe: The Development of Official Statistics and Some Differences in Practice," *J. Roy. Statist. Soc.* 91 (1928): 360.

39. *Evolution of Preventive Medicine* (Baltimore, 1927), p. 115.

40. In addition to 6 and 7 Wm. IV, c. 86; and *Regulations for . . . Superintendent Registrars* (London, 1838), see Farr, "Letter," *27th A.R.R.G.,* pp. 178–80 [PP, 1866, XIX] for a summary of the procedure for registering a death.

41. Little, *History,* p. 119; and Paul Vaughan, *Doctors' Commons: A Short History of the British Medical Association* (London, Melbourne, Toronto, 1959), pp. 11–12. For Farr's summary of the Association's continuing interest see "Draft of Petition of the British Medical Association to be Presented to the House of Commons," *Br. Ann. Med.* 1 (1837): 442–43.

42. Cullen, "The Making," pp. 55–58; and Cullen, *The Statistical Movement,* pp. 53–54. Another claimant for the distinction of suggesting the cause of death be included in the act is F. Bisset Hawkins; see Glass, *Numbering the People,* p. 140, n. 56.

43. Of the 2,193 registrars appointed up to September 30, 1838, 527 were medical men. Glass, *Numbering the People*, p. 140, n. 56.

44. See the editorial "More Task-work from the Poor-Law Commissioners," *London Medical Gazette* 18 (1836): 879–81; and the letter to the editor in response Ibid. 19 (1836–37): 127, portions from both of which are quoted in Cullen, "The Making," p. 58. Farr's journal was also critical although somewhat more restrained. See "National Registration," *Br. Ann. Med.* 1 (1837): 180–81.

45. Benjamin Ward Richardson, *The Health of Nations: A Review of the Works of Edwin Chadwick*, 2 vols. [1887] (London, 1965), 1: xliii–xlv, and 79–80; and S. E. Finer, *The Life*, pp. 154–55.

46. Farr, "Letter," *38th A.R.R.G.*, p. 226 [PP, 1877, XXV].

47. Details of the administration of the G.R.O. may be found in a financial account the office prepared for Parliament in 1847, PP, 1847, XXXIV. See also Cullen, *The Statistical Movement*, pp. 29–30.

48. Humphreys, in Farr, *Vital Statistics*, p. xix.

49. Finer, *The Life*, pp. 154–55.

50. Ibid., p. 143.

51. Maboth Moseley, *Irascible Genius: The Life of Charles Babbage, Inventor* (London, 1964), p. 130.

52. Cullen, *The Statistical Movement*, p. 160, n. 4.

53. *English Sanitary Institutions*, p. 211.

54. Cullen, *The Statistical Movement*, pp. 29–30.

55. *The Medical Dictator and Other Biographical Studies* (London, 1936), pp. 103–04.

56. See two editorials in particular: "National Registration," *Br. Ann. Med.* 1 (1837): 180–82; and "Registration of Diseases," Ibid., p. 664.

57. [Farr], "National Registration," p. 182.

58. July 10 is the date given in Humphreys, in Farr, *Vital Statistics*. p. xii. July 6 is given in "A Return...Registrar General," PP, 1847, XXXIV, p. 5.

59. This account is from a letter of Chadwick to Dr. T. H. Laycock of April 13, 1844, which has been reprinted in Glass, *Numbering the People*, pp. 149–50. See also Finer, *The Life*, p. 143.

60. This suggestion is advanced rather tentatively by Humphreys, in Farr, *Vital Statistics*, p. xii. It is repeated in Greenwood, *Medical Dictator*, p. 98.

61. Greenwood, *Medical Dictator*, p. 98.

62. Humphreys, in Farr, *Vital Statistics*, p. xii; and Finer, *The Life*, p. 143.

63. "A Return...Registrar General," PP, 1847, XXXIV.

64. For details of Farr's later income see Humphreys, in Farr, *Vital Statistics*, p. xvi; Great Britain, Treasury Minute [copy], Feb. 28, 1880 in L. S. E. Farr Collection, XIII, item 12; and Glass, *Numbering the People*, p. 142, n. 70.

65. L. S. E. Farr Collection, II, item 20, ff. 217–21. This memorandum has been recently published in Glass, *Numbering the People*, pp. 168–69.

66. This point is made in the obituary notice "Dr. Farr," *The Review* (April 25, 1883), p. 221.

67. This topic will be discussed later. The most important papers are: William Lucas Sargant, "On Certain Results and Defects of the Reports of the Registrar-General," *J. Statist. Soc. Lond.* 27 (1864): 170–221; William Lucas Sargant, "Inconsistences of the English Census of 1861, with the Registrar-General's Reports: and Deficiencies in the Local Registry of Births," *Ibid.* 28 (1865): 73–124; and William Farr, "On Infant Mortality, and on Alleged Inaccuracies of the Census," Ibid. 28 (1865): 125–49.

68. Finer, *The Life*, p. 143.

69. "Report to the Right Honourable George Sclater-Booth, M.P., President of the Local Government Board, etc., etc.," *40th A.R.R.G.*, p. xl [PP, 1878–79, XIX].

70. C. Fraser Brockington, *Public Health in the Nineteenth Century* (Edinburgh and London, 1965), p. 159.

71. George Graham, letter to William Farr, June 6, 1866, L. S. E. Farr Collection, I, item 45, f. 80.

72. G[eorge] G[raham], letter to William Farr, Oct. 31, 1874, L. S. E. Farr Collection, VIII, item 8. Farr's memorandum and the revised forms he proposed are Ibid., items 7, 9, and 10.

73. Simon, *English Sanitary Institutions*, pp. 211-12.

74. Quoted in Glass, *Numbering the People*, pp. 142-43, n. 70.

75. M. W. Flinn, "Introduction," in Edwin Chadwick, *Report on the Sanitary Condition of the Labouring Population of Gt. Britain* [1842] (Edinburgh, 1965), pp. 30-31.

76. O. R. McGregor, "Social Research," p. 152.

77. Royston Lambert, *Sir John Simon 1816–1904 and English Social Administration* (London, 1963), p. 300, n. 33.

78. William Farr, letter to Edwin Chadwick, Feb. 13, 1837, University College, London University, Edwin Chadwick Mss. The letter has been reprinted in Glass, *Numbering the People*, p. 148. For comments see Cullen, "The Making," p. 59; or Cullen, *The Statistical Movement*, p. 54; and Glass, *Numbering the People*, p. 141, n. 63.

79. "National Registration," pp. 180-82.

80. PP, 1863, XIX.

81. PP, 1854-55, XIII, 188-98 and 204-10.

82. PP, 1857-58 XVIII, 242-47 and app. LXX, 506-07 and LXXII, pp. 516-26.

83. PP, 1868-69, XXXII, 243-48 and 279-91.

84. PP, 1864, XXIV, pt. 2, 154-78.

85. PP, 1852-53, XXI, 297-312.

86. PP, 1861, VII, 161-91.

87. PP, 1877, XV, 1-42.

88. Humphreys in Farr, *Vital Statistics*, p. xviii.

89. 37 and 38 Vic. c. 88 (1874).

90. *1st A.R.R.G.*, p. 77 [PP, 1839, XVI, 58-59]. See also *Regulations for. . .Superintendent Registrars*, pp. 43-45; Graham republished this circular in *7th A.R.R.G.*, pp. 252-53 [PP, 1846, XIX, xviii].

91. "Directions Respecting the Registration of the Causes of Death," *Lancet*, 1842-43, ii, 236-37; and "Notice Relative to Returns of 'Causes of Death,'" *Lond. Med. Gazette* 32 (1842-43): 252.

92. A copy of this form and Graham's report is found in *7th A.R.R.G.*, pp. 254-56. [PP, 1846, XIX, xix-xx].

93. Farr, "Letter," *33rd A.R.R.G.*, p. 408 [PP, 1872, XVII].

94. Farr provided a brief history of the introduction of these forms in Farr, "Letter," *38th A.R.R.G.*, p. 227 [PP, 1877, XXV].

95. T. H. C. Stevenson, *Manual of the International List of Causes of Death, as Adapted for Use in England and Wales* (London, 1912), pp. ix-x.

96. "Suggestions for Important Improvements in the Registration of Births and Deaths," *Lond. Med. Gazette*, n. s. 1 (1845): 212-14.

97. *Lancet*, 1842-43, ii, 278-79; and "The Circular of the Registrar-General," Ibid., 1845, ii, 270-72.

98. *Lancet*, 1845, ii, 272.

99. "Registration of Causes of Death in the Army and in Civil Life," *Lancet*, 1855, ii, 36.

100. Farr, "Letter," *1st A.R.R.G.*, p. 99 [PP, 1839, XVI, 71]. Since this work went to press, a useful account of Farr's nosologies has appeared in Margaret Pelling, *Cholera, Fever and English Medicine 1825-1865* (Oxford, 1978), pp. 91-102.

101. Farr, "Letter," *1st A.R.R.G.*, p. 92 [66-67].

102. For Farr's account of the history of these nosologies see Farr, "Letter," *38th A.R.R.G.*, pp. 227-30 [PP, 1877, XXV].

103. Farr, "Vital Statistics," in McCulloch, 1st ed., pp. 594-99.

104. See for example his comments in "Statistical Nosology," *4th A.R.R.G.*, pp. 189-90 [PP, 1842, XIX, 114].

105. Ibid., p. 147 [93].

106. Farr, "Letter," *1st A.R.R.G.*, pp. 92-99 [PP, 1839, XVI, 66-71].

107. Ibid., p. 93 [67].

108. Ibid.

109., 9 (1840): 351-52.

110. *Report of a Committee of the Royal College of Physicians of Edinburgh, Appointed to Consider the Best Mode of Framing Public Registers of Deaths* (Edinburgh, 1841); and Marc D'Espine, "Essai statistique sur la mortalité du Canton de Genève pendant l'année 1838," *Annales d'hygiène publique et de médecine légale* 23 (1840): 111-26. Alison also restated his case after Farr responded to his initial criticism. See William Pulteney Alison, "Observations on the Best Mode of Registering Deaths," *Northern J. Med.* 1 (1844): 225-32.

111. *Report, B.A.A.S.* 5 (1835): 251-55.

112. D'Espine was an especially able representative of Pierre Louis's numerical methods. See Eduard-Rudolf Müllener, "Pierre-Charles-Alexandre-Louis' (1787-1872) Genfer Schüler und die 'méthode numérique,'" *Gesnerus* 24 (1967): 51-58.

113. Farr, "Letter," *2nd A.R.R.G.*, pp. 78-80 [PP, 1840 XVII, 9]; and "Statistical Nosology," *4th A.R.R.G.*, app., pp. 206-16 [PP, 1842, XIX, 123-27].

114. "Statistical Nosology," *4th A.R.R.G.*, app., pp. 147-205 [PP, 1842, XIX, 93-122]. The section listing the disease entries is pp. 147-65 [93-105].

115. Ibid., 186-205 [112-22]. The zymotic diseases are discussed specifically on pp. 199-205 [119-22].

116. "The Vital Statistics of England," *Br. and For. Med. Rev.* 18 (1844): 198.

117. "Last Report of the Registrar-General," *Lond. Med. Gazette* 31 (1842-43): 792.

118. For an example of such modifications see Farr, "Letter," *13th A.R.R.G.*, pp. 130-31.

119. Will[iam] Farr, "Projet de classification," *Compte rendu de la deuxième session du Congrès International de Statistique* (Paris, 1856), pp. 147-65. Farr also provided an English summary in "Report on the Nomenclature and Statistical Classification of Diseases, for Statistical Returns," *16th A.R.R.G.*, pp. 71-96.

120. Farr, "Report on the Nomenclature," p. 71.

121. Farr, "Letter," *38th A.R.R.G.*, p. 228 [PP, 1877, XXV].

122. Farr, "Projet de classification," pp. 151-53; and Farr, "Report on the Nomenclature," pp. 76-77.

123. Farr, "Statistical Nosology," *4th A.R.R.G.*, pp. 199-205 [PP, 1842, XIX, 119-21]. We will discuss Farr's disease theory in Chapter Five.

124. Farr, "Report on the Nomenclature," p. 75.

125. Marc D'Espine, "Projet de classification des causes de mort . . . "*Compt rendu de la deuxième session du Congrès International de Statistique* (Paris, 1856), pp. 133-46. For a summary of these nosologies and their reception see Henry W. Rumsey, *Essays and Papers on some Fallacies of Statistics . . .* (London, 1875), pp. 122-35.

126. B[ernard] Benjamin, *Elements of Vital Statistics* (London, 1959), p. 88; and Stevenson, *Manual*, p. v (see above, n. 95).

127. James Stark, "Remarks on Dr. Farr's Proposed New Statistical Classification of Diseases for Statistical Returns," *Edinburgh Med. J.* 5 (1860): 1069-82.

128. "Report on the Questions Submitted by Dr. Farr to the Council," *Trans. Epidem. Soc. Lond.*, n. s. 2 (1862-66): app.: 1-30. A summary of the incident and the responses is found in Rumsey, *Essays and Papers*, pp. 139-44. Medical cynicism about the pathological theory underlying the zymotic class may be sampled in an editorial in *Med. Times and Gazette*, 1860, ii, 111; and in Farr's report on a "hard fight" at the Royal College of Physicians in his letter to Florence Nightingale, April 25, 1863, B.M. Add. Mss., 43,399, ff. 111-12.

129. See for example Farr, "Letter," *21st A.R.R.G.*, pp. 205-9 [PP, 1860, XXIX].

130. Barbara Gutmann Rosenkrantz, *Public Health and the State: Changing Views in Massachusetts, 1842-1936* (Cambridge, Mass., 1972), pp. 24 and 27. See also Surgeon General, United States Army, *The Medical and Surgical History of the War of the Rebellion* (Washington, D.C., 1875), 1, pt. 1: xvi-xix.

131. For an early version of the list see Arthur Newsholme, *The Elements of Vital Statistics in Their Bearing on Social and Public Health Problems*, new ed. (New York, 1924), pp. 612-18.

132. James H. Cassedy, "The Registration Area and American Vital Statistics: Development of a Health Research Resource, 1885-1915," *Bull. Hist. Med.* 39 (1965): 221-31; and Fernand Faure, "The Development and Progress of Statistics in France," in *The History of Statistics: Their Development and Progress in Many Countries,* ed. John Koren (New York, 1918), pp. 283-89.

133. I have explored this problem in my article "Mortality Statistics and Victorian Health Policy: Program and Criticism," *Bull. Hist. Med.* 50 (1976): 335-55.

134. Farr, "Letter," *27th A.R.R.G.,* pp. 179-82 [PP, 1866, XIX].

135. Chadwick pointed out the unsavory character of some of the local registrars he encountered. See Cullen, *The Statistical Movement,* pp. 30-31.

136. Four such cases in a group of 2,200 registrars had come to light in 29 years. Farr, "Letter," *27th A.R.R.G.,* p. 180 [PP, 1866, XIX].

137. See in particular Farr's discussion of abstracting deaths returned as due to "dropsy." Farr, "Letter," *30th A.R.R.G.,* p. 208 [PP, 1868-69, XVI].

138. Stevenson, *Manual,* pp. ix-x; Benjamin, *Elements,* p. 85 (see above, n. 126); and Cullen, *The Statistical Movement,* p. 34.

139. Roy M. MacLeod, "The Anatomy of State Medicine," pp. 205-06 and 209-13.

140. Henry Wyldbore Rumsey, *Essays on State Medicine* (London, 1856), pp. 7-12 and 349-53.

141. Rumsey, *Essays and Papers,* dedication.

142. In the dedication Rumsey refers to their friendship of forty years standing. As early as 1837 Farr praised a pamphlet Rumsey wrote for the Provincial Medical and Surgical Association's Committee on Medical Relief of the Poor, "The Provincial Medical and Surgical Association," *Br. Ann. Med.* 2 (1837): 60. We also have evidence of the sad ending of the friendship. Rumsey's wife, F. S. Rumsey, wrote to Farr in August 1875 and April 1876 about her husband's failing health and asking Farr's advice on some financial matters. She mentions she had not seen Farr's younger daughter, Florence, that term, as if those visits were quite routine. F. S. Rumsey, letters to William Farr, 13 Aug. 1875 and 10 April 1876, L. S. E. Farr Collection, I, item 87, ff. 157-58 and item 88, ff. 159-60b. For Farr's tribute to Rumsey see *Br. Med. J.,* 1875, i, 460.

143. "On Certain Deficiences in Our Public Records of Mortality and Sickness, with Suggestions for an Improved and Extended National System of Registration," *Trans. N.A.P.S.S.* (Bradford, 1859), 574-84; and "On Certain Departments of Medico-Sanitary Police and Medico-Legal Inquiry, in Connexion with the Scientific Superintendence of Mortuary Registration," Ibid., pp. 585-95.

144. "The Fallacies and Shortcomings of our Sanitary Statistics," *Social Science Review, and Journal of the Sciences,* n. s. 4 (1865): 234-50, 358-63, 403-14, 481-95; 5 (1866): 21-43, 310-21, 440-47; 6 (1866): 97-110.

145. "On the Value of Life Tables, National and Local, as Evidence of Sanitary Condition," *Trans. Manchr. Statist. Soc.,* (1866-67), 1-15; and "On Certain Fallacies in Local Rates of Mortality, Arising from Defective Information . . .," Ibid. (1871-72), 17-39.

146. London, 1875. Citations of Rumsey's criticisms will be made to this volume.

147. Rumsey, *Essays and Papers,* pp. 107-20 and 150-58.

148. The cause of death was not confidential information in England until 1926. Major P. Granville, "Vital Registration in Europe . . .," *J. Statist. Soc. Lond.* 91 (1928): 360.

149. Rumsey, *Essays and Papers,* p. 150, n. 1.

150. Ibid., p. 154.

151. William Farr, evidence and testimony, *Report from the Select Committee on Public Health Bill, and Nuisances Removal Amendment Bill,* PP, 1854-55, XIII, 192. The idea had been proposed even earlier by Thomas Rowe Edmonds in "On the Laws of Sickness, According to Age, Exhibiting a Double Coincidence between the Laws of Sickness and the Laws of Mortality," *Lancet* 1835-36, i, 858.

152. Rumsey, *Essays and Papers,* pp. 54-55.

153. Benjamin W[ard] Richardson, "Facts and Suggestions on the Registration of Disease," *Trans. N.A.P.S.S.* (Dublin, 1861), pp. 544-47; Gavin Milroy, "Suggestions for Utilising the Statistics of Disease Among the Poor," *Trans. Epidem. Soc. Lond.* (1859-60), pp. 72-74; and Lambert, *John Simon,* pp. 419-21.

154. Rumsey, *Essays and Papers*, pp. 50-53 and 99-103.

155. Jeanne L. Brand, *Doctors and the State*, pp. 60-63. See also Rumsey, *Essays and Papers*, pp. 103-6; and the sections on notification of infectious diseases held by the Social Science Association, *Trans. N.A.P.S.S.* (Dublin, 1881), pp. 532-56, and Ibid. (Northampton, 1882), 448-65.

156. Farr, "Letter," *3rd A.R.R.G.*, pp. 90-97 [PP, 1841, sess. 2, VI, 15-19]; and Farr, "Letter," *19th A.R.R.G.*, pp. 196-205 [PP, 1857-58, XXIII]. He also studied the returns for violent deaths. See in particular Farr, "Letter," 3rd A.R.R.G., pp. 75-90 [PP, 1841, sess. 2, VI, 5-15]; and *6th A.R.R.G.*, pp. 210-66 [PP, 1844, XIX, 149-74].

157. Farr, "Letter," *3rd A.R.R.G.*, p. 91 [PP, 1841, sess. 2, VI, 15].

158. Farr, "Letter," *19th A.R.R.G.*, pp. 204-5 [PP, 1857-58, XXI].

159. Farr, "Letter," *27th A.R.R.G.*, pp. 182-89 [PP, 1866, XIX]. The basic idea was not entirely original and, as Farr and other members of the British medical profession would have known, a similar scheme had been tried or suggested in some places on the Continent. See "Parochial Registration with Reference to Medical Statistics," *Lond. Med. Gazette* 14 (1834): 105, and D'Espine, "Essai Statistique," p. 119.

160. Farr, "Statistical Nosology," *4th A.R.R.G.*, p. 209 [PP, 1842, XIX, 124]; Farr, "Letter," *30th A.R.R.G.*, p. 210 [PP, 1868-69, XVI]; and Farr, "Letter," *31st A.R.R.G.*, pp. 197-98 [PP, 1870, XVI].

161. MacLeod, "The Anatomy of State Medicine," pp. 206-26.

162. Little, *History*, pp. 120-21. Rumsey was familiar with Farr's earlier proposals on the reform of the coroner's office and had reached a conclusion similar to Farr's that special registration officers were needed. See Rumsey, "On Certain Departments of Medico-Sanitary Police," pp. 590-91.

163. Henry W. Rumsey, "Remarks on State Medicine in Great Britain," *Br. Med. J.*, 1867, ii, 197-201. The speech was published separately with additions and was entitled *On State Medicine in Great Britain and Ireland* (London, 1867).

164. Brand, *Doctors and the State*, pp. 8-21 and MacLeod, "The Anatomy of State Medicine," p. 218. For information on the appointment of the Joint Committee and its interest in the registration system see: *Br. Med. J.*, 1868, i, 33, 489, 541-43; and Ibid., 1868, ii, 194-95.

165. 37 and 38 Vict. c. 88 (1874).

166. Farr, "Letter," *33rd A.R.R.G.*, p. 408 [PP, 1872, XVII].

Chapter Four

1. Farr, letter to the Registrar General, March 17, 1840, originally published in the *Official Circulars* of the Poor Law commissioners. Reprinted in Glass, *Numbering the People*, p. 161.

2. Farr, "Letter," *12th A.R.R.G.*, p. lii [not in PP]; Farr, "Letter," *27th A.R.R.G.*, p. 185 [PP, 1866, XIX].

3. W[illiam] Farr, "On the Construction," p. 854; *English Life Table: Tables of Lifetimes, Annuities, and Premiums, with an Introduction by William Farr, M.D., F.R.S., D.C.L.* (London, 1864), pp. cxxxix-cxliv. Farr had appreciated the potential benefit of Babbage's machine when he calculated his first life table two decades earlier. William Farr, "Construction of Life Tables," *5th A.R.R.G.*, p. 352 [PP, 1843, XXI, 167].

4. [Farr], *English Life Table*, p. cxl.

5. David V. Glass, "Some Aspects of the Development of Demography," *J. Roy. Soc. Arts* 104 (1956): 859.

6. "[Presidential] Address," *Report, B.A.A.S.* 34 (1864): 152.

7. One of the rare appearances of a discussion of continuous functions and his use of integral calculus is found in William Farr, "On the Pay of Ministers of the Crown," *J. Statist. Soc. Lond.* 20 (1857): 127. In discussing population growth and the problem of calculating mean population for an interval of time he employed notions of limits and infinitesimals to a curve. See Farr, "On the Modes," p. 569; [Farr], *English Life Table*, pp. xiv-xviii; Farr, "On the Construction," pp. 840-42.

8. W[illiam] Farr, "On the Law of Recovery and Dying in Small-Pox. Article II," *Br. Ann. Med.* 1 (1837): 138-39.

9. Manuscript questions, L. S. E. Farr Collection, XIII, item 7.

10. Draft of an unfinished article on permutations, L. S. E. Farr Collection, II, item 1, ff. 2-4.

11. See the discussion in Greenwood, *Some British Pioneers*, pp. 64-65.

12. *Medical Dictator*, pp. 106-9.

13. Arthur Newsholme, "The Measurement of Progress in Public Health with Special Reference to the Life and Work of William Farr," *Economica* 3 (1923): 196-202.

14. For examples see Westergaard, pp. 152-54, and 208.

15. For general comments on this problem see Farr "[Presidential] Address," pp. 155-57.

16. An early example is found in Farr's attempt to correct the returns for suicides and violent deaths in Farr, "Letter," *3rd A.R.R.G.*, pp. 78-79 [PP, 1841, sess. 2, VI, 8].

17. Rumsey, *Essays and Papers*, p. 184.

18. Farr, "Vital Statistics," in McCulloch, 1st ed., pp. 567-68.

19. Farr's classic treatment of the effect of age on mortality and morbidity is found in Farr, "Letter," *Suppl. 35th A.R.R.G.*, pp. xxi-xxxvii [PP, 1875, XVIII, pt. 2]. Criticism of the G.R.O.'s statistics in the 1850s and 1860s no doubt helped sharpen his appreciation of this problem.

20. "Introduction," *Vital Statistics: A Memorial Volume of Selections from the Reports and Writings of William Farr*, ed. Noel A. Humphreys [1885] (Metuchen, N.J., 1975), p. viii.

21. "Address by W. Farr, M.D., F.R.S. on Public Health," *Trans. N.A.P.S.S.* (Manchester, 1866), pp. 67-78.

22. Farr, "Letter," *Suppl. 25th A.R.R.G.*, pp. iv-v [PP, 1865, XIII].

23. *5th A.R.R.G.*, pp. 31-33 [PP, 1843, XXI, xxiii-xxiv]. This section appears in George Graham's report, but it was undoubtedly written by Farr. See also Farr, "On the Construction," p. 838.

24. Farr, "Letter," *1st A.R.R.G.*, pp. 89-90 [PP, 1839, XVI, 65].

25. W[illiam] Farr, "On the Law of Recovery and Dying," p. 134.

26. Farr, "Address...on Public Health," p. 67.

27. Farr, "On the Construction," p. 842.

28. Farr, "Letter," *Suppl. 35th A.R.R.G.*, p. xxi [PP, 1875, XVIII, pt. 2]. This distinction is also implicit in Farr's healthy district standard which we will discuss shortly; see William Farr [testimony], *Report from the Select Committee on Public Health Bill and Nuisances Removal Amendment Bill*, PP, 1854-55, XIII, 196.

29. In comparing mortality rates for different places Thomas Rowe Edmonds used both modes of expression in the same paragraph; "Statistics of Mortality in England," *Br. Med. Almanack*, Suppl. (1837), 131.

30. Farr, "Letter," *Suppl. 25th A.R.R.G.*, p. v., [PP, 1865, XIII].

31. W[illiam] Farr, "On the Modes," pp. 568-69; [Farr], *English Life Table*, pp. xiv-xx.

32. $Y_x = (k\,P_0/\lambda r)\,(r^x - 1)$ is the formula he used to calculate the years of life for x years where r is the annual rate of increase of the population, λr the logarithm of r, p_0 the population at the beginning of the period and k the modulus of the common logarithm. Farr was indebted to T. R. Edmonds for this formula. See Farr, "On the Construction," pp. 844-46. In [Farr], *English Life Table*, pp. xiv-xx he gave equivalent formulas found by calculating the area under the curve in each of these four cases.

33. I have discussed the general outlines of the controversy in my article "Mortality Statistics," pp. 335-55.

34. *Report on the Sanitary Condition of the Labouring Population of Gt. Britain* [1842], ed. M. W. Flinn (Edinburgh, 1965), esp. pp. 219-76; and "On the Best Modes of Representing Accurately, by Statistical Returns, the Duration of Life, and the Pressure and Progress of the Causes of Mortality amongst Different Classes of the Community, and amongst the Populations of Different Districts and Counties," *J. Statist. Soc. Lond.* 7 (1844): 1-40.

35. William Farr, "The 'Annual Mortality' and the 'Mean Age at Death': A Comparison of the Methods Which Have Been Employed at Various Times for Determining the Relative Salubrity and Mortality of Different Classes of the Population," *6th A.R.R.G.*, pp.

570-77 [PP, 1844, XIX, 315-18]; F. G. P. Neison, "On a Method Recently Proposed for Conducting Inquiries into the Comparative Sanatory Conditions of Various Districts, with Illustrations, Derived from Numerous Places in Great Britain at the Period of the Last Census, *J. Statist. Soc. Lond.* 7 (1844): 40-68; W[illiam] A. Guy, "Vital Statistics," *The Cyclopaedia of Anatomy and Physiology*, ed. Robert B. Todd (London, 1849-52), 4, pt. 2: 1469-75. For Chadwick's response to Neison's attack see Chadwick, letter to T. H. Laycock, April 13, 1844, in Glass, *Numbering the People*, pp. 149-50.

36. *5th A.R.R.G.*, pp. 38-48 [PP, 1843, XXI, xxviii-xxxiii].

37. Farr's testimony, *Report from the Select Committee on Public Health Bill, and Nuisances Removal Amendment Bill*, PP, 1854-55, XIII, 196-97; Farr, "Letter," *20th A.R.R.G.*, pp. 174-76 [PP, 1859, sess. 2, XII]; and John Simon, "Introductory Report by the Medical Officer of the Board," *Papers Relating to the Sanitary State of the People of England*, PP, 1857-58, XXIII, iii-iv.

38. Farr's testimony, *Report from the Select Committee on Public Health Bill*, p. 204. A variation was to calculate the excess deaths caused by the prevailing degree of insalubrity. See Farr, "Letter," *Suppl. 25th A.R.R.G.*, pp. xxvi-xxvii [PP, 1865, XIII].

39. *5th A.R.R.G.*, p. 37 [PP, 1843, XXI, xxvi-xxvii].

40. Ibid.

41. Ibid., pp. 21-22 [xvi].

42. For brief histories of actuary practice see Glass, *Numbering the People*, pp. 120-26; [Joshua Milne], "Annuities," *Encyclopaedia Britannica*, 7th ed. (1842), 3: 198-210; Newsholme, *Vital Statistics*, new ed. (1924), pp. 231-37; and George M. Low, "The History of Actuarial Science in Great Britain," *Troisième congrès international d'actuaires* (Paris, 1901), pp. 848-75.

43. "An Estimate of the Degrees of Mortality of Mankind, Drawn from Curious Tables of the Births and Funerals at the City of Breslaw; with an Attempt to Ascertain the Price of Annuities upon Lives," *Phil. Trans.* 17 (1693): 596-610. For short historical evaluations see Meitzen, *History*, pp. 31-33.

44. For Price's career as an actuary see Glass, *Numbering the People*, pp. 121 and 123; and Maurice Edward Ogborn, *Equitable Assurances: The Story of Life Assurance in the Experience of the Equitable Life Assurance Society 1762-1962* (London, 1962), pp. 90-97.

45. Meitzen, *History*, pp. 32-33; and E. Grebenik, "The Development of Demography in Great Britain," in *The Study of Population: An Inventory and Appraisal*, eds. Philip M. Hauser and Otis Dudley Duncan (Chicago and London, 1959), pp. 190-91.

46. *A Treatise on the Valuation of Annuities and Assurances on Lives and Survivorships; on the Construction of Tables of Mortality; and on the Probabilities and Expectations of Life*, 2 vols. (London, 1815).

47. The scope of his reading may be seen in the works he recommended to his audience in the introduction to his own national life tables: Farr, "Letter," *6th A.R.R.G.*, pp. 524-26 [PP, 1844, XIX, 296-97]; and Farr, "Letter," *12th A.R.R.G.*, pp. iii-vi [not in PP].

48. *Life Tables, Founded upon the Discovery of a Numerical Law Regulating the Existence of Every Human Being* (London, 1832). Edmonds also published a series of a dozen articles in the *Lancet* in the middle thirties, of which the following were the most important to Farr: "On the Laws of Collective Vitality," *Lancet*, 1834-35, ii, 5-8; "On the Mortality of the People of England," Ibid., 310-16; "On the Law of Mortality in Each County of England," Ibid., 1835-36, i, 364-71 and 408-16; "On the Mortality of Infants in England," Ibid., 690-94; "On the Laws of Sickness, According to Age, Exhibiting a Double Coincidence between the Laws of Sickness and the Laws of Mortality," Ibid., 855-58; and "Statistics of the London Hospital, with Remarks on the Law of Sickness," Ibid., 1835-36, ii, 778-83. See also his "Statistics of Mortality in England," *Br. Med. Almanack*, Suppl. 1837), pp. 130-35. Farr regularly cited Edmonds as an actuary authority.

49. C. H. Driver, "Thomas Rowe Edmonds," *Encyclopaedia of the Social Sciences*, (New York, 1937), 3: 399; C. H. Driver, "A Forgotten Sociologist," *J. Adult Ed.* 3 (1929): 134-54; and M[ax] Beer, *A History of British Socialism* (London, 1919-1920) 1: 230-36.

50. Edmonds, "On the Laws of Collective Vitality," p. 6; and Edmonds, "Statistics of Mortality in England," p. 131.

51. For short summaries of their construction see T. R. Edmonds, "On the Mortality at Glasgow, and on the Increasing Mortality in England," *Lancet*, 1835-36, ii, 358-59; and Edmonds, "On the Law of Mortality in Each County," pp. 370-71.

52. Edmonds, "On the Law of Mortality in Each County," p. 369; and Edmonds, "On the Mortality of Infants," pp. 692-94.

53. Benjamin Gompertz, "On the Nature of the Function Expressive of the Law of Human Mortality, and on a New Mode of Determining the Value of Life Contingencies," *Phil. Trans.* 115 (1825): 513-83.

54. See in particular articles and letters by Edmonds, Gompertz, Augustus DeMorgan, and T. B. Sprague in *Assurance Mag. and J. Institute Actuaries* 9 (1860-61): 86-89, 170-84, 214-15, 288-98, 327-41; and Ibid. 10 (1861-62): 32-44, 104-13.

55. Glass, *Numbering the People,* pp. 120 and 133, n. 14.

56. Edmonds, "On the Law of Mortality in Each County," pp. 365 and 411.

57. Ibid., p. 365.

58. Edmonds, "On the Laws of Collective Vitality," p. 5.

59. Ibid., and Edmonds, "On the Law of Mortality in Each County," p. 364. Compare these to [Farr], "Vital Statistics," *Br. Ann. Med.* 1 (1837): 353-54.

60. Farr, "Vital Statistics," in McCulloch, 1st ed., pp. 567-72 and 585.

61. Edmonds, "Statistics of the London Hospital," p. 778.

62. T. R. Edmonds, letters to William Farr, 6 April 1859 and 25 May 1860, L. S. E. Farr Collection, I, items 23 and 24, ff., 44-47 (b).

63. Farr, "Construction of Life Tables," pp. 345-46 [PP, 1843, XXI, 163]. At about the time the controversy took place, Farr claimed Edmonds had "extended" Gompertz's discovery. Farr, "On the Construction," p. 844.

64. *5th A.R.R.G.*, pp. 16-52 and 342-67 [PP, 1843, XXI, xii-xxxv and 161-78] and *6th A.R.R.G.*, App. pt. 2, pp. 517-666 [PP, 1844, XIX, 290-358]. The *Fifth Annual Report* contained the basic tables and accounts of the construction of life tables and a popular discussion of the general principles and uses of these tables. The *Sixth Annual Report* gave many more tables and included much discussion of actuary applications.

65. "English Life Table, No. 2, Males," *12th A.R.R.G.*, App., pp. 73-152 [not in PP]; and "English Life Table, No. 2, Females," *20th A.R.R.G.*, 177-203 [PP, 1859, sess. 2, XII].

66. *English Life Tables: Tables of Lifetimes, Annuities, and Premiums, with an Introduction by William Farr, M.D., F.R.S., D.C.L.* (London, 1864).

67. Farr, "On the Construction," pp. 860-61.

68. Farr, *English Life Table* [no. 3], pp. lxxvi-lxxxix.

69. Farr, "On the Construction," pp. 839-61; and Farr, *English Life Table* [No. 3], pp. xiv-xxviii. See also *5th A.R.R.G.*, pp. 342-67 [PP, 1843, XXI, 161-77] and *6th A.R.R.G.*, pp. 524-46 [PP, 1844, XIX, 296-305]. Another useful, slightly more modern account which is written within the statistical tradition Farr helped to create is in Newsholme, *The Elements*, 3rd ed. (1899), pp. 255-89. Farr acknowledged his debt to his actuarial predecessors in Farr, "Construction of Life Tables," pp. 345-46 and 349 [163 and 165].

70. Farr's life table notation presents several difficulties to historians. His usage evolved over his career. In his first two national life tables Farr labeled the columns that he would later designate as "l," "d," and "L," with "D," "C," and "N," respectively. There is one further source of confusion about notation. Farr changed standard life table labels. The columns that actuaries had labeled "L" and "T," he changed to "P" and "Q," respectively.

71. In his later works Farr described his formula for mean afterlifetime as an approximation only. Farr, *English Life Table* [No. 3], pp. xxxiii-xxxv.

72. Ibid., xxxvii-xxxviii.

73. Farr, "Construction of Life Tables," p. 349 [165]; and Farr, "Letter," *Suppl. 25th A.R.R.G.*, pp. iii-iv [PP, 1865, XIII].

74. Farr, "On the Construction," pp. 844-48.

75. Ibid., p. 848. See also Farr, "Construction of Life Tables," pp. 344-47 [162-64].

76. Farr, "Construction of Life Tables," p. 344 [162]; and Farr, "On the Construction," pp. 847-48. Newsholme gave a clear derivation of this formula in *The Elements*, 3rd ed. (1899), pp. 259-60.

77. Farr, "Construction of Life Tables," pp. 347–48 [164].

78. Farr, *English Life Table* [No. 3], p. xxvi.

79. Farr, [*English Life Table* No. 1], *6th A.R.R.G.*, p. 524 [PP, 1844, XIX, 296].

80. W[illiam] Farr, "English Reproduction Table," *Phil. Trans.* 171 (1880): 281–88.

81. Farr, *English Life Table* [No. 3], p. xxxv.

82. W[illiam] Farr, "Address . . . on Public Health," *Trans. N.A.P.S.S.* (Manchester, 1866), p. 68; Farr, "Letter," *Suppl. 35th A.R.R.G.*, pp. xii–xiv [PP, 1875, XVIII, pt. 2]. Newsholme gives a numerical expression for this relationship which I have not been able to locate in Farr's writings. Newsholme, *The Elements*, 3rd ed. (1899), p. 301. It was Newsholme's form of Farr's law that Lotka commented on. Alfred J. Lotka, "The Relation between Birth Rate and Death Rate in a Normal Population and the Rational Basis of an Empirical Formula for the Mean Length of Life Given by William Farr," *Q. Pub. Am. Statist. Assn.*, n. s. 16 (1918): 121–30; and Alfred J. Lotka, "A Simple Graphic Construction for Farr's Relation between Birth-Rate, Death-Rate, and Mean Length of Life," Ibid., n. s. 17 (1921): 998–1,000.

83. William Farr, "On the Pay of Ministers of the Crown," *J. Statist. Soc. Lond.* 20 (1857): 107–8 and 125–27.

84. Farr, [*English Life Table* No. 1], *6th A.R.R.G.*, pp. 549–52 [not in PP].

85. Ibid., 651–52 [not in PP].

86. *5th A.R.R.G.*, p. 19 [PP, 1843, XXI, xv].

87. "On the Value of Life Tables," p. 1; reprinted in Rumsey, *Essays and Papers*, p. 218.

88. *5th A.R.R.G.*, p. 31 [PP, 1843, XXI, xxiv].

89. *5th A.R.R.G.*, pp. 23, 25, 36, 46–48. [PP, 1843, XXI, xvii, xix, xxvi, xxvii, xxxiii–xxiv].

90. *7th A.R.R.G.*, pp. 334–37 [not in PP].

91. William Farr, "The Northampton Table of Mortality," *8th A.R.R.G.*, pp. 278–93 and 332–33 [PP, 1847–48, XXV, 290–97].

92. Ibid., pp. 293–320 [pp. 297–310].

93. W[illiam] Farr, "On the Construction," pp. 837–78. See also *33rd A.R.R.G.*, pp. 441–57 [PP, 1872, XVII].

94. William Ogle formally introduced the standarized death rates: John Brownlee, *The Use of Death-Rates*, pp. 10–13. For more modern discussions see Raymond Pearl, *Introduction to Medical Biometry and Statistics*, 3rd ed. (Philadelphia and London, 1940), pp. 269–81; and Abraham M. Lilienfeld, *Foundations of Epidemiology* (New York, 1976), pp. 60–64.

95. Farr, "Letter," *Suppl. 25th A.R.R.G.*, pp. xxvi–xxviii; [PP, 1865, XIII]; William Farr, evidence and testimony, "Report of the Commissions Appointed to Inquire into the Condition of All Mines in Great Britain to Which the Provisions of the Act 23 and 24 Vict., Cap. 151, Do not Apply with Reference to the Health and Safety of Persons Employed in Such Mines," app. B, PP, 1864, XXIV, pt. 2, 154–78.

96. "The Late Dr. Farr," *The Insurance Record* (May 4, 1883), in L. S. E. Farr Collection, XI, item 20.

97. [Review of Farr, "Letter," *12th A.R.R.G.*] *Assurance Magazine* 4 (1854): 266–68; [review of Farr, *English Life Table* [No. 3], Ibid. 12 (1864–65): 109–10; and Marcus N. Adler, "Some Considerations on the Government Life Annuities and Life Assurances Bill," Ibid. 12 (1864–65): 3–32.

98. James Chisholm, "On the Arrangement of Commutation, or D and N, Tables," *Assurance Magazine* 14 (1868): 208–9 and 211–12; and Thomas Bond Sprague, "On the Limitation of Risks: Being an Essay towards the Determination of the Maximum Amount of Risk to Be Retained by a Life Insurance Company on a Single Contingency," Ibid. 8 (1866): 21–22n.

99. "The Late Dr. Farr," *Insurance Record* (May 4, 1883), in L. S. E. Farr Collection, XI, item 20, and Hare, *William Farr*, p. 5 [galley].

100. T. E. Young, "Can a Law of Mortality Be Represented in a Mathematical Form?," *Assurance Magazine* 22 (1880): 139–40.

101. For Farr's criticism see [William Farr], "Life Assurance Offices," *Br. Ann.*

Med. 2 (1837): 249-51 and 281-83; William Farr, "On Benevolent Funds," pp. 701-04 and 817-23, esp. 820-21; Farr, "Letter," *12th A.R.R.G.*, pp. iii-xxv [not in PP].

102. Maurice Edward Ogborn, *Equitable Assurances: The Story of Life Assurance in the Experience of the Equitable Life Assurance Society 1762-1962* (London, 1962), pp. 229-39.

103. PP, 1852-53, XXI, 297-312; and William Farr, *A System of Life Insurance Which May Be Carried out under the Control of the Government and Would (1) Be Equitable in Its Operations: (2) Afford the Best Security, and Be in the Best Condition to Fulfill Its Future Engagements: (3) Be Well Adapted to the Wants of the People, as it Would Afford All the Advantages of an Insurance Office, and Some of Those of a Bank: and (4) Operate at Less Risk, Less Expense, and Lower Premiums than Small Offices. (5) It Might Also Be Made a Considerable Source of National Revenue* (London, 1853). The British Museum catalogue gives the date of publication as 1861; 1853, however, seems more likely and is the date given in the library catalogue at the London School of Economics and by Humphreys in Farr, *Vital Statistics*, p. xvii. See also Farr, "Letter," *12th A.R.R.G.*, pp. xvi-lii [not in PP].

104. Farr, *A System of Life Insurance*, pp. 3-8.

105. Ibid., pp. 8-16.

106. Ibid., pp. 16-20; and Farr, "Letter," *12th A.R.R.G.*, pp. xlv-xlviii [not in PP].

107. For brief accounts of the savings banks see George Christopher Trout Bartley, Thomas Allan Ingram, and Bradford Rhodes, "Savings Banks," *Encyclopaedia Britannica*, 11th ed., 24: 243-45; and Thomas Allan Ingram, "Post and Postal Service," Ibid., 27: 187.

108. Humphreys in Farr, *Vital Statistics*, p. xvii; and "William Farr, C.B., F.R.S., M.D., D.C.L.," *Lancet*, 1883, i, 801.

109. Farr, "Letter," *12th A.R.R.G.*, pp. xxxv-xliii [not in PP].

110. Ibid., p. xxxvi.

111. Ibid., p. xliii.

112. Farr, "On Benevolent Funds," p. 822.

113. William Farr, "General Cattle Mutual Insurance Fund," *J. Roy. Agric. Soc. Engl.*, 2nd ser. 2 (1866): 455-71. Farr had already interested Kay Shuttleworth in such a scheme; Farr, letter to Florence Nightingale, Nov. 22, 1865, B.M. Add. Mss. 43400, f. 84.

114. Farr, "Letter," *31st A.R.R.G.*, pp. 206-9 [PP, 1870, XVI].

115. "Statistics of the Civil Service of England, with Observations on the Constitution of Funds, to Provide for Fatherless Children and Widows," *J. Statist. Soc. Lond.* 12 (1849): 103-50.

116. Ibid., pp. 124-50.

117. *Remarks on a Proposed Scheme for the Conversion of the Assessments Levied on Public Salaries, Under Act 4 and 5 Will. IV. Cap. 24. into a "Provident Fund" for the Support of the Widows and Orphans of Civil Service Servants of the Crown* (London, [1849]).

118. Farr, "On the Pay of Ministers," pp. 116-20.

119. Manuscript notes of questions and Farr's answers are preserved in L. S. E. Farr Collection, II, item 14, ff. 169-85. W. Willis wrote to Farr to thank him on behalf of the committee, Ibid., I, item 105, ff. 186-86(b).

120. William Farr, letter to Henry Lord Brougham, Aug. 4, 1857, University College, Brougham Mss.

121. William Farr, letter to George Leveson-Gower, 2nd Earl Granville, May 2, 1871 [draft], L. S. E. Farr Collection, I, item 28, ff. 52-53(b).

122. William Farr, letters to Florence Nightingale: July 23, 1863, and Aug. 26, 1863, B.M. Add. Mss. 43,399, ff. 122-23 and 144-45.

123. Humphreys in Farr, *Vital Statistics*, p. xvii. Farr sent a copy of that paper to Nightingale; Farr, letter to Florence Nightingale, Jan. 26, 1865, B.M. Add. Mss. 43400, f. 10.

124. L. S. E. Farr Collection, XIII, items 1 and 4; and Ibid., I, items 7 and 17.

125. L. S. E. Farr Collection, X, f. 4.

126. Ibid., I, item 73, f. 135; and XIII, item 2.

127. New York State, Insurance Department, *Circular No. 39, of the New York*

State Insurance Department. Containing an Index and Explanation of the Life Insurance Symbols of Dr. William Farr (Albany, 1868).

128. William Farr, *Net Premiums for Insurance Against Fatal Accident. According to Age and Sex* (London, 1880).

129. Humphreys in Farr, *Vital Statistics*, p. xxiii.

130. Hare, *William Farr*, p. 5 [of galleys].

131. "The Late Dr. Farr," *Insurance Record* (May 4, 1883), in L. S. E. Farr Collection, XI, item 20.

132. For a brief description of consols see "Consols," *Encyclopaedia Britannica*, 11th ed., 6: 979–80 and William Blain and Edward Walter Hamilton, "National Debt," Ibid., 19: 270.

133. "The Late Dr. Farr."

134. George Scott, letter to James Thompson, July 10, 1863, L. S. E. Farr Collection, I, item 92, ff. 167–68.

135. "An Explanatory Word from Shaw," in Florence Farr, Bernard Shaw, W. B. Yeats, *Letters*, ed. Clifford Bax (New York, 1942), p. ix.

136. We know for example that a mortgage Farr gave in 1857 was transferred to his estate after his death in 1883. See exchange of letters between How and Son; Janson, Cobb and Pearson; and Joseph Whithall, June 8, 1883; June 12, 1883; and June 13, 1883, in L. S. E. Farr Collection, I, items 53 and 59, ff. 98–99 and 108–9. Farr was also one of the trustees of the Bromby and West Kent Mutual Benefit Building Society, Business Card in L. S. E. Farr Collection, XIII, item 5.

137. Farr's most explicit views on this subject are found in his "On the Valuation of Railways, Telegraphs, Water Companies, Canals, and Other Commercial Concerns, with Prospective, Deferred, Increasing, Decreasing, or Terminating Profits," *J. Statist. Soc. Lond.* 39 (1876): 465–72.

138. Ibid., p. 471.

139. Ibid., p. 470.

140. Ibid., p. 467.

141. W[illiam] Farr, "The Application of Statistics to Naval and Military Matters," *J. United Services Institution*, (1859), pp. 220, in L. S. E. Farr Collection, IV, item 1.

142. William Farr, "The Income and Property Tax," *J. Statist. Soc. Lond.* 16 (1853): 3.

143. Farr, "On the Valuation of Railways," [1876]; and W[illiam] Farr "On the Valuation of Railways," *J. Statist. Soc. Lond.* 36 (1873): 256–59.

144. Farr, "On the Valuation of Railways," [1873], pp. 256–57.

145. Ibid., p. 257–58.

146. Farr, "On the Valuation of Railways," [1876], pp. 513–30.

147. William Farr, "[Presidential] Address [to Section F]" *Report, B.A.A.S.* 34 (1864): 158.

148. B. F. Kiker, *Human Capital: In Retrospect. Essays in Economics*, No. 16 (Columbia, S.C., 1968), esp. 5–11.

149. Ibid., pp. x–xi and 1–5.

150. Ibid., pp. viii–ix, 5–11, 112–17, 123 and 133. See also Rashi Fein, "On Measuring Economic Benefits of Health Programmes," in *Medical History and Medical Care*, ed. Gordon McLachlan and Thomas McKeown (London, New York, Toronto, 1971), pp. 187–88.

151. Farr, "The Income and Property Tax," pp. 1–44.

152. Ibid., p. 38.

153. Ibid., p. 2.

154. Ibid., p. 38.

155. For the present study Farr used data on wages and living expenses of agricultural laborers at different ages taken from a Parliamentary investigation of the new Poor Law, Ibid., pp. 42–44. He had explained how to calculate the present value of future earnings in his first national life table, *6th A.R.R.G.*, pp. 653–54 [not in PP].

156. Farr, "Income and Property Tax," pp. 39–40.

157. Ibid., p. 43.

158. Farr, "Letter," *Suppl. 35th A.R.R.G.*, p. xlii [PP, 1875, XVIII, pt. 2].

159. Kiker, *Human Capital*, pp. 1-2.

160. Lambert A. J. Quetelet, *A Treatise on Man and the Development of his Faculties*, trans. R. Knox (Edinburgh, 1842), p. 28.

161. Farr, "Letter," *31st A.R.R.G.*, pp. 205-6 [PP, 1870, XVI].

162. Farr, "Reports of the Official Delegates, p. 413.

163. Edwin Chadwick, *Report on the Sanitary Condition of the Labouring Population of Great Britain* [1842] (Edinburgh, 1965), pp. 254-76. McCulloch's estimate is referred to: Ibid., p. 274.

164. William Farr, testimony, Report of the *Commissioners Appointed to Inquire into the Regulations Affecting the Sanitary Condition of the Army*, PP, 1857-58, XVIII, 517.

165. [Farr], "Vital Statistics," in McCulloch, 1st ed., 2: 574-78; Farr, "Vital Statistics," in McCulloch, 4th ed., 2: 579-86; and [William] Farr, "The Health of the British Army, and the Effects of Recent Sanitary Measures on its Mortality and Sickness," *J. Statist. Soc. Lond.* 24 (1861): 472-83.

166. Farr, "Vital Statistics," in McCulloch, 1st ed., 2: 587.

167. Farr, "Letter," *25th A.R.R.G.*, pp. 177-78 [PP, 1864, XVII].

168. Farr, "Statistics of Insanity," pp. 137-40.

169. Ibid., and Farr, "Letter," *1st A.R.R.G.*, p. 107 [PP, 1839, XVI, 76].

170. Farr, "Vital Statistics," in McCulloch, 1st ed., 2: 568.

171. William Farr, "Mortality of Children in the Principal States of Europe," *J. Statist. Soc. Lond.* 29 (1866): 1.

172. Farr, "Note," p. 354.

Chapter Five

1. "Anticontagion between 1821 and 1867," *Bull. Hist. Med.* 22 (1948): 562-93.

2. *Cholera, Fever and English Medicine 1825-1865* (Oxford, 1978), esp. Chapter Two. See also pp. 297-301 for criticism of Ackerknecht's approach.

3. This division was used by both extremists such as Maclean and Southwood Smith and by moderates like Henry. See: Charles Maclean, *Evils of Quarantine Laws, and Non-Existence of Pestilential Contagion* (London, 1824), pp. 202-6; [Southwood Smith], "Contagion and Sanitary Laws," *Westminster Rev.* 3 (1825): 134-35 and 138-46; and William Henry, "Report on the State of Our Knowledge of the Laws of Contagion," *Report, B.A.A.S.* 4 (1834): 67-94.

4. [Southwood Smith], "Contagion and Sanitary Laws," p. 146.

5. Such standard objections to the doctrine of contagion as follows in the text are raised in Maclean, *Evils*, pp. 217-28; [Southwood Smith], "Contagion and Sanitary Laws," pp. 147-48; and [Southwood Smith], "Plague—Typhus Fever—Quarantine," *Westminster Rev.* 3 (1825): 516-19.

6. Henry, "Report on the State," p. 85.

7. Southwood Smith, *A Treatise on Fever* [1830] (Philadelphia, 1831), p. 205.

8. Ibid., pp. 205-13.

9. Ibid., p. 214.

10. [Southwood Smith], "Plague—Typhus Fever—Quarantine," pp. 520-21.

11. This point is argued in Pelling, *Cholera*, pp. 68-70.

12. Maclean, *Evils*, pp. 212-14.

13. Southwood Smith, *The Common Nature of Epidemics*, ed. T. Baker (London, 1866), p. 25.

14. Ibid., 30; and Chadwick's testimony to the Metropolitan Sewage Manure Company Committee in 1846 [PP, 1846, X, 651] cited in S. E. Finer, *The Life*, p. 298.

15. Pelling, *Cholera*, p. 145.

16. William Farr, letter to Florence Nightingale, February 17, 1859, B.M. Add. Mss. 43398, f. 112.

17. [William Farr], "Causes of the High Mortality," pp. 416-17 [205-06].

18. Farr, "Letter," *2nd A.R.R.G.*, pp. 93-94 [PP, 1840, XVII, 18].

19. Farr, "Letter," *3rd A.R.R.G.*, App., pp. 102-9 [PP, 1841, sess. 2, VI, 22 and 24-28].

20. Farr, "Letter," *2nd A.R.R.G.*, App. pp. 91-92 [PP, 1840, XVII, 16].

21. Ibid., p. 88 [14].

22. [Farr], "Statistical Nosology," pp. 199-205 [119-22]; and [Farr], "Causes of the High Mortality in Town Districts," pp. 411-19 [203-7].

23. [Farr], "Causes of the High Mortality," pp. 411-15 [203-5]. He returned to the question of population density and income later in the same report, pp. 419-26 [207-10].

24. This section of the report was reprinted as "Mr. Farr on the Causes of Mortality in Town Districts," *Prov. Med. J.* 7 (1843-44): 439-41.

25. [Farr], "Causes of the High Mortality," 411-15 [203-5].

26. Ibid., pp. 415-19 [205-7].

27. Ibid., p. 418 [206-7].

28. [Farr], "Statistical Nosology," pp. 199-205 [119-22].

29. Ibid., pp. 197-200 [118-20].

30. Ibid., p. 201 [120].

31. J. K. Crellin, "The Dawn of the Germ Theory: Particles, Infection and Biology," in *Medicine and Science in the 1860's: Proceedings of the Sixth British Congress on the History of Medicine,* ed. F. N. L. Poynter (London, 1968), p. 61; and Phyllis Allen Richmond, "Some Variant Theories in Opposition to the Germ Theory of Disease," *J. Hist. Med.* 9 (1954): 295-96. Richmond's comments on Farr should be taken with caution. For an indication of how widespread the use of the term was and the fact that Farr was usually seen as its originator see: George Gregory, "Lecture on the Laws Which Govern the Mode and Rate of Decay in the Human Frame," *Lancet,* 1842-43, ii, 8; E[dward] Headlam Greenhow, "Illustrations of the Necessity for a More Analytical Study of the Statistics of Public Health," *Trans. N.A.P.S.S.* (Birmingham, 1857), 368-69; and Rumsey, *Essays and Papers,* pp. 126-27.

32. Farr, "Statistical Nosology," 205 [122].

33. Ibid., pp. 199-200 [119].

34. Farr, "Address on Public Health," pp. 75-76.

35. [Farr], "Causes of the High Mortality," p. 418 [207].

36. [Farr], "Statistical Nosology," pp. 200 and 201 [119 and 120].

37. Ibid., pp. 200 and 201 [120].

38. Farr, "Address on Public Health," p. 75.

39. Farr, "Letter," *17th A.R.R.G.*, p. 99 [not in PP].

40. William Farr, "Report on the Nomenclature and Statistical Classification of Diseases, for Statistical Returns," *16th A.R.R.G.*, pp. 76-77 and 82-85 [not in PP].

41. Crellin, "The Dawn of the Germ Theory," esp. pp. 58-66.

42. [William Farr], *Report on the Cholera Epidemic of 1866 in England, Suppl. 29th A.R.R.G.*, pp. lxv-lxx [PP, 1867-68, XXXVII].

43. Ibid., pp. lxix-lxx.

44. Farr, "Letter," *Suppl. 35th A.R.R.G.*, pp. iv and lxv [PP, 1875, XVIII, pt. 2].

45. Farr, "Letter," *22nd A.R.R.G.*, p. 183 [PP, 1861, XVIII].

46. Farr, "Letter," *30th A.R.R.G.*, pp. 216-17 [PP, 1868-69, XVI].

47. Farr, "Letter," *2nd A.R.R.G.*, App., p. 95 [PP, 1840, XVII, p. 18]. See also Rosen, "Jacob Henle and William Farr," pp. 585-89.

48. [Farr], *Report on Cholera, 1866,* pp. lxv-lxvi; and Farr, "Letter," *30th A.R.R.G.*, pp. 217-18 [PP, 1868-69, XVI].

49. Farr, "Letter," *30th A.R.R.G.*, p. 217 [PP, 1868-69, XVI].

50. Farr, "Letter," *30th A.R.R.G.*, p. 211; and Farr, *Report on the Cholera Epidemic of 1866,* p. lxvi.

51. Farr, "Letter," *31st A.R.R.G.*, p. 198 [PP, 1870, XVI].

52. Farr, "Letter," *34th A.R.R.G.*, p. 221 [PP, 1873, XX].

53. Farr, "Letter," *Suppl. 35th A.R.R.G.*, p. lix [PP, 1875, XVIII, pt. 2].

54. Farr, "Letter," *39th A.R.R.G.*, p. 226 [PP, 1878, XXII].

55. Charles-Edward Amory Winslow. *The Conquest of Epidemic Disease: A Chapter in the History of Ideas* (Princeton, 1944), pp. 259-66.

56. Henry I. Bowditch, *Brief Memories of Louis and Some of His Contemporaries in the Parisian School of Medicine of Forty Years Ago* (Boston, 1872), p. 10.

57. Rosen, "Jacob Henle and William Farr," p. 586.

58. "On the Laws of Sickness," pp. 855-58; and "Statistics of the London Hospital," pp. 778-83.

59. Edmonds, "On the Laws of Sickness," p. 858.

60. Ibid.

61. Farr, "Vital Statistics," in McCulloch, 1st ed., 2: 585; William Farr, "On Benevolent Funds," pp. 703-4; and Farr, "Vital Statistics," in McCulloch, 4th ed., 2: 595.

62. We have seen that Edmonds cited Farr's figures in the *Br. Med. Almanack*, Edmonds, "Statistics of the London Hospital," p. 778.

63. "On a Method of Determining the Danger," pp. 72-79; "On the Law of Recovery and Dying," pp. 134-43; and "On Prognosis," *Br. Med. Almanack* (1838), pp. 199-216.

64. Farr, "On a Method of Determining the Danger," p. 76.

65. Farr, "On the Law of Recovery and Dying," pp. 138-40.

66. Farr, "On a Method of Determining the Danger," p. 75.

67. Ibid., p. 73.

68. William Farr, "On Cholera," *Br. Med. Almanack* (1839), pp. 204-9. This paper under the title "On the Law of Recovery and Mortality in Cholera Spasmodica" was read by Farr's friend Robert Dundas Thomson to the British Association and appeared in abstract in *Lancet*, 1838-39, i, 26-29.

69. Farr, "On a Method of Determining the Danger," pp. 75-76; and Farr, "On Cholera," pp. 204-5.

70. Farr, "On a Method of Determining the Danger," pp. 72 and 75-76; and Farr, "On the Law of Recovery and Mortality," p. 27.

71. Farr, "On a Method of Determining the Danger," pp. 75-76.

72. "A Method of Determining the Effects of Systems of Treatment in Certain Diseases," *Br. Med. J.*, 1862, ii, 193-95; and Ibid., *Lancet*, 1862, ii, 157-58. The tables appear only in the *Br. Med. J.* paper.

73. "Statistics of Insanity," 1 (1837): 648-53, 679-83, 744-48, 811-14; Ibid. 2 (1837): 137-40, 171-74, 204-7, 235-39, 357-61; and "Report upon the Mortality of Lunatics," *J. Statist. Soc. Lond.* 4 (1841): 17-33.

74. Farr, "Report upon the Mortality," pp. 27-28.

75. Robert D[undas] Thomson, "On Mr. Farr's Law of Recovery and Mortality in Cholera," *Report, B.A.A.S.* 8 (1838), transactions of the sections: pp. 126-27.

76. *Report on the Mortality of Cholera in England, 1848-49* (London, 1852), pp. xliii-xliv.

77. *Report on Cholera, 1866*, p. lx.

78. Farr, "Letter," *25th A.R.R.G.*, pp. 175-78 [PP, 1864, XVII].

79. Farr, *Vital Statistics*, pp. 317-92.

80. John Brownlee, "Historical Note," p. 250.

81. Farr, "Letter," *2nd A.R.R.G.*, App., 91-98 [PP, 1840, XVII, pp. 16-20].

82. Ibid., p. 96 [19].

83. Ibid., p. 97 [19].

84. Ibid., p. 92 [16].

85. Ibid., p. 96 [19].

86. Farr, "Note," p. 352.

87. W[illiam] Farr, "Mr. Lowe and the Cattle Plague," *Daily News* (London), Feb. 19, 1866, pp. 5-6. For a discussion of Farr's method see Brownlee, "Historical Note," pp. 250-52; and Greenwood, *The Medical Dictator*, pp. 115-19.

88. Brownlee, "Historical Note," p. 251; and Greenwood, *The Medical Dictator*, p. 117.

89. I have discussed these cholera studies elsewhere and their relation to Farr's theory of disease. John M. Eyler, "William Farr on the Cholera: The Sanitarian's Disease Theory and the Statistician's Method," *J. Hist. Med.* 28 (1973): 79-100.

90. *Report on Cholera, 1848-49*. Farr's name is not attached to the long introduction, although George Graham's prefatory letter states Farr had supervision of the report.

Farr published a paper in which he summarized what he believed were the most important results of this study, "Influence of Elevation on the Fatality of Cholera," *J. Statist. Soc. Lond.* 15 (1852): 155–83. My citations are to the longer work.

91. Farr, *Report on Cholera, 1848–49*, xxxix–xliv.

92. Ibid., pp. xlvi–xlviii and plates II, III, and IV.

93. Ibid., pp. xlix.

94. Ibid., pp. l–lii.

95. Ibid., pp. lviii–lxviii.

96. Ibid., p. lxiii.

97. Alexander D. Langmuir, "Epidemiology of Airborne Infection," *Bacteriological Reviews* 25 (1961): 174.

98. Farr, *Report on Cholera, 1848–49*, p. lxv.

99. John Snow, *On the Mode of Communications of Cholera* (London, 1849).

100. Farr, *Report on Cholera, 1848–49*, pp. lxxvi–lxxviii, lviii–lxii, lii, and lxix–lxx.

101. Ibid., lix–lx.

102. For details of the change in water supply in South London that created this test condition and the research that followed see: John Simon, *Report on the Last Two Cholera-Epidemics of London as Affected by the Consumption of Impure Water; Addressed to the Rt. Hon. the President of the General Board of Health by the Medical Officer of the Board,* PP, 1856, LII, 1–35; and John Snow, *On the Mode of Communication of Cholera*, 2nd ed. (London, 1855), in Wade Hampton Frost, ed., *Snow on Cholera: Being a Reprint of Two Papers by John Snow, M.D.* (New York and London, 1936), pp. 68–69 and 76–91.

103. *Statutes at Large,* 15 and 16 Vic, c. 84 (1852).

104. N[eil] Arnott, et. al., *Report of the Committee for Scientific Inquiries in Relation to the Cholera-Epidemic of 1854,* PP, 1854–55, XXI, 623.

105. Farr, "Letter," *17th A.R.R.G.*, pp. 74–99 [not in PP].

106. Ibid., p. 82.

107. Ibid., pp. 91–94.

108. John Simon, *English Sanitary Institutions,* p. 260n.

109. Farr, "Letter," *17th A.R.R.G.*, p. 99.

110. Ibid., p. 95.

111. N. Arnott, et. al., *Report of the Committee,* p. 48.

112. Simon, *Report on the Last Two Cholera-Epidemics,* p. 15.

113. *Report on Cholera, 1866,* pp. xiii–xv and lxv–lxxii.

114. Ibid., pp. lv–lxi.

115. *Lancet,* 1868, ii, 223.

116. For further information on the following summary see Farr, *Report on Cholera, 1866,* pp. xv–xxxiii.

117. Ibid., pp. xii and xvii–xx. For a recent assessment see W. Luckin, "The Final Catastrophe—Cholera in London, 1866," *Med. Hist.* 21 (1977): 32–42.

118. Farr, *Report on Cholera, 1866,* pp. xxxi–xxxiii.

119. Ibid., pp. xv–xvii and lxxx.

120. Ibid., pp. lxii–lxiii.

121. Snow, 2nd ed. in Frost, *Snow on Cholera,* pp. 97–98.

122. Farr, "Letter," *17th A.R.R.G.*, pp. 88–90 [not in PP]; and Arnott, et. al., *Report of the Committee,* pp. 13–16.

123. For the following explanation of how the elevation law could be preserved see Farr, *Report on Cholera, 1866,* pp. liii–lv.

124. Ibid., pp. xiv and xx.

125. This and other features of the water supply are summarized in John Sutherland's report in Benjamin Hall, *Letter of the President of the General Board of Health, to the Right Honourable the Viscount Palmerston . . . Accompanying a Report from Dr. Sutherland on Epidemic Cholera in the Metropolis in 1854,* PP, 1854–55, XLV, 40–45.

Chapter Six

1. Farr, "Letter," *Suppl. 35th A.R.R.G.*, p. iii [PP, 1875, XVIII, pt. 2].

2. For illustrations of Farr's studies of occupational mortality see: *Report of the Commissioners Appointed to Inquire into the Condition of All Mines in Great Britain to Which the Provisions of the Act 23 and 24 Vict. Cap. 151, Do not Apply with Reference to the Health and Safety of Persons Employed in Such Mines,* App. B., PP, 1864, 24, pt. 2, 154-78; and Farr, "Letter," *Suppl. 35th A.R.R.G.*, pp. lii-lviii [PP, 1875, XVIII, pt. 2]. For his comments on the effectiveness of vaccination see Farr, "Letter," *34th A.R.R.G.*, pp. 219-21 [PP, 1873, XX]; and also criticism by the opponent of vaccination, George S. Gibbs: *Smallpox and Vaccination. A Letter Addressed to Major Graham* (Darlington, 1873).

3. Farr, "Letter," *1st A.R.R.G.*, pp. 88-89 [PP, 1839, XVI, 64-65]. Most of this paragraph is also reprinted in Cullen, *The Statistical Movement,* pp. 36-37.

4. Ibid., p. 38; see also pp. 36-37.

5. D.E.C. Eversley, *Social Theories of Fertility and the Malthusian Debate* (Oxford, 1959), pp. 35-41. For a discussion of the conditions in the early eighteenth century that supported the conclusion that cities were unhealthy places, see M. Dorothy George, *London Life in the Eighteenth Century* [1925] (New York and Evanston, 1965), pp. 21-61.

6. For the following figures on population growth see: M. W. Flinn (ed.), "Introduction," p. 4; and Arthur Newsholme, *The Elements of Vital Statistics,* 3rd ed. (London, 1899), p. 149.

7. For able discussions of the consequences of urban growth see Flinn, "Introduction," pp. 3-18; George Rosen, "Disease, Debility, and Death," *The Victorian City: Images and Realities,* ed. H. J. Dyos and Michael Wolff (London and Boston, 1973), 2: 625-67.

8. Flinn, "Introduction," pp. 13-14.

9. Farr, "Letter," *5th A.R.R.G.*, p. 419 [PP, 1843, XXI, 207].

10. For a summary of this controversy of 1840 and a reprinting of the relevant documents see Glass, *Numbering the People,* pp. 146 and 150-67.

11. Farr, "The Influence of Scarcities," pp. 158-74.

12. Farr, "Letter," *5th A.R.R.G.*, pp. 410-11 and 425 [PP, 1843, XXI, 202-3 and 210].

13. Farr, "Vital Statistics," in McCulloch, 1st ed., 2: 577.

14. [Farr], [English Life Table No. 1], *6th A.R.R.G.*, pp. 661-62 [not in PP].

15. Farr, "Letter," *1st A.R.R.G.*, pp. 111-13 [PP, 1839, XVI, 78-79], and Farr, "Letter," *2nd A.R.R.G.*, App. pp. 84-85 [PP, 1840, XVII, 12].

16. Farr, "Letter," *2nd A.R.R.G.*, App. pp. 84-85 [PP, 1840, XVII, 12]. See also [William Farr], "Causes of the High Mortality," p. 430 [PP, 1843, XXI, 212]. Cullen, *The Statistical Movement,* p. 37, claims Chadwick took up this idea without acknowledging Farr. Chadwick's biographer, however, found the origin of Chadwick's idea of recovering the cost of the sewage system by selling the sewage manure in his observation of the success of Scottish farmers in using Edinburgh's sewage and in the relevations of Liebig's *Animal Chemistry.* S. E. Finer, *The Life,* pp. 223-24.

17. Farr, "Vital Statistics," in McCulloch, 1st ed., 2: 601.

18. Farr, "Vital Statistics," in McCulloch, 4th ed., 2: 569.

19. See for example Farr, "Letter," *1st A.R.R.G.*, p. 102 [PP, 1839, XVI, 73]; William Farr, "Note," p. 354; Farr, "Letter," *30th A.R.R.G.*, p. 213 [PP, 1868-69, XVI]; Farr, "Letter," *34th A.R.R.G.*, pp. 219-21 [PP, 1873, XX]; and Farr, "Letter," *Suppl. 35th A.R.R.G.*, pp. lxv-lxvii [PP, 1875, XVIII, pt. 2].

20. "National Board of Health," *Br. Ann. Med.* 1 (1837): 760.

21. Farr, "Letter," *1st A.R.R.G.*, p. 89 [PP, 1839, XVI, 65].

22. Farr, "Letter," *Suppl. 35th A.R.R.G.*, p. iv [PP, 1875, XVIII, pt. 2].

23. "Registration of Sickness," *All the Year Round,* Dec. 15, 1860, p. 228.

24. Benjamin Ward Richardson, "A Biographical Dissertation," in *The Health of Nations,* 1: xlvi.

25. *1st A.R.R.G.*, pp. 108-18 [PP, 1839, XVI, 76-81].

26. Ibid., pp. 108-9 [76-77].

27. Ibid., pp. 110-11 [77-78]. He lists the principal towns that compose the urban districts in *5th A.R.R.G.*, p. 406 [PP, 1843, XXI, 200].

28. "Statistical Nosology," *1st A.R.R.G.*, p. 93 [PP, 1839, XVI, 67].

29. "Diseases of Towns and of the Open County," *1st A.R.R.G.*, p. 108 [PP, 1839, XVI, 76].

30. Ibid., pp. 111-12 [78].

31. Ibid., pp. 112-16 [78-80].

32. *2nd A.R.R.G.*, App., pp. 80-81 [PP, 1840, XVII, 9-10]; and *3rd A.R.R.G.*, App., pp. 98-99 [PP, 1841, sess. 2, VI, 20].

33. *2nd A.R.R.G.*, App., p. 83 [PP, 1840, XVII, 11].

34. *3rd A.R.R.G.*, App., p. 99 [PP, 1841, sess. 2, VI, 20].

35. Ibid.

36. Ibid., p. 101 [22].

37. Cullen, *The Statistical Movement*, p. 40. See also pp. 38-39.

38. Farr, letter to Florence Nightingale, April 25, 1860, B.M. Add. Mss. 43398, f. 178.

39. *5th A.R.R.G.*, pp. 397-405 [PP, 1843, XXI, 194-99].

40. Ibid., pp. 406-7 [200].

41. Ibid., pp. 410-19 [202-7].

42. Ibid., pp. 419-26 [207-10].

43. For the following explanation see Ibid., pp. 409, 419-20, and 424 [201-2, 207, and 209].

44. Ibid., pp. 422-23 [209].

45. Ibid., pp. 424-25 [210].

46. Farr's popular introduction to the principles and uses of a life table and his first warning about the use of the mean age at death occur in Graham's letter, Ibid., pp. 16-49 [xii-xxxv]. A more technical discussion and the basic tables are found in Farr's Letter, Ibid., pp. 342-67 [161-78]. The remaining portions of English life table number one appeared in *6th A.R.R.G.*, pp. 517-666 [PP, 1844, XIX, 290-358].

47. *5th A.R.R.G.*, pp. 23, 25, 29, 36, and 46-48 [PP, 1843, XXI, xvii, xix, xxi, xxvi, xxvii, xxxiii-xxxiv].

48. Ibid., pp. 50-52 [xxxvi-xxxviii].

49. *2nd A.R.R.G.*, App., p. 82 [PP, 1840, XVII, 10].

50. *5th A.R.R.G.*, p. 408 [PP, 1843, XXI, 201].

51. Farr, "Letter," *7th A.R.R.G.* [not in PP], pp. 330-39, and Farr, 'Letter," *8th A.R.R.G.*, pp. 278-93 and 332-33 [PP, 1847-48, XXV, 290-97 and 318].

52. *5th A.R.R.G.*, p. 48 [PP, 1843, XXI, xxxv].

53. Gt. Britain, *Statutes at Large*, 11 and 12 Vic. c. 63, "An Act for promoting the Public Health."

54. Edward Headlam Greenhow, "The Results of an Inquiry into the Different Proportions of Death Produced by Certain Diseases in Different Districts in England," *Papers Relating to the Sanitary State of the People of England*, PP, 1857-58, XXIII, 1-164. Simon's introduction is found, Ibid., pp. iii-xlviii. Greenhow provided a popular introduction and prefatory comment to this report: "Illustrations," pp. 365-87. For a discussion of the background and significance of this report see C. Fraser Brockington, *Public Health in the Nineteenth Century* (Edinburgh and London, 1965), pp. 195-200.

55. Greenhow, "Illustrations," pp. 365-66; and Greenhow, "Results," p. 16 (see above, n. 54).

56. Greenhow, "Illustrations," p. 368; and Greenhow, "Results," pp. 17-18.

57. Brockington, *Public Health*, pp. 208-14.

58. For an example of this sort of study, which Simon sponsored, see "Dr. Greenhow's Reports on the Prevalence and Causes of Diarrhoea at Coventry, Birmingham, Wolverhampton. . . ," *2nd Rep. Med. Off. Privy Council*, PP, 1860, XXIX, 65-160. Simon's introduction is found on pp. 57-64.

59. Royston Lambert, *Sir John Simon 1816-1904 and English Social Administration* (London, 1963), pp. 264-65.

60. Eyler, "Mortality Statistics," pp. 348-55.

61. "The Value of Death-Rates as a Test of Sanitary Condition," *J. Statist. Soc. Lond.* 37 (1874): 438.

62. *5th A.R.R.G.*, pp. 22-52 [PP, 1843, XXI, xvi-xxxv]; *2nd A.R.R.G.*, App., p. 83 [PP, 1840, XVII, 11]; and *9th A.R.R.G.*, App., p. 160 [PP, 1849, XXI, 5-8].

63. A[lfred] Aspland, "Inaugural Address at the Opening of Session 1863-64," *Trans. Manchr. Statist. Soc.* (1863-64), p. viii.

64. William Farr, [evidence and testimony], *Report from the Select Committee on Public Health Bill, and Nuisances Removal Amendment Bill,* PP, 1854-55, XIII, 196-97 and 204. Several years later Farr provided a similar explanation in Farr, "Letter," *20th A.R.R.G.*, pp. 174-75 [PP, 1859, sess. 2, XII]. John Simon acknowledged the value of this standard in "Introductory Report," *Papers Relating to the Sanitary State of the People of England,* PP, 1857-58, XXIII, iii-iv.

65. See Farr's testimony in *Report from the Select Committee on Public Health Bill, and Nuisances Removal Amendment Bill,* PP, 1854-55, XIII, 204.

66. Farr, "On the Construction," pp. 869-78.

67. Farr, "Letter," *20th A.R.R.G.*, p. 174 [PP, 1859, sess. 2, XII].

68. PP, 1865, XIII; and PP, 1875, XVIII, pt. 2.

69. Farr, "Letter," *Suppl. 25th A.R.R.G.*, pp. xxxv-xxxvi [PP, 1865, XIII]; and Farr, "Letter," *Suppl. 35th A.R.R.G.*, pp. lii-lviii [PP, 1875, XVIII, pt. 2].

70. Farr, "Letter," *Suppl. 25th A.R.R.G.*, pp. xxi-xxiii [PP, 1865, XIII].

71. Farr, "Letter," *Suppl. 35th A.R.R.G.*, pp. ix-xx, and xxxviii-lii [PP, 1875, XVIII, pt. 2].

72. Farr, "Letter," *Suppl. 25th A.R.R.G.*, pp. v-xxi [PP, 1865, XIII]; and Farr, "Letter," *Suppl. 35th A.R.R.G.*, pp. xxi-xxii and xxv-xxxiv [PP, 1875, XVIII, pt. 2].

73. Farr, "Letter," *Suppl. 35th A.R.R.G.*, pp. xxxv-xxxvii; and tables 7-15.

74. Farr, "Letter," *Suppl. 25th A.R.R.G.*, pp. xxvi-xxvii [PP, 1865, XIII].

75. Ibid.

76. Ibid., pp. xxvii-xxviii.

77. Farr, "Letter," *Suppl. 35th A.R.R.G.*, pp. xxi-xxii [PP, 1875, XVIII, pt. 2].

78. "On Certain Results," pp. 170-221; and "Inconsistencies of the English Census of 1861," pp. 73-124. See esp. "Inconsistencies of the English Census," pp. 108-9.

79. "On Infant Mortality," pp. 125-49.

80. "A Note on the Under-Registration," p. 72n.

81. *16th A.R.R.G.*, pp. 144-53.

82. PP, 1852-53, LXXXV, 1.

83. Ibid., facing xlix.

84. Farr, "Letter," *Suppl. 25th A.R.R.G.*, pp. xxxii-xxxv [PP, 1865, XIII].

85. Farr, "Letter," *Suppl. 35th A.R.R.G.*, pp. xxiii-xxv [PP, 1875, XVIII, pt. 2].

86. m: (d)$^{.12}$ :: m:(d$'$)$^{.12}$, Ibid., p. xxiv. The exponent .12 was really an approximation for the one Farr used (.11998).

87. *General Report, Census of England and Wales for the Year 1871,* PP, 1873, LXXI, pt. 2: xxviii; Farr, "Letter," *40th A.R.R.G.*, pp. 331-46 [PP, 1878-79, XIX]; and William Farr, "Density or Proximity," pp. 530-35. Farr first used this approach in the *Census of 1851. Numbers of the Inhabitants in the Years 1801, 1811, 1821, 1831, 1841 and 1851,* PP, 1852-53, LXXXV, diagram facing p. 1.

88. $e' = e\,(p'/p)^{.24}$ where e and e$'$ are the mean durations of life in two districts having mean proximities p and p$'$.

89. We may write this approximation $e = 1/d - 1/3\,(1/d - 1/b)$, where e is the mean duration of life; d, the death rate; and b, the birth rate. See Farr, "Letter," *40th A.R.R.G.*, p. 235 [PP, 1878-79, XIX]; and Farr, "Density or Proximity," p. 532.

90. Farr, "Letter," *5th A.R.R.G.*, pp. 411-30 [PP, 1843 XXI, 203-13].

91. Ibid., 423-24 and 426-27 [209-10 and 211]; and Farr, "Letter," *40th A.R.R.G.*, pp. 245-46 [PP, 1878-79, XIX].

92. For recent historical comment on the purposes of such projects see H. J. Dyos, "Urban Transformation: A Note on the Objects of Street Improvement in Regency and Early Victorian London," *Int. Rev. Soc. Hist.* 2 (1957): 259-65.

93. See for example the popular exposition given in Arthur Ransome, *On the Distri-*

bution of Death and Disease (Manchester and London, 1884), pp. 24-31.

94. "The Vital Statistics of Peabody Buildings and other Artisans' and Labourers' Block Dwellings," *J. Statist. Soc. Lond.* 54 (1891): 70.

95. Ibid., pp. 85-89 and 110-11.

96. Ibid., p. 89.

97. Ibid., pp. 101, 105, and 108-9.

98. (London, 1935), pp. 299-302.

99. Farr, "Letter," *5th A.R.R.G.*, pp. 422-23 [PP, 1843, XXI, 209].

100. Farr, "Letter," *1st A.R.R.G.*, p. 113 [PP, 1839, XVI, 80].

101. Farr, "Letter," *Suppl. 25th A.R.R.G.*, pp. xxxiv-xxxv [PP, 1865, XIII].

102. Farr, "Density or Proximity," pp. 532-33.

103. Farr, "Letter," *5th A.R.R.G.*, p. 426 [PP, 1843, XXI, 211].

104. Farr, "Letter," *1st A.R.R.G.*, p. 113 [PP, 1839, XVI, 80]; and Farr, "Letter," *2nd A.R.R.G.*, App., p. 85 [PP, 1840, XVII, 12].

105. Farr, "Letter," *5th A.R.R.G.*, pp. 430-32 [PP, 1843, XXI, 213-14].

106. Ibid., p. 427 [211].

107. Farr, "Letter," *Suppl. 35th A.R.R.G.*, p. lxxi [PP, 1875, XVIII, pt. 2].

108. See for example W. T. Gairdner, *Public Health in Relation to Air and Water* (Edinburgh, 1862), pp. 33-34, 62-64, and 122-24.

109. For Farr's understanding of Malthus's position see Farr, "Medical Reform. An Oration," pp. 107-8; and *General Report. Census of England and Wales for the Year 1861*, PP, 1863, LIII, pt. 1:24. See also Quetelet, *A Treatise on Man*, p. 57.

110. Eversley, *Social Theories*, p. 74.

111. William Farr, "Population," *4th A.R.R.G.*, p. 140 [PP, 1842, XIX, 88-89].

112. Farr, "On Some Doctrines of Population," p. 570; and Farr, "Letter," *Suppl. 35th A.R.R.G.*, pp. xv-xvi [PP, 1875, XVIII, pt. 2].

113. Farr, "Population," pp. 133-43 [85-90]; and Farr, "Medical Reform. An Oration," pp. 108-9.

114. Farr, "Letter," *Suppl. 35th A.R.R.G.*, pp. xv-xvi and xx [PP, 1875, XVIII, pt. 2]; Farr, "Letter," *30th A.R.R.G.*, p. 210 [PP, 1868-69, XVI]; and *Census of 1861, General Report*, pp. 25-26. For an anticipation of these arguments see *Census of 1851, Ages, Civil Condition. Occupations, and Birth-Place of the People*, PP, 1852-53, LXXXVIII, pt. 1, lxiii-lxviii.

115. *Census of 1851, Ages, Civil Conditions . . .*, p. lxv (see above, n. 114); *Census of 1861, General Report*, p. 25; and William Farr, manuscript notes, L. S. E. Farr Collection, II, item 9. See also S. E. Finer, *The Life*, pp. 23-24.

116. Farr, "Population," pp. 134-39 [86-88]; and *Census of 1871, General Report*, pp. xv-xvi.

117. Farr, "Population," p. 139 [88].

118. Ibid.

119. pp. xii-xiii [PP, 1875, XVIII, pt. 2].

120. Eversley, *Social Theories*, pp. 59-60, 74-75, 92-95, 130-31, and 169-70.

121. Farr, "Letter," *Suppl. 35th A.R.R.G.*, p. xiv [PP, 1875, XVIII, pt. 2].

122. Farr, "Letter," *30th A.R.R.G.*, pp. 210-11 [PP, 1868-69, XVI].

123. Farr, "Vital Statistics," in McCulloch, 4th ed., 2: 603.

124. Farr, "Medical Reform. An Oration," p. 108.

125. Farr, "Letter," *30th A.R.R.G.*, p. 210. [PP, 1868-69, XVI].

126. For Victorian attitudes on contraception see J. A. Banks, *Prosperity and Parenthood: A Study of Family Planning among the Victorian Middle Classes* (London, 1954), pp. 139-69.

127. Farr, "On Some Doctrines of Population," pp. 576-77; and *General Report: Census of 1861*, p. 20.

128. *General Report, Census of 1871*, pp. xvi-xvii.

129. Ibid., p. xvii.

130. Farr, "Population," pp. 140-42 [89-90]; and *General Report, Census of 1871*, p. xv. For the classical views referred to see Eversley, *Social Theories*, pp. 29-31.

131. Farr, "Letter," *Suppl. 35th A.R.R.G.*, p. xii [PP, 1875, XVIII, pt. 2].

132. For the opposition of eugenicists to the notions of the inheritance of acquired characteristics and of the long term value of environmental reform see Karl Pearson, *The Groundwork of Eugenics* (London, 1909), pp. 12-21.

133. Victor L. Hilts, "William Farr (1807-1883) and the 'Human Unit,'" *Vict. Stud.* 14 (1970): 143-50.

134. Farr, "Letter," *1st A.R.R.G.*, p. 90 [PP, 1839, XVI, 65] and Farr, "Letter," *2nd A.R.R.G.*, App., p. 86 [PP, 1840, XVII, 13-14].

135. Farr, "Letter," *Suppl. 35th A.R.R.G.*; p. xxvii [PP, 1875, XVIII, pt. 2].

136. Humphreys in Farr, *Vital Statistics*, pp. x-xi.

137. Harald Westergaard, *Contributions*, pp. 224-26. Anthropometry had been studied earlier, of course. See, for example, Quetelet, *A Treatise on Man*, pp. vi-vii and 57-72.

138. *Report of the Proceedings of the Fourth Session of the International Statistical Congress, Held in London July 16th, 1860, and the Five Following Days* (London, 1861), p. 175.

139. Farr, "Address on Public Health," p. 82.

140. "Report of the Anthropometric Committee," *Report B.A.A.S.* 46 (1876): 266; Ibid. 47 (1877): 231-32; Ibid. 48 (1878), 152-53; Ibid. 49 (1879): 175-209; and Ibid. 50 (1880): 120-59.

141. Ibid. 50 (1880): 121-40; and Ibid. 51 (1881): 225-70.

142. For Nightingale's attitudes see Edwin W. Kopf, "Florence Nightingale as Statistician," *Pub. Am. Statist. Assn.* 15 (1916-17): 398-99; and Edward Cook, *The Life of Florence Nightingale* (London, 1913), 2: 440.

143. See for example how the term "race" is used in the two censuses over which Farr had the most influence: *General Report, Census of 1871*, p. ix; and *General Report, Census of 1861*, p. 7.

144. Farr, "Letter," *Suppl. 25th A.R.R.G.*, pp. xiii-xiv [PP, 1865, XIII]. The idea that cities were both unhealthy and infertile was, of course, an old one. See, for example, Eversley, *Social Theories*, pp. 35-42; and John Saville, *Rural Depopulation in England and Wales 1851-1951* (London, 1957), pp. 125-26.

145. [Farr] *Report on Cholera, 1848-49*, p. xci; see also p. ciii; or Farr, "Influence of Elevation," pp. 171 and 182-83.

146. Farr, *Report on Cholera, 1848-49*, p. xcvii; or Farr, "Influence of Elevation," pp. 177-78.

147. Farr, "Lecture Introductory to a Course on Hygiene," p. 241.

148. Farr, "Medical Reform. An Oration," p. 107.

149. Farr, "Lecture Introductory to a Course on Hygiene," p. 244.

150. Farr, "Vital Statistics," in McCulloch, 1st ed., 2: 569.

151. Farr, "Mortality of Children," pp. 11-12.

152. William Farr, "Influence of Marriage on the Mortality of the French People," *Trans. N.A.P.S.S.* (Liverpool, 1858), p. 508.

153. *Br. Med. J.*, 1869, ii, 267.

154. Farr, "The Application," p. 213, found in L. S. E. Farr Collection, IV, item 1.

155. Farr, *Report on Cholera, 1848-49*, pp. xcvi-xcvii; or Farr, "Influence of Elevation," p. 177.

156. Farr, "Statistics of Insanity," p. 649.

157. Farr, "On Some Doctrines of Population," p. 578.

158. For a concise statement of Galton's views see Francis Galton, "The Possible Improvement of the Human Breed under the Existing Conditions of Law and Sentiment," *Nature* 64 (1901): 663-65.

159. Farr, "Letter," *30th A.R.R.G.*, p. 210 [PP, 1868-69, XVI].

160. Farr, "Mortality of Children," p. 12.

Chapter Seven

1. The party was given in the autumn of 1856 by Colonel Alexander M. Tulloch, Cook, *The Life*, 1: 315.

2. Farr, letter to Florence Nightingale [Feb. 14, 1857], B.M. Add. Mss. 43,398, f. 7.

3. Most of Nightingale's letters to Farr are preserved in the Wellcome Institute for the History of Medicine, London. Typescript copies of these letters plus the originals of a few of her letters to Farr as well as Farr's letters to her are found in the British Museum. Add. Mss. 43,398, 43,399, and 43,400. Several Nightingale letters to Farr are also preserved in L. S. E. Farr Collection, I, items 75-77. We know there were more letters from her.

4. There is ample evidence that the G.R.O. staff did statistical work for her publications. See, for instance, a letter she wrote to Farr June 13, 1859, sending presentation copies and asking him to express her thanks to his assistants for help in preparing material for her *Notes on Hospitals,* Wellcome Collection, item 8, or copy B.M. Add. Mss. 43,398, f. 129.

5. See for example his letters of August 2, 1858 and [Nov. ?], 1858, B.M. Add. Mss. 43,398, ff. 70-71 and 96-97.

6. Examples may be found in Farr, letters to Florence Nightingale, Oct. 5 and Oct. 15, 1858, B.M. Add. Mss. 43,398, ff. 82-84; and Farr, letters to Florence Nightingale [July 27], Aug. 18, and Oct. 9, 1863, B.M. Add. Mss. 43,399, ff. 126-27, 136-37, and 149-50.

7. Farr, letters to Florence Nightingale, Nov. 16 and 17, 1858, B.M. Add. Mss. 43,398, ff. 92-94.

8. Jan. 2, 1865, B.M. Add. Mss. 43,400, f. 1; and Dec. 24, 1868, Ibid., ff. 208-9.

9. Nightingale letters to William Farr, Nov. 12, 1870 and Nov. 27, 1871, copies B.M. Add. Mss. 43,400, ff. 245 and 268; [not in Wellcome] and Nightingale letter to F[lorence] Farr, May 3, 1883, Ibid., f. 281.

10. Nightingale, letter to William Farr, Sept. 16, 1860, Wellcome Collection, item 26, or copy B.M. Add. Mss. 43,398, f. 204; and Nightingale, letter to William Farr, Dec. 11, 1871, copy B.M. Add. Mss. 43,400, f. 270.

11. Nightingale, letter to William Farr, August 31, 1859, Wellcome Collection, item 10, or copy B.M. Add. Mss. 43,398, f. 135.

12. Nightingale, letters to William Farr, February 9 and 25, 1865, Wellcome Collection, items 80 and 83, or copies B.M. Add. Mss. 43,400 ff. 14-15 and 19-20.

13. For the collaboration of Nightingale and Sutherland see Zachary Cope, *Florence Nightingale and the Doctors* (London, 1958), pp. 27-41.

14. Nightingale, letter to William Farr, Feb. 5, 1858, Wellcome Collection, item 1, or copy B.M. Add. Mss. 43,398, f. 41.

15. Nightingale, letter to William Farr, Nov. 27, 1871, copy B.M. Add. Mss. 43,400, f. 269. [original not in Wellcome].

16. Nightingale, letters to William Farr, [March 1858] and Jan. 9, 1864, Wellcome Collection, items 2 and 68, or copies B.M. Add. Mss. 43,398, f. 47, and 43,399, f. 170.

17. Kopf, "Florence Nightingale," p. 392; and Cook, *The Life,* 1: 376-77.

18. Nightingale, letter to William Farr, Dec. 4, 1862, Wellcome Collection, item 59, or copy B.M. Add. Mss. 43,399, f. 95.

19. Nightingale, letter to William Farr, Feb. 23, 1874, Wellcome Collection, item 123, or draft B.M. Add. Mss. 43,400, f. 276.

20. Cook, *The Life,* 1:480-82; and Pearson, *The Life,* 2: 414-15.

21. Farr, letter to Florence Nightingale, Jan. 7, 1860, B.M. Add. Mss. 43,398, f. 162; and Nightingale, letter to William Farr, Jan. 9, 1860, Wellcome Collection, item 15, or copy B.M. Add. Mss. 43,398, f. 164.

22. Nightingale, draft of a letter, [March 1861], B.M. Add. Mss. 43,399, ff. 6-7.

23. Nightingale has been labeled a passionate statistician before. See Pearson, *The Life,* 2: 414.

24. For an account of the appointment and management of the commission see Cook, *The Life,* 1: 321-34, 343-48, and 353-63.

25. See especially Farr, letters to Florence Nightingale, May 7, May 16, [June 21?] and July 19, 1857, B.M. Add. Mss. 43,398, ff. 8-9, 10-11, 13, 14-15.

26. *Report of the Commissioners Appointed to Inquire into the Regulations Affecting the Sanitary Condition of the Army, the Organization of Military Hospitals, and the Treatment of the Sick and Wounded,* PP, 1857-58, XVIII, 242-47, and 506-7.

27. Ibid., 516-26 and following tables and diagrams.

28. Cook, *The Life,* 1: 360-61.

29. *Report*, Army Sanitary Commission, p. 516. See above, n. 26.

30. Ibid., p. 516–17 and diagrams A–D.

31. Ibid., p. 517 and diagram G.

32. Ibid., p. 519 and diagram K.

33. Ibid., p. 517.

34. Ibid., p. 520 and diagrams I and K.

35. Ibid., p. 518.

36. See Ibid., diagrams A–I, K, and Z following p. 526.

37. See also *5th A.R.R.G.*, pp. 50–52 [PP, 1843, XXI, xxxvi–xxxviii].

38. *Report*, Army Sanitary Commission, p. 517. See above, n. 26.

39. *Report on Cholera, 1848–49*, plates 4 and 5.

40. *Report*, Army Sanitary Commission, p. 520. See above, n. 26.

41. *Census of 1851, Numbers of the Inhabitants in the Years 1801, 1811, 1821, 1831, 1841, and 1851*. PP, 1852–53, LXXXV, facing p. 1.

42. *Report*, Army Sanitary Commission, pp. 520–21. See above, n. 26.

43. For the appointment, work, and effect of this committee see Cook, *The Life*, 1: 389; and Cope, *Florence Nightingale*, p. 62.

44. *Report of the Committee on the Preparation of Army Medical Statistics, and on the Duties to Be Performed by the Statistical Branch of the Army Medical Department*, PP, 1861, XXXVII.

45. Ibid., pp. 32, 70–78, and 85–91.

46. At the request of the Government Tulloch prepared a series of reports on the health of British troops abroad: *Statistical Report on the Sickness, Mortality, and Invaliding among the Troops in the West Indies*, PP, 1837–38, XL; *Statistical Reports on the Sickness, Mortality, and Invaliding among the Troops in the United Kingdom, the Mediterranean and British America*, PP, 1839, XVI; *Statistical Reports of the Sickness, Mortality, and Invaliding among the Troops in Western Africa, St. Helena, Cape of Good Hope, and Mauritius*, PP, 1840, XXX; and *Statistical Reports of the Sickness, Mortality, and Invaliding among Her Majesty's Troops Serving in Ceylon, the Tenasserim Provinces, and the Burmese Empire*, PP, 1842, XXVII.

47. *Report of the Committee on Army Medical Statistics*, pp. 48–49. See above, n. 44.

48. Farr, letter to Florence Nightingale, May 27, 1861, B.M. Add. Mss. 43,399, f. 24.

49. Cook, *The Life*, 2: 18–38.

50. Ibid., 2: 44–53. As a civilian she had a peculiar relationship with the War Office, functioning at times as a sanitary consultant; Ibid., pp. 60–62.

51. Nightingale, letter to William Farr, Aug. 8, 1862, Wellcome Collection, item 54, or copy B.M. Add. Mss. 43,399, ff. 70–71.

52. Farr, letter to Florence Nightingale, Aug. 9, 1862, B.M. Add. Mss. 43,399, ff. 72–73.

53. There are several references to this assistance in the correspondence. See for example Farr, letter to Florence Nightingale, Jan. 9, 1860, B.M. Add. Mss. 43,398, f. 164.

54. For their correspondence on Colonel Tulloch's testimony see: Nightingale, letter to William Farr, July 12, 1861, copy, B.M. Add. Mss. 43,399, f. 32; and Farr, letter to Florence Nightingale [July 13 or 14, 1861], B.M. Add. Mss. 43,399, f. 33.

55. Nightingale, letters to William Farr, Sept. 17, 1861; Oct. 2, 1861; and July 13, 1862, Wellcome Collection, items 43, 45, and 53, or copies B.M. Add. Mss. 43,399, ff. 46–47; 54–55; and 68.

56. Farr, letter to Florence Nightingale, July [?] 1862, B.M. Add. Mss. 43,399, f. 69.

57. *Report of the Commissioners Appointed to Inquire into the Sanitary State of the Army in India*, PP, 1863, XIX, see esp. pp. 15–48 and 172–97.

58. Farr, letter to Florence Nightingale, June 17, 1862, B.M. Add. Mss. 43,399, f. 66.

59. The annual rates of mortality per 1,000 in India were: English troops 69, English Officers 38, English civil servants 20, and native troops 18. *Report*, Indian Sanitary Commission, pp. 36 and 41. See above, n. 57.

60. "Mortality and Diseases of Armies," *Br. Med. Almanack*, 1836, 109–11; and

Farr, "Vital Statistics," in McCulloch, 1st ed., 2: 580. His treatment of the mortality of soldiers and sailors in the fourth edition of the latter work (1854) was considerably longer, Farr, "Vital Statistics," in McCulloch, 4th ed., 2: 554-65.

61. Farr, "Vital Statistics," in McCulloch, 1st ed., 2: 572-73.

62. In the preceding decades English belief in the inherent unhealthiness of the tropics had grown as a result of colonial experience in West Africa. See P[hilip] D. Curtin, "'The White Man's Grave:' Image and Reality, 1780-1850," *J. Br. Stud.* 1 (1961): 102-6.

63. "The Health of the British Army," pp. 472-83; "Report of the Fifth Section on the Vital Statistics of the Army," *Report of the Proceedings of the Fourth Session of the International Statistical Congress* . . . (London, 1861), pp. 142-43; and "Reports of the Official Delegates, 1, Report of Dr. William Farr," pp. 414-15.

64. Farr, letter to Florence Nightingale, Feb. 3, 1863, B.M. Add. Mss. 43,399, ff. 103-4.

65. For summaries of evidence and recommendations see *Report,* Indian Sanitary Commission, pp. 160-71. See above, n. 57.

66. Farr, letter to Florence Nightingale, June 3, 1863, B.M. Add. Mss. 43,399, ff. 117-18.

67. Farr, letter to Florence Nightingale, Dec. 22, 1863, B.M. Add. Mss. 43,399, f. 162.

68. Farr, letter to Florence Nightingale, Nov. 24, 1863, B.M. Add. Mss. 43,399, f. 155.

69. For a summary of her suggestions see Nightingale, letter to William Farr, May 10, 1865, copy B.M. Add. Mss., 43,400, ff. 44-46. For summaries of the points at issue see *Lancet,* 1865, i, 572-73; and *Br. Med. J.,* 1865, ii, 478. William Clode of the G.R.O. presented Farr's case in a letter to the editor, *Br. Med. J.,* 1865, ii, 568. The issue was also aired before the British Association; see James Bird, "On the Vital and Sanitary Statistics of our European Army in India, Compared with Those of French Troops under Like Conditions of Climate and Locality," *J. Statist. Soc. Lond.* 26 (1863): 390-96.

70. "Statistics of the English Hospitals," *Br. Med. Almanack,* (1836), pp. 114-23.

71. Ibid., p. 117.

72. Farr, "On a Method of Determining the Danger," pp. 72-79; Farr, "On the Law of Recovery and Dying," pp. 134-43; and Farr, "Statistics of Insanity," 1 (1837): 648-53, 679-83, 744-48, 811-14, and 2 (1837): 137-40, 171-74, 204-7, 235-39, and 357-61.

73. "Report of the Committee on Hospital Statistics," *J. Statist. Soc. Lond.* 5 (1842): 168-76; "Second Report of the Committee of the Statistical Society of London on Hospital Statistics," Ibid. 7 (1844): 214-31. For a brief summary of the committee's work see Cullen, *The Statistical Movement,* p. 98.

74. "Report of the Committee on Hospital Statistics," pp. 175-76; and "Second Report . . .," pp. 218-31. See above, n. 73.

75. See also his note accompanying printed tables in B.M. Add. Mss. 43,399, f. 223.

76. "Report of the Committee on Hospital Statistics," pp. 171-72, "Second Report . . .," pp. 216-17. See above, n. 73.

77. "A Register of the Cases of Disease Observed at the London and Metropolitan Free Hospitals . . . .," *Lancet,* 1855, ii, 211-16.

78. B.M. Add. Mss., 43,398, ff. 3-4. On this occasion he calculated mortality on cases treated, not on the basis of average patient population.

79. This work was first presented as two papers to the second meeting of the Social Science Association, "Notes on the Sanitary Condition of Hospitals, and on Defects in the Construction of Hospital Wards, Parts I and II," *Trans. N.A.P.S.S.* (Liverpool, 1858), 462-73 and 473-82. They were published the following year as a book.

80. See, for example, Grace Goldin, "Building a Hospital of Air: The Victorian Pavilions of St. Thomas' Hospital, London," *Bull. Hist. Med.* 49 (1975): 512-35.

81. See, for example, Farr, letter to Florence Nightingale, April 3, 1860, B.M. Add. Mss. 43,398, f. 172.

82. *Report of the Proceedings of the Fourth Session of the International Statistical Congress* . . . (London, 1861), pp. 247-304.

83. "Hospital Statistics and Hospital Plans," *Trans. N.A.P.S.S.* (Dublin, 1861), 554-60.

84. For the standard treatment of this incident see Cook, *The Life,* 1: 429–30, and 433.

85. For a late statement of their appreciation see Nightingale, letter to William Farr, April 8, 1865, copy B.M. Add. Mss. 43,400, f. 32; and Farr, letter to Florence Nightingale, April 10, 1865, B.M. Add. Mss. 43,400, ff. 33–35.

86. [William H. Stone], "Hospital Registration," *Med. Times and Gazette,* 1860, ii, 110–11 and 188–90. Stone identifies himself as the author of this article in a letter to the editor, Ibid., p. 342. See also letters to the editor by John W. Tripe, Ibid., pp. 221–22 and 388.

87. *Med. Times and Gazette,* 1860, ii, 189.

88. Ibid., pp. 316–17 and 387.

89. Ibid., p. 317.

90. Nightingale, letters to William Farr, Oct. 20, 1860, and Oct. 22, 1860, Wellcome Collection, items 29 and 30, or copies B.M. Add. Mss. 43,398, ff. 208–9 and 210.

91. Nightingale, letter to William Farr, Nov. 15, 1862, Wellcome Collection, item 58, or copy B.M. Add. Mss. 43,399, f. 90.

92. Florence Nightingale, *Notes on Hospitals,* 3rd ed. (London, 1863), pp. 159–80.

93. Ibid., p. 3.

94. *24th A.R.R.G.,* pp. 174–210, and 229–31 [PP, 1863, XIV]. The table in question is from p. 205.

95. Nightingale, *Notes on Hospitals,* 3rd ed., p. 4.

96. Ibid., pp. 4–7.

97. See pp. 129–30.

98. *Med. Times and Gazette,* 1864, i, 186–88.

99. *Lancet,* 1864, i, 248–50.

100. The comments in the *Lancet,* 1864, i, appeared under the title "Mortality in Hospitals" as follows: Holmes, March 19, pp. 338–39; Holmes, March 26, pp. 365–66; Farr, April 9, pp. 420–22; Holmes, April 16, pp. 451–52; J. S. Bristowe, April 16, p. 452; and Farr, April 23, p. 469. The ensuing comments in the *Medical Times and Gazette* are: Bristowe, Feb. 20, p. 211; Farr, Feb. 27, pp. 242–43; "M.D.," March 5, pp. 264–65; Charles Grieg, March 5, p. 272; J. Burney Yeo, March 12, p. 296; Bristowe, March 12, pp. 296–97; Bristowe, April 9, p. 405; Bristowe, April 30, pp. 491–92.

101. Nightingale, *Notes on Hospitals,* 3rd ed., pp. 8–10 and 22. See also Nightingale, "Notes on the Sanitary Condition," pp. 466–68.

102. *Med. Times and Gazette,* 1864, i, 129.

103. *Lancet,* 1864, i, 250.

104. *Med. Times and Gazette,* 1864, i, 188.

105. J. Burney Yeo, "Hospital Mortality," Ibid., p. 296; and T. Holmes, "Hospital Mortality," Ibid., pp. 349–50.

106. *Congrès International de Bienfaisance de Londres,* 2: 124, cited in *Lancet,* 1864, i, 249.

107. Nightingale, *Notes on Hospitals,* 3rd ed., p. 2.

108. *Med. Times and Gazette,* 1864, i, 129.

109. Ibid., p. 187.

110. Ibid., p. 129.

111. *Lancet,* 1864, i, 365.

112. Ibid., p. 339.

113. For an early example see Farr, "Letter," *5th A.R.R.G.,* pp. 428–29 [PP, 1843, XXI, 212]. After a tour of the new Herbert Hospital he complimented her on its design, Farr, letter to Florence Nightingale, June 24, 1865, B.M. Add. Mss. 43,400, ff. 66–67.

114. Farr, "Letter," *24th A.R.R.G.,* p. 231 [PP, 1863, XIV].

115. Richardson's original observation on the low rate of mortality after surgery, especially lithotomy, in the Norwich Hospital occurred in his medical history of Norwich, *Med. Times and Gazette,* 1864, i, 40–43 and 67. The ensuing correspondence is found, Ibid., 74–75, 217, 243–44, 262–63, 294–96, 318–19, and 349–50.

116. Ibid., p. 243.

117. Nightingale, *Notes on Hospitals,* 3rd ed., pp. 26–32.

118. Lambert, *Sir John Simon,* pp. 344–45, and 478–83. For a different assessment

of the value the Nightingale wards at St. Thomas's see Goldin, "Building a Hospital," pp. 512-35.

119. This report appeared somewhat later: John Seyer Bristowe and Timothy Holmes, "Report on the Hospitals of the United Kingdom," App. no. 15, *Sixth Report of the Medical Officer of the Privy Council,* PP, 1864, XXVIII. For the section most relevant to the controversy with Farr and Nightingale see pp. 512-68.

120. Nightingale, letter to William Farr, February 23, 1864, Wellcome Collection, item 71, or copy B.M. Add. Mss. 43,399, ff. 193-94.

121. B.M. Add. Mss. 43,399, f. 198.

122. *Lancet,* 1864, i, 420-22.

123. Ibid., pp. 451-52.

124. Ibid., p. 469.

125. *Med. Times and Gazette,* 1864, i, 492.

126. E. M. Sigsworth, "Gateways to Death? Medicine, Hospitals and Mortality, 1700-1850," in *Science and Society 1600-1900,* ed. Peter Mathias (Cambridge, 1972), pp. 102-3; and Lambert, *Sir John Simon,* p. 345.

127. *Med. Times and Gazette,* 1864, i, 491.

128. Ibid., p. 186.

129. Arthur Newsholme, "William Farr," [a lecture at the Johns Hopkins University] in L. S. E. Farr Collection, IX, item 5, p. 217.

130. Farr, letter to Florence Nightingale, Aug. 10, 1858, B.M. Add. Mss. 43,398, ff. 72-74.

131. Farr, letter to Florence Nightingale, Dec. 11, 1871, B.M. Add. Mss. 43,400, ff. 272-73.

132. Farr, letter to Florence Nightingale, Feb. 10, 1859, B.M. Add. Mss. 43,398, f. 110.

133. John Simon, letter to William Farr, Nov. 21 [1879], L. S. E. Farr Collection, I, item 94.

134. Cook, *The Life,* 391-92; and Nightingale, letter to William Farr, Feb. 25, 1859, Wellcome Collection, item 5 or copy B.M. Add. Mss. 43,398, f. 117.

135. Nightingale, letter to Florence Nightingale, Sept. 29, 1866, Wellcome Collection, item 104, or copy B.M. Add. Mss. 43,400, ff. 109-10.

136. Ibid.

137. Nightingale, letter to William Farr, April 2, 1860, Wellcome Collection, item 17 or copy B.M. Add. Mss. 43,398, f. 169.

138. Cope, *Florence Nightingale,* pp. 116-18; and Lambert, *Sir John Simon,* p. 345.

139. Lambert, *Sir John Simon,* pp. 521-23.

140. Farr, letter to Florence Nightingale, April 3, 1860, B.M. Add. Mss. 43,398, f. 171.

141. Farr, letter to Florence Nightingale [c. July 23, 1857], B.M. Add. Mss. 43,398, f. 21.

142. See for example Farr, letters to Florence Nightingale, Nov. 22, 1865, and Sept. 5, 1868, B.M. Add. Mss. 43,400, ff. 84 and 202.

143. Farr, letter to Florence Nightingale, Feb. 17, 1859, B. M. Add. Mss. 43,398, f. 112. See also ff. 113-14.

144. Undated postscript B.M. Add. Mss. 43,399, f. 19. The assigned date, April 1861, is unlikely. April 1859 seems more probable from the contents.

145. Cope, *Florence Nightingale,* pp. 14-16.

146. In 1879 Nightingale wrote to Lord Beaconsfield urging Farr's appointment as Graham's successor to the post of registrar general. A year later she urged the Government to make Farr C.B., see Cook, *The Life,* 2: 289.

147. Nightingale, letter to Florence Farr, May 3, 1883, copy, B.M. Add. Mss. 43,400, f. 281.

Chapter Eight

1. "Report of the Council for the Financial Year ended 31st December 1879, and for the Sessional Year ending 30th June, 1880," *J. Statist. Soc. Lond.* 43 (1880): 411; *Br. Med.*

J., 1880, i, 527; Ibid., 1880, ii, 299; and Cook, *The Life,* 2: 289n.

2. Great Britain, Treasury Minute [copy], Feb. 28, 1880, in L. S. E. Farr Collection, XIII, item 12.

3. Farr was survived by three unmarried daughters, a married daughter, and a married son. For details see letter of August 30, 1883, by an unnamed correspondent of the Statistical Society of London to F. H. Janson, the solicitor of the Farr Estate, L. S. E. Farr Collection, I, item 100. See also Hare, *William Farr,* p. 8 in L. S. E. Farr Collection, XI, item 30. Farr's best known child was his youngest child, Florence, who became an actress. See explanatory comments by Shaw, George Yeats, and the editor in Florence Farr, Bernard Shaw, and W. B. Yeats, *Letters,* ed. Clifford Bax (New York, 1942), pp. v–xii and 47–50.

4. For the Farr Testimonial Fund see *Br. Med. J.,* 1880, i, 378, 418, 456, and 721; Ibid., 1880, ii, 238, 309, 727; or *Lancet,* 1880, i, 382, 423, 459, 617, 733; Ibid., 1880, ii, 220, 308, and 715; Ibid., 1881, i, 847; and Ibid., 1881, ii, 190. Noel Humphreys provided a detailed account in Farr, *Vital Statistics,* pp. 553–56. For the closing of the fund see R. L. Antrobus [for Derby], letter to William Farr, Esq., R.N., April 23, 1883, L. S. E. Farr Collection, I, item 4; Horance Seymour [for Gladstone] letters to William Farr, R.N., April 25, 1883 and May 2, 1883, Ibid., I, items 43 and 44; and Florence Nightingale, letter to F. H. Janson, June 25, 1883, Ibid., I, item 78; and F. H. Janson, letter to Joseph Whittall (n.d.), Ibid., I, item 61.

5. Flinn, "Introduction," p. 27.

6. "The New Registrar-General," *The Times* (London), Jan. 8, 1880, p. 11; Hare, *William Farr,* p. 7; and "Sketch of Dr. William Farr," *Popular Science Monthly* 23 (1883): 406.

7. D. V. Glass, *Numbering the People,* p. 142, n. 70; and E. Grebenik, "The Sources and Nature of Statistical Information in Special Fields of Statistics: Population and Vital Statistics," *J. Roy. Statist. Soc.,* Ser. A. 118 (1955): 452.

8. *D.N.B.,* 6: 1090. See also Hare, *William Farr,* p. 7.

9. Lambert, *Sir John Simon,* p. 512, and Brockington, *Public Health,* p. 201.

10. Farr had tried to convince the government years earlier to make Graham K. C. B. Farr, letter to W. Cowper, Feb. 8, 1864, B.M. Add. Mss. 43,399, ff. 186–89.

11. "Dr. Farr," *Br. Med. J.,* 1880, i, 69.

12. *Br. Med. J.,* 1880, i, 69, 140, 183, 223–24, 262, 264, 299, and 378; and *Lancet,* 1880, i, 227 and 381.

13. Great Britain, *Hansard's Parliamentary Debates* 250 (1880): 148–49, 585–88, and 1,193.

14. "Dr. William Farr and the Office of Registrar-General," *Br. Med. J.,* 1880, i, p. 182.

15. "William Farr, C.B., M.D.," *Lancet,* 1880, i, 537.

16. Lambert, *Sir John Simon,* pp. 501–34; Brand, *Doctors and the State,* pp. 15–31; and Roy M. MacLeod, "The Frustration of State Medicine 1880-1899," *Med. Hist.* 11 (1967): 16–17 and 32–33. For Simon's account of these events see his *English Sanitary Institutions,* pp. 322–92.

17. *Lancet,* 1880, i, 19.

18. *The Times* [London] (April 23, 1883), p. 10.

19. *Trans. Sanitary Institute of Gt. Brit.,* 5 (1883–84): 74–76; and Gairdner, *Public Health,* pp. 18–19. Gairdner played a role in encouraging the publication of Farr's memorial volume. W[illiam] Gairdner, letters to Joseph Whittall, Aug. 16, 1883, and Dec. 8, 1883, in L. S. E. Farr Collection, I, items 39 and 40; and "Preface," in Farr, *Vital Statistics,* pp. v–vi.

20. *Br. Med. J.,* 1883, i, p. 783.

21. Edward Headlam Greenhow, "The Results of an Inquiry into the Different Proportions of Death Produced by Certain Diseases in Different Districts in England," *Papers Relating to the Sanitary State of the People of England,* PP, 1857-58, XXIII, 1–164.

22. *9th A.R.R.G.,* App., p. 160 [PP, 1849, XXI, 5–8].

23. *24th A.R.R.G.,* pp. 174–210 and 229–31 [PP, 1863, XIV].

24. Farr, "Letter," *Suppl. 35th A.R.R.G.,* p. xxiv [PP, 1875, XVIII, pt. 2].

25. "The Value of Death-Rates," p. 438.

26. Greenhow, "Results to an Inquiry." See above, n. 21.

27. Farr, letter to Florence Nightingale, Aug. 10, 1858, B.M. Add. Mss. 43,398, ff. 73-74.

28. Rumsey, "On the Value of Life Tables," pp. 7, 9-10, and 14-15.

29. Farr, letter to Florence Nightingale, Dec. 11, 1871, B.M. Add. Mss. 43,400, f. 272.

30. *Fifty Years in Public Health: A Personal Narrative with Comments* (London, 1935), p. 273.

31. Newsholme, "William Farr," in L. S. E. Farr Collection, IX, item 5, p. 203. Newsholme, "The Measurement of Progress," pp. 186, 189, 190, and 194.

32. Greenwood, *Some British Pioneers,* p. 79. See also Greenwood, *The Medical Dictator,* p. 91.

33. Brownlee, "Historical Note," pp. 250-52.

34. Brownlee, *The Use of Death-Rates.* Brownlee's contemporaries in the Statistical Society were skeptical of his commitment to the use of life table death rates. See "Discussion of the Value of Life-Tables in Statistical Research," *J. Roy. Statist. Soc.* 85 (1922): 537-60.

35. Brownlee, *The Use of Death-Rates,* p. 28.

36. Abraham M. Lilienfeld, *Foundations of Epidemiology* (New York, 1976), p. 23; David E. Lilienfeld and Abraham M. Lilienfeld, "Epidemiology: A Retrospective Study," *Am. J. Epidemiol.* 106 (1977): 449; and Alexander D. Langmuir, "Epidemiology of Airborne Infection," *Bact. Rev.* 25 (1961): 173-74.

37. Susser and Adelstein, "Introduction," *Vital Statistics,* p. iii; Alexander D. Langmuir, "William Farr: Founder of Modern Concepts of Surveillance," *Int. J. Epidemiol.* 5 (1976): 13-18; and Alexander D. Langmuir, "The Surveillance of Communicable Diseases of National Importance," *New Engl. J. Med.* 268 (1963): 182.

38. Susser and Adelstein, "Introduction," *Vital Statistics,* p. xiii.

39. Farr, letter to Florence Nightingale, Sept. 2, 1864, B.M. Add. Mss. 43,399, f. 206.

40. Farr, letter to Florence Nightingale, Nov. 24, 1863, B.M. Add. Mss. 43,399, f. 154.

41. Erwin H. Ackerknecht, "Anticontagionism between 1821 and 1867," *Bull. Hist. Med.* 22 (1948): 567 and 589-93.

42. Farr, "Note," p. 353.

43. Farr, "Letter," *Suppl. 25th A.R.R.G.*, p. xiii [PP, 1865, XIII].

44. I have discussed this use of death rates in Eyler, "Mortality Statistics," pp. 335-39.

45. W[illiam] Farr, "Address on Public Health," *Trans. N.A.P.S.S.* (Manchester, 1866), p. 70.

46. Finer, *The Life,* pp. 381-89 and 412-20; and R. M. MacLeod, "Law, Medicine and Public Opinion: The Resistance to Compulsory Health Legislation 1870-1907," *Public Law* (Summer and Autumn, 1967), pp. 107-28 and 189-211.

47. Cullen, *The Statistical Movement,* pp. 135-49.

48. Guy, "On the Value," pp. 25-47; Griffin and Griffin, *Observations;* and *Br. and For. Med. Rev.* 22 (1841): 1-21.

49. Cullen, *The Statistical Movement,* p. 35.

50. Farr, letter to Florence Nightingale, Feb. 3, 1863, B.M. Add. Mss. 43,399, ff. 103-4.

51. For explanation of how the ideas of the statistical movement must be understood as a compromise between the "demands of science and politics" see Hilts, "Aliis exterendum," pp. 21-43.

SELECTED BIBLIOGRAPHY

I. Manuscript Collections

Brougham Papers. University College, London.
Chadwick Papers. University College, London.
Farr Papers. London School of Economics.
Farr/Quetelet Letters [microfilm No. 11]. American Philosophical Society Library, Philadelphia. Originals from Bibliothéque Royale de Belgique, Brussels.
Edward Jarvis Papers. Francis A. Countway Library of Medicine, Boston.
Nightingale Papers. Wellcome Institute for the History of Medicine, London.
Nightingale Papers. British Library [British Museum], Add. Mss. 43,398, 43,399, and 43,400.

II. British Parliamentary Papers other than those by William Farr

1833, XIV   *Report from the Select Committee on Parochial Registration.*

1837–38, XXVIII   *Report of Commissioners on the State, Custody, and Authenticity of Registers or Records of Births or Baptisms, Deaths or Burials, and Marriages in England and Wales, other than the Parochial Registers.*

1847, XXXIV   *A Return of the Number of Persons Employed at the Office of the Registrar General.*

1850, XXI   *Report of the General Board of Health on the Epidemic of Cholera of 1848 and 1849.*

1852–53, XXI   *Report from the Select Committee on Assurance Associations.*

1852–53, LXXXV   *Census of Britain, 1851. Population Tables. I. Numbers of the Inhabitants in the Years 1801, 1811, 1821, 1831, 1841, and 1851.*

1852–53, LXXXVIII, pt. 1   *Census of 1851, Ages, Civil Conditions, Occupations and Birth-Place of the People.*

1854, XXXV   *Report of the General Board of Health on the Administration of the Public Health Act and the Nuisances Removal and Diseases Prevention Acts, from 1848 to 1854.*

1854–55, XIII   *Report from the Select Committee on Public Health Bill, and Nuisances Removal Amendment Bill.*

1854–55, XXI   *Report of the Committee for Scientific Inquiries in Relation to the Cholera-Epidemic of 1854.*

1854–55, XLV   *Letter of the President of the General Board of Health, to The Right Honourable the Viscount Palmerston, Secretary of State for the Home Department, etc., etc., Accompanying a Report from Dr. Sutherland on Epidemic Cholera in the Metropolis in 1854.*

1856, LII   *Report on the Last Two Cholera-Epidemics of London, as Affected by the Consumption of Impure Water; Addressed to the Rt. Hon. the President of the General Board of Health by the Medical Officer of the Board.*

241

1857–58, XVIII–XIX   *Report of the Commissioners Appointed to Inquire into the Regulations Affecting the Sanitary Condition of the Army, the Organization of Military Hospitals, and the Treatment of the Sick and Wounded.*

1857–58, XXIII   *Papers Relating to the Sanitary State of the People of England.* John Simon, "Introductory Report by the Medical Officer of the Board," pp. iii–xlviii. Edward Headlam Greenhow, "The Results of an Inquiry into the Different Proportions of Death Produced by Certain Diseases in Different Districts in England," pp. 1–164.

1860, XXIX   *Second Report of the Medical Officer of the Privy Council.* [Edward Headlam] Greenhow, "Dr. Greenhow's Reports on the Prevalence and Causes of Diarrhoea at Coventry, Birmingham . . ., pp. 65–160.

1861, VII   *Report from the Select Committee Appointed to Inquire into the Present Mode of Assessing and Collecting the Income and Property Tax, and whether any Mode of Levying the Same, so as to Render the Tax More Equitable, Can Be Adopted.*

1861, XXXVII   *Report of the Committee on the Preparation of Army Medical Statistics, and on the Duties to Be Performed by the Statistical Branch of the Army Medical Department.*

1863, XIX   *Report of the Commissioners Appointed to Inquire into the Sanitary State of the Army in India.*

1863, LIII, pt. 1   *Census of England and Wales for the Year 1861, General Report.*

1864, XXIV, pt. 2   *Report of the Commissioners Appointed to Inquire into the Condition of All Mines in Great Britain to Which the Provisions of the Act 23 & 24 Vict. Cap. 151, Do Not Apply with Reference to the Health and Safety of Persons Employed in Such Mines.*

1864, XXVIII   Sixth Report of the Medical Officer of the Privy Council. App. 15: John Seyer Bristowe and Timothy Holmes, " Report on the Hospitals of the United Kingdom."

1865, XXVI   *Seventh Report of the Medical Officer of the Privy Council.* John Simon, "Medical Officer's Report," pp. 1–30.

1867, XXXVII   *Ninth Report of the Medical Officer of the Privy Council.* John Simon, "Medical Officer's Report, pp. 7–35.

1868–69, XXXII   *First Report of the Royal Sanitary Commission.*

1873, LXXI, pt. 2   *Census of England and Wales for the Year 1871, General Report.*

1877, XV   *Report from the Select Committee on Police Superannuation Funds.*

III. British Statutes at Large

6 & 7 Wm. IV, c. 85 (1836).   "An Act for Marriages in England."

6 & 7 Wm. IV, c. 86 (1836).   "An Act for Registering Births, Deaths, and Marriages in England."

11 & 12 Vict., c. 63 (1847–48).   "An Act for Promoting the Public Health."

15 & 16 Vict., c. 84 (1852).   "An Act to Make Better Provision Respecting the Supply of Water to the Metropolis."

17 & 18 Vict., c. 80 (1854).   "An Act to Provide for the Better Registration of Births, Deaths, and Marriages in Scotland."

18 & 19 Vict., c. 29 (1854-55).   "An Act to Make Further Provision for the Registration of Births, Deaths, and Marriages in Scotland."

26 & 27 Vict., c. 11 (1863)   "An Act for the Registration of Births and Deaths in Ireland."

26 & 27 Vict., c. 27 (1863)   "An Act to Amend the Law Relating to Marriages in Ireland."

37 & 38 Vict., c. 88 (1874)   "An Act to Amend the Law Relating to the Registration of Births and Deaths in England, and to Consolidate the Law Respecting the Registration of Births and Deaths at Sea."

IV. Published Works by William Farr

"Address," *Br. Med. Almanack* (1835), pp. 3-6.

"[Presidential] Address [to Section F, Economic Science and Statistics]," *Report, B.A.A.S.* 34 (1864): 151-63.

"Address by W. Farr, M.D., F.R.S. on Public Health," *Trans. N.A.P.S.S.* (Manchester, 1866), 67-83.

"An Address Delivered in the Section of State Medicine, at the Annual Meeting of the British Medical Association, in Leeds, July 1869," *Br. Med. J.,* 1869, ii, 265-67.

"The 'Annual Mortality' and the 'Mean Age at Death': A Comparison of the Methods Which Have Been Employed at Various Times for Determining the Relative Salubrity and Mortality of Different Classes of the Population," *6th A.R.R.G.,* pp. 570-77 [PP, 1844, XIX, 315-18].

"Apothecaries' Company an Anomaly—Necessity for Its Reform, and Conversion into a College of Pharmacy," *Br. Ann. Med.* 1 (1837): 340-43.

"Apothecaries' Hall," *Br. Ann. Med.* 2 (1837): 248-49.

"The Application of Statistics to Naval and Military Matters," *J. United Service Institution* (August 1859), pp. 209-24.

"Bills of Mortality. Registration of Births, Deaths, and Diseases," *Br. Med. Almanack,* 1836, 125-33.

"Causes of the High Mortality in Town Districts," *5th A.R.R.G.,* pp. 406-35 [PP, 1843, XXI, 200-15].

"Chronological History of Medicine," *Br. Med. Almanack,* 1836, pp. 9, 11, 13, 15, 17, 19, 21, 23, 25, 27, 29, 31-33.

"Chronological History of Medicine," *Br. Med. Almanack,* (1837), pp. 9, 11, 13, 15, 17, 19, 21, 23, 25, 27, 29, 31-35.

"Chronological History of Medicine," *Br. Med. Almanack,* (1838), pp. 7, 9, 11, 13, 15, 17, 19, 21, 23, 25, 27, 29-31.

"The College of Physicians—Its Tyranny," *Br. Ann. Med.* 1 (1837): 405-7.

"The College of Physicians vs. Scotch Graduates," *Br. Ann. Med.* 1 (1837): 662-3.

"Concours—Trial of Mr. Nice—Practical Knowledge not Indentures the Passport to Practise," *Br. Ann. Med* 1 (1837): 468-70.

"Considerations, in the Form of a Draft Report, Submitted to Committee, Favourable to the Maintenance of Section F," *J. Statist. Soc. Lond.* 40 (1877): 473-76.

"Construction of Life Tables," *5th A.R.R.G.,* pp. 342-67 [PP, 1843, XXI, 161-78].

"Contribution to the Natural History of Quackery," *Br. Ann. Med.* 1 (1837): 314-15.

"Coroners' Inquests," *Br. Ann. Med.* 1 (1837): 182-84.

"A Cure for Sore Nipple," *Lancet,* 1841-42, ii, 154-55.

"Curricula," *Br. Ann. Med.* 1 (1837): 430-32.

"Density or Proximity of Population: Its Advantages and Disadvantages," *Trans. N.A.P.S.S.* (Cheltenham, 1878), pp. 530-35.

"Directions Respecting the Registration of the Causes of Deaths," *Lancet,* 1842-43, ii, 236-37.

"Dr. Farr on the Duties of the New Medical Officers of Health," *Lancet,* 1856, i, 19.

"Dr. Farr on the Registration Clauses of the Vaccination Bill," *Lancet,* 1867, i, 721-22.

"Dr. Rumsey," *Br. Med. J.,* 1875, i, 460.

"Education at Oxford," *Br. Ann. Med.* 1 (1837): 275-76.

[English Life Table No. 1], *5th A.R.R.G.*, pp. 354-58 and 366-67 [PP, 1843, XXI, 168-72 and 178] and *6th A.R.R.G.*, pp. 517-666 [PP, 1844, XIX, 290-358].

"English Life Table, No. 2, Females," *20th A.R.R.G.*, App., pp. 177-203 [PP, 1859, sess. 2, XII].

"English Life Table, No. 2, Males," *12th A.R.R.G.*, App. pp. 73-152.

English Life Table: Tables of Lifetimes, Annuities, and Premiums, with an Introduction by William Farr, M.D., F.R.S., D.C.L. (London, 1864).

"English Reproduction Table," *Phil. Trans.* 171 (1880): 281-88.

"General Cattle Mutual Insurance Fund," *J. Roy. Agric. Soc. Engl.,* 2nd ser., 2 (1866): 455-71.

"The Great Powers," *Assurance Mag. and J. Institute Actuaries* 6 (1857): 147-59.

"The Health of the British Army, and the Effects of Recent Sanitary Measures on Its Mortality and Sickness," *J. Statist. Soc. Lond.* 24 (1861): 472-83.

"Healthy District Life Table, with Tables of Annuities, and Premiums," *33rd A.R.R.G.*, pp. 441-57 [PP, 1872, XVII].

"History of the Medical Profession, and Its Influence on Public Health, in England," *Br. Med. Almanack,* suppl. (1839), pp. 113-78.

"Hospital Mortality," *Med. Times and Gazette,* 1864, i, 242-43.

"Hospital Registration," *Med. Times and Gazette,* 1860, ii, 316-17 and 387.

"Inaugural Address," *J. Statist. Soc. Lond.* 34 (1871): 409-23.

"Inaugural Address," *J. Statist Soc. Lond.* 35 (1872): 417-30.

"The Income and Property Tax," *J. Statist. Soc. Lond.* 16 (1853): 1-44.

"Influence of Elevation on the Fatality of Cholera," *J. Statist. Soc. Lond.* 15 (1852): 155-83.

"Influence of Marriage on the Mortality of the French People," *Trans. N.A.P.S.S.* (Liverpool, 1858), 504-13.

"The Influence of Scarcities and of the High Prices of Wheat on the Mortality of the People of England," *J. Statist. Soc. Lond.* 9 (1846): 158-74.

"Is the Medical Profession Represented in Parliament?" *Br. Ann. Med.* 2 (1837): 216-18.

"Lecture Introductory to a Course on Hygiene, or the Preservation of the Public Health," *Lancet,* 1835–36, i, 240–45.

"Lecture on the History of Hygiene," *Lancet,* 1835–36, i, 773–80.

"Letter to the Registrar-General on the Mortality in the Registration Districts of England during the 10 Years 1851–60," *Suppl. 25th A.R.R.G.* [PP, 1865, XIII].

"Letter to the Registrar-General on the Mortality in the Registration Districts of England during the Years 1861–70," *Suppl. 35th A.R.R.G.* [PP, 1875, XVIII, pt. 2].

Letters to the Registrar General on the Causes of Death in England [title varies]. *Annual Report of the Registrar-General of Birth, Deaths, and Marriages in England,* vols. 1–41.

"Life Assurance Offices," *Br. Ann. Med.* 2 (1837): 249–51 and 281–83.

"Medical Competition," *Br. Ann. Med.* 2 (1837): 116.

"Medical Reform. An Oration Delivered at the Last Anniversary Meeting of the British Medical Association," *Lancet,* 1839–40, i, 105–11.

"Medical Reform. Representative Bodies v. the Corporations," *Br. Ann. Med.* 1 (1837): 563–66.

"Medical Relief of Paupers," *Br. Ann. Med.* 1 (1837): 243–45.

"A Method of Determining the Effects of Systems of Treatment in Certain Diseases," *Br. Med. J.,* 1862, ii, 193–95.

"A Method of Determining the Effects of Systems of Treatment in Certain Diseases, *Lancet* 1862, ii, 157–58.

"Miss Nightingale's 'Notes on Hospitals,'" *Med. Times and Gazette* 1864, i, 186–87.

"Mr. Lowe and the Cattle Plague," *Daily News* (London), (Feb. 19, 1866), pp. 5–6.

"Mortality and Diseases of Armies," *Br. Med. Almanack* (1836), 109–11.

"Mortality in Hospitals," *Lancet,* 1864, i, 420–22, 469.

"Mortality of Children in the Principal States of Europe," *J. Statist. Soc. Lond.* 29 (1866): 1–35.

"National Board of Health," *Br. Ann. Med.* 1 (1837): 372–75, 758–60.

"National Registration," *Br. Ann. Med.* 1 (1837): 180–82.

Net Premiums for Insurance against Fatal Accident, according to Age and Sex (London, 1880).

"The New Classification of the People according to Their Employments," *Census of England and Wales for the Year 1861, General Report, App.* [PP, 1863, LIII, pt. 1, 225–48].

"The Northampton Table of Mortality," *8th A.R.R.G.,* pp. 278–349 [PP, 1847–48, XXV, 290–325].

"Note on the Present Epidemic of Small-Pox, and on the Necessity of Arresting Its Ravages," *Lancet,* 1840–41, i, 351–54.

"Notice Relative to Returns of 'Cause of Death,'" *Lond. Med. Gazette,* 1842–43, ii, 252.

"Observation," *Br. Ann. Med.* 1 (1837): 692–95.

"On a Method of Determining the Danger and the Duration of Diseases at Every Period of Their Progress., Article I.," *Br. Ann. Med.* 1 (1837): 72–79.

"On Benevolent Funds and Life Assurance in Health and Sickness," *Lancet*, 1837-38, i, 701-4 and 817-23.

"On Cholera," *Br. Med. Almanack* (1839), pp. 204-9.

"On Infant Mortality, and on Alleged Inaccuracies of the Census," *J. Statist. Soc. Lond.* 28 (1865): 125-49.

"On Prognosis," *Br. Med. Almanack* (1838), pp. 199-216.

"On Some Doctrines of Population. A Paper Read in Section F of the British Association, at Plymouth, in August Last," *J. Statist. Soc. Lond.* 40 (1877): 568-79.

"On Some Points Connected with the Inquiry into the Present State of the Poor," *Br. Ann. Med.* 1 (1837): 455-62.

"On the Construction of Life-Tables, Illustrated by a New Life-Table of the Healthy Districts of England," *Phil. Trans.* 149 (1859): 837-78.

"On the Law of Recovery and Dying in Small-Pox, Article II," *Br. Ann. Med.* 1 (1837): 134-43.

"On the Law of Recovery and Mortality in Cholera Spasmodica," *Lancet*, 1838-39, i, 26-29.

"On the Modes of Calculating the Death-Rate of a Population," *Lancet*, 1862, i, 568-69.

"On the Pay of Ministers of the Crown," *J. Statist. Soc. Lond.* 20 (1857): 102-31.

"On the Valuation of Railways," *J. Statist. Soc. Lond.* 36 (1873): 256-59.

"On the Valuation of Railways, Telegraphs, Water Companies, Canals, and Other Commercial Concerns, with Prospective, Deferred, Increasing, Decreasing, or Terminating Profits," *J. Statist. Soc. Lond.* 39 (1876): 464-530.

"Physiology—Mode of Studying It," *Br. Ann. Med.* 1 (1837): 727-28.

"Poor-Law—Steam-Boiler Explosions—Coroners' Inquests," *Br. Ann. Med.* 1 (1837): 790-92.

"Population," *4th A.R.R.G.*, App., pp. 133-43 [PP, 1842, XIX, 85-90].

"Progress of Medicine," *Br. Ann. Med.* 1 (1837): 663-64.

"Progress of the Medical Profession—Obstructions in the Way," *Br. Ann. Med.* 1 (1837): 629-31.

"Projet de classification [des causes de mort physiologiques, accidentelles et morbides]," *Compte rendu de la deuxième session du Congrès International de Statistique* (Paris, 1856), pp. 147-65.

"Proportion of Sickness at Different Ages," *Br. Med. Almanack* (1836), 111-13.

"The Provincial Medical and Surgical Association," *Br. Ann. Med.* 2 (1837): 59-61.

"Quackery. Inflammation of the Bowels caused by Morrison's Pills," *Lancet*, 1835-36, ii, 109-10.

"Registration of Diseases," *Br. Ann. Med.* 1 (1837): 664.

"Registration of the Causes of Death," *4th A.R.R.G.*, App., pp. 144-47 [PP, 1842, XIX, 91-93].

Remarks on a Proposed Scheme for the Conversion of the Assessments Levied on Public Salaries, Under Act 4 and 5 Will. IV. Cap. 24. into a "Provident Fund" for the Support of the Widows and Orphans of Civil Servants of the Crown. (London, [1849]).

"Remedy for Sore Nipple. Tincture of Catechu," *Lancet*, 1841-42, ii, 523-24.

"Remuneration of Medical Men. Pay of Surgeons in the Army Contrasted with the Pay of Surgeons in the Unions," *Br. Ann. Med.* 1 (1837): 553-55.

"Report of Dr. Farr on the Progress of Government Statistics in Great Britain," *J. Statist. Soc. Lond.* 21 (1858): 13-16.

"Report of the International Statistical Congress, Held at Vienna, September, 1855, App. B., Invitation to Hold the Congress of 1859 in London," *J. Statist. Soc. Lond.* 21 (1858): 16-17.

Report on the Cholera Epidemic of 1866 in England. Suppl. 29th A.R.R.G. [PP, 1867-68, XXXVII].

Report on the Mortality of Cholera in England, 1848-49 (London, 1852).

"Report on the Nomenclature and Statistical Classification of Diseases, for Statistical Returns," *16th A.R.R.G.*, App., pp. 71-96.

"Report to the International Statistical Congress Held at the Hague in 1869," *31st A.R.R.G.*, pp. 235-68 [PP, 1870, XVI].

"Report to the Registrar-General on the International Statistical Congress held at Paris in 1855," *16th A.R.R.G.*, App., pp. 106-25.

"Report to the Registrar General on the International Statistical Congress at Vienna," *19th A.R.R.G.*, App., pp. 206-22 [PP, 1857-58, XXIII].

"Report upon the Mortality of Lunatics," *J. Statist. Soc. Lond.* 4 (1841): 17-33.

"Reports of the Official Delegates from England at the Meeting of the International Statistical Congress, Berlin, September, 1863. 1. Report of Dr. William Farr, F.R.S., F.S.S.," *J. Statist. Soc. Lond.* 26 (1863): 412-16.

"The Rise and Progress of the Provincial Medical and Surgical Association," *Br. Med. Almanack* (1837), pp. 121-30.

"The State of Medical Science," *Br. Ann. Med.* 1 (1837): 22-26.

"Statistical Nosology," *4th A.R.R.G.*, App., pp. 147-216 [PP, 1842, XIX, 93-127].

"Statistics of Insanity—County Lunatic Asylums," *Br. Ann. Med.* 1 (1837): 648-53, 679-83, 744-48, 811-14; 2 (1837): 137-40, 171-74, 204-7, 235-39, 357-61.

"Statistics of the Civil Service of England, with Observations on the Constitution of Funds, to Provide for Fatherless Children and Widows," *J. Statist. Soc. Lond.* 12 (1849): 103-50.

"Statistics of the English Hospitals," *Br. Med. Almanack* (1836), pp. 114-23.

A System of Life Insurance Which May Be Carried out under the Control of the Government and Would (1) Be Equitable in Its Operations: (2) Afford the Best Security, and Be in the Best Condition to Fulfill its Future Engagements: (3) Be Well Adapted to the Wants of the People, as it Would Afford All the Advantages of an Insurance Office, and Some of Those of a Bank: and (4) Operate at Less Risk, Less Expense, and Lower Premiums than Small Offices. (5) It Might Also Be Made a Considerable Source of National Revenue (London [1853]).

"Vital Statistics," *Br. Ann. Med.* 1 (1837): 353-60.

"Vital Statistics," in J[ohn] R[amsay] McCulloch (ed.), *A Descriptive and Statistical Account of the British Empire: Exhibiting Its Extent, Physical Capacities, Population, Industry, and Civil and Religious Institutions*, 4th ed. (London, 1854), 2: 541-625.

Vital Statistics: A Memorial Volume of Selections from the Reports and Writings of William Farr, M.D., D.C.L., C.B., F.R.S., ed. Noel A. Humphreys (London, 1885).

"Vital Statistics of Sweden," *Br. Med. Almanack,* suppl. (1838), 216-23.

"Vital Statistics; or, the Statistics of Health, Sickness, Diseases, and Death," in J[ohn] R[amsay] McCulloch (ed.), *A Statistical Account of the British Empire: Exhibiting Its Extent, Physical Capacities, Population, Industry, and Civil and Religious Institutions* (London, 1837), 2: 567-601.

V. Published Works by Other Authors

Abrams, Philip. *The Origins of British Sociology: 1834-1914.* Chicago and London, 1968.

Ackerknecht, Erwin H. "Anticontagionism between 1821 and 1867." *Bull. Hist. Med.* 22 (1948): 562-93.

Alison, William Pulteney, "Observations on the Best Mode of Registering Deaths." *Northern J. Med.* 1 (1844): 225-32.

_____. *Observations on the Epidemic Fever of MDCCCXLIII in Scotland, and Its Connection with the Destitute Condition of the Poor.* Edinburgh, 1844.

Anderson, J. G. *The Birthplace and Genesis of Life Assurance and other Essays,* 2nd ed. London, 1940.

Ashton, T. S. *Economic and Social Investigations in Manchester, 1833-1933: A Centenary History of the Manchester Statistical Society.* London, 1934.

Aspland. Alfred. "An Examination of the Report of the Commissioners to Enquire into the Mortality of the Army." *Trans. Manchr. Statist. Soc.* (1859), pp. 69-108.

_____. "Inaugural Address at the Opening of Session 1863-64." *Trans. Manchr. Statist. Soc.* (1863-64), pp. i-xxvi.

Banks, J. A. *Prosperity and Parenthood: A Study of Family Planning among the Victorian Middle Classes.* London, 1954.

Barnes, Robert. "A Register of the Cases of Disease Observed at the London and Metropolitan Free Hospitals during the Month of August, 1855; with Clinical Remarks on the Etiology and Characters of the Current Diseases, and on the Importance of Publishing a Periodical Register of Prevailing Diseases." *Lancet,* 1855, ii, 211-16.

Barrett, C.R.B. *The History of the Society of Apothecaries of London.* London, 1905.

Beer, M[ax]. *A History of British Socialism,* 2 vols. London, 1919-20.

Bettany, George Thomas. "Farr, William, 1807-1883." *D.N.B.,* 6: 1,090-91.

Bowditch, Henri I. *Brief Memories of Louis and Some of His Contemporaries in the Parisian School of Medicine of Forty Years Ago.* Boston, 1872.

Brand, Jeanne L. *Doctors and the State: The British Medical Profession and Government Action in Public Health, 1870-1912.* Baltimore, 1965.

Bristowe, J. S. "Hospital Mortality," *Med. Times and Gazette,* 1864, i, 491-92.

_____. "The Mortality in General Hospitals," *Med. Times and Gazette,* 1864, i, 296-97.

_____. "Mortality in Hospitals." *Lancet,* 1864, i, 452.

_____. "Miss Nightingale on Hospitals," *Med. Times and Gazette,* 1864, i, 211.

British Association for the Advancement of Science, Anthropometric Committee. "Report of the Anthropometric Committee." *Report, B.A.A.S.* 46 (1876): 266; Ibid. 47 (1877): 231-32; Ibid. 48 (1878): 152-53; Ibid. 49 (1879): 175-209; Ibid. 50 (1880): 120-59; and Ibid. 51 (1881): 225-72.

British Association for the Advancement of Science, Edinburgh Subcommittee on Registration. "Report on the Registration of Deaths." *Report, B.A.A.S.* 5 (1835): 251-55.

Brockington, C. Fraser. *Public Health in the Nineteenth Century.* Edinburgh and London, 1965.

Brownlee, John. "Historical Note on Farr's Theory of the Epidemic." *Br. Med. J.* 1915, ii, 250-52.

_____. *The Use of Death-Rates as a Measure of Hygienic Conditions.* London, 1922.

Cassedy, James H. *Demography in Early America: Beginnings of the Statistical Mind, 1600–1800.* Cambridge, Mass., 1969.

_____. "The Registration Area and American Vital Statistics: Development of a Health Research Resource, 1885-1915." *Bull. Hist. Med.* 39 (1965): 221-31.

Chadwick, Edwin. "On the Best Modes of Representing Accurately, by Statistical Returns, the Duration of Life, and the Pressure and Progress of the Causes of Mortality amongst Different Classes of the Community, and amongst the Populations of Different Districts and Countries." *J. Statist. Soc. Lond.* 7 (1844): 1-40.

Cook, Edward. *The Life of Florence Nightingale,* 2 vols. London, 1913.

Cope, Zachary. *Florence Nightingale and the Doctors.* London and Colchester, 1958.

Creighton, Charles. *A History of Epidemics in Britain,* 2 vols. Cambridge, 1891-94.

Crellin, J. K. "Airborne Particles and the Germ Theory: 1860-1880," *Annals of Science* 22 (1966): 49-60.

_____. "The Dawn of the Germ Theory: Particles, Infection and Biology," in *Medicine and Science in the 1860s: Proceedings of the Sixth British Congress on the History of Medicine,* ed. F. N. L. Poynter. London, 1968, pp. 57-76.

Cullen, M. J. "The Making of the Civil Registration Act of 1836." *J. Ecclesiastical Hist.* 25 (1974): 39-59.

_____. *The Statistical Movement in Early Victorian Britain: The Foundations of Empirical Social Research.* New York, 1975.

D'Espine, Marc. "Essai statistique sur la mortalité du Canton de Genève pendant l'année 1838." *Annales d'hygiène publique et de médecine légale* 23 (1840): 5-130.

_____. "Projet de classification des causes de mort physiologiques, accidentelles et morbides, à l'usage de la statistique mortuaire de tous les pays; préparé pour le Congres International de Statistique de Paris," *Compte rendu de la duexième session du Congrès International de Statistique.* Paris, 1856, pp. 133-46.

Dewhurst, Kenneth. *Dr. Thomas Sydenham (1624–1689): His Life and Writing.* Berkeley and Los Angeles, 1966.

Dyos, H. J. "Urban Transformation: A Note on the Objects of Street Improvement in Regency and Early Victorian London." *Int. Rev. Soc. Hist.* 2 (1957): 259–65.

Edmonds, T. R. "Laws of Human Mortality." *Br. Med. Almanack* (1836), pp. 104–9.

————. *Life Tables, Founded upon the Discovery of a Numerical Law Regulating the Existence of Every Human Being.* London, 1832.

————. "On the Law of Mortality in Each County of England." *Lancet,* 1835–36, i, 364–71, and 408–16.

————. "On the Laws of Collective Vitality." *Lancet,* 1834–35, ii, pp. 5–8.

————. "On the Laws of Sickness, according to Age, Exhibiting a Double Coincidence between the Laws of Sickness and the Laws of Mortality." *Lancet,* 1835–36, i, 855–58.

————. "On the Mortality at Glasgow, and on the Increasing Mortality in England," *Lancet,* 1835–36, ii, 353–59.

————. "On the Mortality of Infants in England." *Lancet,* 1835–36, i, 690–94.

————. "On the Mortality of the People in England." *Lancet,* 1834–35, ii, 310–16.

————. "Statistics of Mortality in England." *Br. Med. Almanack,* suppl. (1837), pp. 130–35.

————. "Statistics of the London Hospital, with Remarks on the Law of Sickness." *Lancet,* 1835–36, ii, 778–83.

Elesh, David. "The Manchester Statistical Society: A Case Study of a Discontinuity in the History of Empirical Social Research." *J. Hist. Behavioral Sci.* 8 (1972): 280–301 and 407–17.

Epidemiological Society of London. *The Commemoration Volume, containing an Account of the Foundation of the Society and of the Commemoration Dinner, together with an Index of the Papers Read at Its Meetings between 1855 and 1900.* [London, 1900].

————. "Report on the Questions, Submitted by Dr. Farr to the Council, Concerning the Classification of Epidemic Diseases." *Trans. Epidem. Soc. Lond.,* n. s. 2 (1862–66): app.

Eversley, D.E.C. *Social Theories of Fertility and the Malthusian Debate.* Oxford, 1959.

Eyler, John M. "Mortality Statistics and Victorian Health Policy: Program and Criticism." *Bull. Hist. Med.* 50 (1976): 335–55.

————. "William Farr on the Cholera: The Sanitarian's Disease Theory and the Statistician's Method." *J. Hist. Med.* 28 (1973): 79–100.

Fein, Rashi. "On Measuring Economic Benefits of Health Programmes," in *Medical History and Medical Care,* eds. Gordon McLachlan and Thomas McKeown. London, New York, Toronto, 1971, pp. 181–217.

Finer, S. E. *The Life and Times of Sir Edwin Chadwick.* London, 1952.

Flinn, M. W. "Introduction," in Edwin Chadwick, *Report on the Sanitary Condition of the Labouring Population of Gt. Britain* [1842], ed. M. W. Flinn. Edinburgh, 1965, pp. 1–73.

_____. *Public Health Reform in Britain*. New York, 1968.

Forbes, Thomas Rogers. *Chronicle from Aldgate: Life and Death in Shakespeare's London*. New Haven and London, 1971.

Frost, Wade Hampton. "Introduction," in *Snow on Cholera: Being a Reprint of Two Papers by John Snow, M.D. Together with a Biographical Memoir by B. W. Richardson, M.D. and an Introduction by Wade Hampton Frost, M.D.* New York and London, 1936.

Gairdner, W. T. *Public Health in Relation to Air and Water*. Edinburgh, 1862.

Galton, Francis. "Considerations adverse to the Maintenance of Section F (Economic Science and Statistics), Submitted by Mr. Francis Galton to the Committee Appointed by the Council to Consider and Report on the Possibility of Excluding Unscientific or Otherwise Unsuitable Papers and Discussions from the Sectional Proceedings of the Association." *J. Statist. Soc. Lond.* 40 (1877): 468–73.

_____. *Memories of My Life*. London, 1908.

_____. "The Possible Improvement of the Human Breed under the Existing Conditions of Law and Sentiment." *Nature* 64 (1901): 659–65.

Gibbs, George S. *"Fortification by Disease," and its Effect on Infant Life*. Brixton, 1877.

_____. *Smallpox and Vaccination. A Letter Addressed to Major Graham, Registrar General of Births, Marriages, and Deaths in England and Wales. . . .* Darlington, 1873.

_____. *The Somerset House "Statistics" on Vaccination*. Brixton, 1877.

_____. *Vaccination Useless and Injurious. A Remonstrance respecting the Vaccination Bill of 1866, Addressed to the Rt. Hon. Henry A. Bruce, M.P.*, 2nd ed. London [1866].

Glass, D. V. "A Note on the Under-Registration of Births in Britain in the Nineteenth Century." *Population Studies* 5 (1952): 70–88.

_____. *Numbering the People: The Eighteenth-Century Population Controversy and the Development of Census and Vital Statistics in Britain*. Farnborough, Hants, 1973.

_____. "Some Aspects of the Development of Demography." *J. Roy. Soc. Arts* 104 (1956): 854–68.

Glazer, Nathan. "The Rise of Social Research in Europe," in *The Human Meaning of the Social Sciences*, ed. Daniel Lerner. Cleveland and New York, 1959, pp. 43–72.

Goldin, Grace. "Building a Hospital of Air: The Victorian Pavilions of St. Thomas' Hospital, London." *Bull. Hist. Med.* 49 (1975): 512–35.

Gompertz, Benajmin. "On the Nature of the Function Expressive of the Law of Human Mortality, and on a New Mode of Determining the Value of Life Contigencies." *Phil. Trans.* 115 (1825): 513–83.

Great Britain, General Register Office. *Regulations for the Duties of Superintendent Registrars*. London, 1838.

Grebenik, E. "The Development of Demography in Great Britain," in *The Study of Population: An Inventory and Appraisal*, eds. Philip M. Hauser and Otis Dudley Duncan. Chicago, 1959, pp. 124–79.

_____. "The Sources and Nature of Statistical Information in Special Fields of

Statistics: Population and Vital Statistics." *J. Roy. Statist. Soc.*, Ser. A 118 (1955): 452–62.

―――――. "Vital Statistics." *International Encyclopaedia of the Social Sciences,* 16: 340–43.

Greenhow, E. Headlam. "Illustrations of the Necessity for a More Analytical Study of the Statistics of Public Health." *Trans. N.A.P.S.S.* Birmingham, 1857, pp. 365–87.

Greenwood, Major. *The Medical Dictator and Other Biographical Studies.* London, 1936.

―――――. *Medical Statistics from Graunt to Farr.* Cambridge, 1948.

―――――. *Some British Pioneers of Social Medicine.* London, New York, Toronto, 1948.

Griffin, Daniel, and William Griffin. *Observations on the Application of Mathematics to the Science of Medicine.* London, 1843.

Griffith, G. Talbot. *Population Problems of the Age of Malthus,* 2nd ed. London, 1967.

Guy, William A. "On the Original and Acquired Meaning of the Term 'Statistics' and on the Proper Functions of a Statistical Society: also on the Question Whether There Be a Science of Statistics; and, if so, What Are Its Nature and Objects, and What Is Its Relation to Political Economy and 'Social Science.'" *J. Statist. Soc. Lond.* 28 (1865): 478–93.

―――――. "On the Value of the Numerical Method as Applied to Science, but Especially to Physiology and Medicine." *J. Statist. Soc. Lond.* 2 (1839): 25–47.

―――――. "Vital Statistics." *The Cyclopaedia of Anatomy and Physiology,* ed. Robert B. Todd. London, 1852, 4, pt. 2: 1469–75.

Halley, Edmond. "An Estimate of the Degrees of the Mortality of Mankind, Drawn from Curious Tables of the Births and Funerals at the City of Breslaw; with an Attempt to Ascertain the Price of Annuities upon Lives." *Phil. Trans.* 17 [no. 196] (1693): 596–610.

[Hare, F.A.C.] *William Farr, F.S.S., M.D., F.R.S., C.B., etc., etc.* London, 1883, in L.S.E. Farr Collection, XI, item 30.

Hawkins, F. Bisset. *Elements of Medical Statistics; Containing the Substance of the Gulstonian Lectures Delivered at the Royal College of Physicians: With Numerous Additions, Illustrative of the Comparative Salubrity, Longevity, Mortality, and Prevalence of Diseases in the Principal Countries and Cities of the Civilized World.* London, 1829.

Henry, William. "Report on the State of Our Knowledge of the Laws of Contagion," *Report, B.A.A.S.* 4 (1834): 67–94.

Hilts, Victor L. "Aliis exterendum, or, the Origins of the Statistical Society of London," *Isis* 69 (1978): 21–43.

―――――. "William Farr (1807–1883) and the 'Human Unit,'" *Vict. Stud.* 14 (1970): 143–50.

Holloway, S.W.F., "The Apothecaries' Act, 1815: A Reinterpretation." *Med. Hist.* 10 (1966): 107–29 and 221–36.

―――――. "Medical Education in England, 1830–1858: A Sociological Analysis." *History* 49 (1964): 299–324.

Holmes, T. "Hospital Mortality," *Med. Times and Gazette,* 1864, i, 349–50.

_____. "Mortality in Hospitals." *Lancet,* 1864, i, 338-39, 365-66, 451-52.

_____. "The Mortality in the Norwich and London Hospitals," *Med. Times and Gazette,* 1864, i, 295-96.

_____. "The Relative Mortality in London and County Hospitals," *Med. Times and Gazette,* 1864, i, 243-44.

_____. "Town and Country Hospitals," *Med. Times and Gazette,* 1864, i, 74-75.

Humphreys, Noel A. "Biographical Sketch of William Farr," in William Farr, *Vital Statistics: A Memorial Volume of Selections from the Reports and Writings of William Farr, M.D., D.C.L., C.B., F.R.S.,* ed. Noel A. Humphreys. London, 1885, pp. vii-xxiv.

_____. "How Far May the Average Death-Rate of a Population Be Considered an Efficient Test of Its Sanitary Condition." *Trans. N.A.P.S.S.* (Birmingham, 1884), pp. 485-96.

_____. "The Value of Death-Rates as a Test of Sanitary Condition." *J. Statist. Soc. Lond.* 37 (1874): 437-71.

International Statistical Congress. *Compte rendu de la deuxième session du Congrès International de Statistique.* Paris, 1856.

_____. *Programme of the Fourth Session of the International Statistical Congress, to Be Held in London on July 16, 1860, and Five Following Days.* London, 1860.

_____. *Report of the Proceedings of the Fourth Session of the International Statistical Congress, Held in London July 16th, 1860, and the Five Following Days.* London, 1861.

John, V., "The Term 'Statistics.' Translated from a Work by Dr. V. John, Professor of the University of Berne, entitled 'Der Name Statistik—Eine Etymologisch-historische Skizze,' Berne: Verlag von K. J. Weiss, 1883." *J. Statist. Soc. Lond.* 46 (1883): 656-79.

Kiker, B. F. *Human Capital: In Retrospect,* Essays in Economics, No. 16. Columbia, S.C., 1968.

Kopf, Edwin W. "Florence Nightingale as Statistician." *Pub. Am. Statist.. Assn.* 15 (1916-17): 388-404.

Koren, John (ed.). *The History of Statistics: Their Development and Progress in Many Countries.* New York, 1918.

Krause, J. T. "The Changing Adequacy of English Registration, 1690-1837," in *Population in History: Essays in Historical Demography,* eds. D. V. Glass and D. E. C. Eversley. London, 1965, pp. 379-93.

Lambert, Royston. *Sir John Simon 1816-1904 and English Social Administration.* London, 1963.

Langmuir, Alexander D. "Epidemiology of Airborne Infection." *Bact. Rev.* 25 (1961): 173-81.

_____. "The Surveillance of Communicable Diseases of National Importance." *New Engl. J. Med.* 268 (1963): 182-92.

_____. "William Farr: Founder of Modern Concepts of Surveillance." *Int. J. Epidemiol.* 5 (1976): 13-18.

Lazarsfeld, Paul F. "Notes on the History of Quantification in Sociology—Trends, Sources and Problems." *Isis* 52 (1961): 277-333.

Lewes, C. L. *Dr. Southwood Smith: A Retrospect.* Edinburgh and London, 1898.

Lilienfeld, David E., and Abraham M. Lilienfeld. "Epidemiology: A Retrospective Study." *Am. J. Epidemiol.* 166 (1977): 445–59.

Little, Ernest Muirhead. *History of the British Medical Association 1832–1932.* London, [1932].

Logan, W.P.D., "Medical Significance of the Census." *Br. Med. J.,* 1951, i, 720–22.

Lorimer, Frank. "The Development of Demography," in *The Study of Population: An Inventory and Appraisal,* eds. Philip M. Hauser and Otis Dudley Duncan. Chicago, 1959, pp. 124–79.

Lotka, Alfred J. "The Relation between Birth Rate and Death Rate in a Normal Population and the Rational Basis of an Empirical Formula for the Mean Length of Life Given by William Farr." *Q. Pub. Am. Statist. Assn.,* n. s. 16 (1918): 121–30.

_____. "A Simple Graphic Construction for Farr's Relation between Birth-Rate, Death-Rate, and Mean Length of Life." *Q. Pub. Am. Statist. Assn.,* n. s. 17 (1921): 998–1,000.

Low, George M. "The History of Actuarial Science in Great Britain." *Troisième Congrès International d'Actuaires.* Paris, 1901, pp. 848–75.

Luckin, W., "The Final Catastrophe—Cholera in London, 1866." *Med. Hist.* 21 (1977): 32–42.

MacDonagh, Oliver. "The Nineteenth-Century Revolution in Government: A Reappraisal." *Hist. J.* 1 (1958): 52–67.

McDonald, J. C. "The History of Quarantine in Britain during the 19th Century." *Bull. Hist. Med.* 25 (1951): 22–44.

McGregor, O. R. "Social Research and Social Policy in the Nineteenth Century." *Br. J. Sociology* 8 (1957): 146–57.

Mack, Mary P. *Jeremy Bentham: An Odyssey of Ideas 1748–1792.* London, Melbourne, Toronto, 1962.

Maclean, Charles. *Evils of Quarantine Laws, and Non-Existence of Pestilential Contagion: Deduced from the Phaenomena of the Plague of the Levant, the Yellow Fever of Spain, and the Cholera Morbus of Asia.* London, 1824.

MacLeod, Roy M. "The Anatomy of State Medicine: Concept and Application," in *Medicine and Science in the 1860s: Proceedings of the Sixth British Congress on the History of Medicine,* ed. F.N.L. Poynter. London, 1968, pp. 199–227.

_____. "The Frustration of State Medicine, 1880–1899." *Med. Hist.* 11 (1967): 15–40.

_____. "Law, Medicine and Public Opinion: The Resistance to Compulsory Health Legislation 1870–1907." *Public Law* (Summer and Autumn, 1967), pp. 107–28 and 189–211.

McMenemey, W. H. "Education and the Medical Reform Movement," in *The Evolution of Medical Education in Britain,* ed. F.N.L. Poynter. London, 1966, pp. 135–54.

_____. *The Life and Times of Sir Charles Hastings: Founder of the British Medical Association.* Edinburgh and London, 1959.

Meitzen, August. *History, Theory, and Technique of Statistics,* trans. Roland P. Falkner. Philadelphia, 1891.

Milne, Joshua. "Annuities." *Encyclopaedia Britannica,* 7th ed. (1842), 3: 198–234.

_____. *A Treatise on the Valuation of Annuities and Assurances on Lives and Survivorships; on the Construction of Tables of Mortality; and on the Probabilities and Expectations of Life,* 2 vols. London, 1815.

Moseley, Maboth. *Irascible Genius: The Life of Charles Babbage, Inventor.* London, 1964.

Müllener, Eduard-Rudolf. "Pierre-Charles-Alexandre Louis' (1787-1872) Genfer Schüler und die méthode numérique." *Gesnerus* 24 (1967): 46-74.

Neison, F.G.P. "On a Method Recently Proposed for Conducting Inquiries into the Comparative Sanatory Condition of Various Districts, with Illustrations, Derived from Numerous Places in Great Britain at the Period of the Last Census." *J. Statist. Soc. Lond.* 7 (1844): 40-68.

Newman, Charles. *The Evolution of Medical Education in the Nineteenth Century.* London, etc., 1957.

Newsholme, Arthur. *The Elements of Vital Statistics,* 3rd ed. London, 1899.

_____. *The Elements of Vital Statistics in Their Bearing on Social and Public Health Problems,* new ed. New York, 1924.

_____. *Evolution of Preventive Medicine.* Baltimore, 1927.

_____. *Fifty Years in Public Health: A Personal Narrative with Comments.* London, 1935.

_____. "The Measurement of Progress in Public Health with Special Reference to the Life and Work of William Farr." *Economica* 3 (1923): 186-202.

_____. "The Vital Statistics of Peabody Buildings and Other Artisans' and Labourers' Block Dwellings." *J. Statist. Soc. Lond.* 54 (1891): 70-99.

_____. "William Farr" [a lecture given at the Johns Hopkins University, n.d.] in L. S. E. Farr Collection, IX, item 5.

Nightingale, Florence. *Notes on Hospitals,* 3rd ed. London, 1863.

_____. "Hospital Statistics and Hospital Plans." *Trans. N.A.P.S.S.* (Dublin, 1861), 554-60.

_____. "Notes on the Sanitary Condition of Hospitals, and on Defects in the Construction of Hospital Wards, Parts I and II." *Trans. N.A.P.S.S.* Liverpool, 1858), 462-82.

Noble, Daniel. *Facts and Observations Relative to the Influence of Manufactures upon Health and Life.* London, 1843.

_____. "Fluctuations in the Death Rate." *Trans. Manchr. Statist. Soc.* (1863-64).

_____. "On certain Popular Fallacies concerning the Production of Epidemic Diseases." *Trans. Manchr. Statist. Soc.* (1859-60), pp. 1-22.

_____. "Thoughts on the Value and Significance of Statistics." *Trans. Manchr. Statist. Soc.* (1865-66), pp. 17-27.

Novak, Steven J. "Professionalism and Bureaucracy: English Doctors and the Victorian Public Health Administration." *J. Social Hist.* 6 (1973): 440-62.

Ogborn, M. E. "The Actuary in the Eighteenth Century." *Proceedings of the Centenary Assembly of the Institute of Actuaries* 3 (1950): 357-73.

_____. *Equitable Assurances: The Story of Life Assurance in the Experience of the Equitable Life Assurance Society 1762-1962.* London, 1962.

Parris, Henry. "The Nineteenth-Century Revolution in Government: A Reappraisal Reappraised." *Hist. J.* 3 (1960): 17-37.

Pearson, Karl. *The Groundwork of Eugenics.* London, 1909.

————. *The Life, Letters and Labours of Francis Galton,* 3 vols. in 4. Cambridge, 1914-30.

Pelling, Margaret. *Cholera, Fever and English Medicine 1825–1865.* Oxford, 1978.

Peterson, M. Jeanne. *The Medical Profession in Mid-Victorian London.* Berkeley, Los Angeles, and London, 1978.

Quetelet, Lambert A. J. *A Treatise on Man and the Development of his Faculties,* trans. R. Knox [1842]. Gainesville, Florida, 1969.

R[ichardson], B[enjamin] W[ard]. "Commentary on Hospital Mortality," *Med. Times and Gazette,* 1864, i, 262-63.

————. "Facts and Suggestions on the Registration of Disease." *Trans. N.A.P.S.S.* Dublin, 1861, pp. 534-47.

————. "Note on Hospital Mortality," *Med. Times and Gazette,* 1864, i, 318-19.

————. *The Health of Nations: A Review of the Works of Edwin Chadwick,* 2 vols. [1887]. London, 1965.

————. "The Medical History of England: The Medical History of Norwich." *Med. Times and Gazette,* 1864, i, 19-21, 40-43, 67-71, and 97-102.

Richmond, Phyllis Allen. "Some Variant Theories in Opposition to the Germ Theory of Disease." *J. Hist. Med.* 9 (1954): 290-303.

Rodgers, Brian. "The Social Science Association, 1857-1886." *Manchester School of Economic and Social Studies* 20 (1952): 283-310.

Rosen, George. "Cameralism and the Concept of Medical Police." *Bull. Hist. Med.* 27 (1953): 21-42.

————. "Disease and Social Criticism: A Contribution to a Theory of Medical History." *Bull. Hist. Med.* 10 (1941): 5-15.

————. "Disease, Debility, and Death," *The Victorian City: Images and Realities,* eds. H. J. Dyos and Michael Wolff. London and Boston, 1973, 2: 625-67.

————. "The Fate of the Concept of Medical Police, 1780-1890." *Centaurus* 5 (1957): 97-113.

————. "Jacob Henle and William Farr." *Bull. Hist. Med.* 9 (1941): 585-89.

————. "Problems in the Application of Statistical Analysis to Questions of Health: 1700-1880." *Bull. Hist. Med.* 29 (1955): 27-45.

————. "What is Social Medicine? A Genetic Analysis of the Concept." *Bull. Hist. Med.* 21 (1947): 674-733.

Rosenberg, Charles E., "Cholera in Nineteenth-Century Europe: A Tool for Social and Economic Analysis." *Comp. Stud. Soc. Hist.* 8 (1965-66): 452-63.

Rosenkrantz, Barbara Gutmann. *Public Health and the State: Changing Views in Massachusetts, 1842-1936.* Cambridge, Mass., 1972.

Royal College of Physicians of Edinburgh, Committee on Registration. *Report of a Committee . . . Appointed to Consider the Best Mode of Framing Public Registers of Death.* Edinburgh, 1841.

Royal Statistical Society. *Annals of the Royal Statistical Society 1834–1934.* London, 1934.

Rumsey, H. St. John. "Henry Wyldbore Rumsey, 1809-1876: A Pioneer of State Medicine." *Practitioner* 172 (1954): 570-72.

Rumsey, Henry W. *Essays and Papers on Some Fallacies of Statistics Concerning*

Life and Death, Health and Disease with Suggestions Towards an Improved System of Registration. London, 1875.

————. *Essays on State Medicine.* London, 1856.

————. "The Fallacies and Shortcomings of Our Sanitary Statistics." *Social Science Review, and Journal of the Sciences,* n. s. 4 (1865): 234-50, 358-63, 403-14, 481-95; 5 (1866): 21-43, 310-21, 440-47; 6 (1866): 97-110.

————. "On Certain Deficiencies in our Public Records of Mortality and Sickness, with Suggestions for an Improved and Extended National System of Registration." *Trans. N.A.P.S.S.* Bradford, 1859, 574-84.

————. "On Certain Departments of Medico-Sanitary Police and Medico-Legal Inquiry, in Connexion with the Scientific Superintendence of Mortuary Registration." *Trans. N.A.P.S.S.,* (Bradford, 1859), 585-95.

————. "On Certain Fallacies in Local Rates of Mortality, Arising from Defective Information—(i) as to the Influence of Class and Occupation, (ii) as to Movements of Population, (iii) as to Public Institutions—with Some Remarks on Hospital Mortality." *Trans. Manchr. Statist. Soc.,* (1871-72), pp. 17-39.

————. "On the Value of Life Tables, National and Local, as Evidence of Sanitary Condition." *Trans. Manchr. Statist. Soc.,* 1866-67, pp. 1-15.

————. "Remarks on State Medicine in Great Britain." *Br. Med. J.,* 1867, ii, 197-201.

Sargant, William Lucus. "Inconsistencies of the English Census of 1861, with the Registrar-General's Reports: and Deficiencies in the Local Registry of Births." *J. Statist. Soc. Lond.* 28 (1865): 73-124.

————. "On Certain Results and Defects of the Reports of the Registrar-General." *J. Statist. Soc. Lond.* 27 (1864): 170-221.

Shoen, Harriet H. "Prince Albert and the Application of Statistics to Problems of Government." *Osiris* 5 (1938): 276-318.

Shryock, Richard Harrison. *The Development of Modern Medicine: An Interpretation of the Social and Scientific Factors Involved* [1947]. Philadelphia and London, 1969.

————. "The History of Quantification in Medical Science." *Isis* 52 (1961): 215-37.

Sigsworth, E. M. "Gateways to Death? Medicine, Hospitals and Mortality, 1700-1850," in *Science and Society 1600-1900,* ed. Peter Mathias. Cambridge, 1972, pp. 97-110.

Simon, Sir John. *English Sanitary Institutions, Reviewed in Their Course of Development, and in Some of Their Political and Social Relations.* London, Paris, New York, and Melbourne, 1890.

Smith, Frank *The Life and Work of Sir James Kay-Shuttleworth.* London, 1923.

Smith, [Thomas] Southwood. *The Common Nature of Epidemics, and Their Relation to Climate and Civilization,* ed. T. Baker. London, 1866.

————. "Contagion and Sanitary Laws." *Westminster Rev.* 3 (1825): 134-67.

————. "Plague—Typhus Fever—Quarantine." *Westminster Rev.* 3 (1825): 499-530.

————. *A Treatise on Fever* [1830]. Philadelphia, 1831.

Snow, John. *On the Mode of Communication of Cholera.* London, 1849.

_____. *On the Mode of Communication of Cholera.* 2nd ed. London, 1855.

Sprigge, S. Squire. *The Life and Times of Thomas Wakley.* London, New York, and Bombay, 1899.

Stark, James. "Remarks on Dr. Farr's Proposed New Statistical Classification of Diseases for Statistical Returns." *Edinburgh Med. J.* 5 (1860): 1,069-82.

Statistical Society of London, "Introduction." *J. Statist. Soc. Lond.* 1 (1838): 1-5.

Statistical Society of London, Committee on Hospital Statistics. "Report of the Committee on Hospital Statistics." *J. Statist. Soc. Lond.* 5 (1842): 168-76.

_____. "Second Report of the Committee of the Statistical Society of London on Hospital Statistics." *J. Statist. Soc. Lond.* 7 (1844): 214-31.

Statistical Society of London. "Sixth Annual Report of the Council of the Statistical Society of London. Session 1839-40." *J. Statist. Soc. Lond.* 3 (1840): 1-13.

Susser, Mervyn, and Abraham Adelstein. "Introduction," *Vital Statistics: A Memorial Volume of Selections from the Reports and Writings of William Farr,* ed. Noel A. Humphreys [1885]. Metuchen, N.J., 1975, pp. iii-xiv.

Thomson, Robert D. "On Mr. Farr's Law of Recovery and Mortality in Cholera." *Report, B.A.A.S.* 8 (1838): 126-27.

Welton, T. A. "On the Classification of the People by Occupations; and on Other Subjects Connected with Population Statistics of England." *J. Statist. Soc. Lond.* 32 (1869): 271-87.

Westergaard, Harald. *Contributions to the History of Statistics* [1932]. New York, 1968.

Willcox, Walter F. "The Development of Military Sanitary Statistics." *Q. Pub. Am. Statist. Assn.* 16 (1918-19): 907-20.

Williams, Orlo. *Lamb's Friend the Census-Taker: Life and Letters of John Rickman.* London, 1912.

Winslow, Charles-Edward Amory. *The Conquest of Epidemic Disease: A Chapter in the History of Ideas.* Princeton, 1944.

INDEX

The Johns Hopkins University Press

This book was composed in Compugraphic English text and display type by Britton Composition from a design by Susan Bishop. It was printed on 55-lb. Number 66 Eggshell Offset paper and bound in Arrestox linen cloth by Universal Lithographers, Inc.